Killer Commodities

Killer Commodities

Public Health and the Corporate Production of Harm

Edited by Merrill Singer and Hans Baer

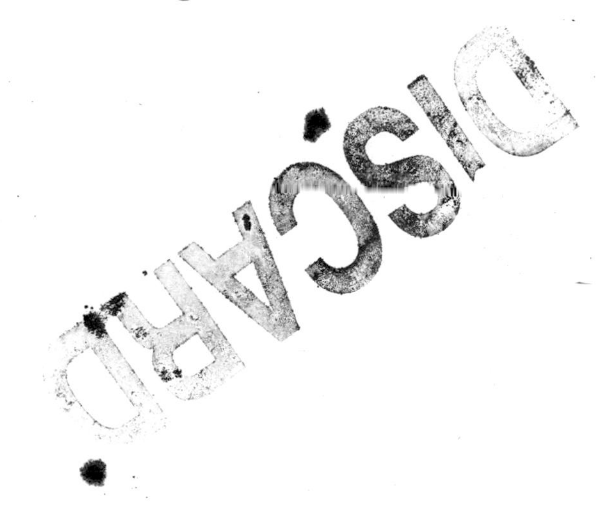

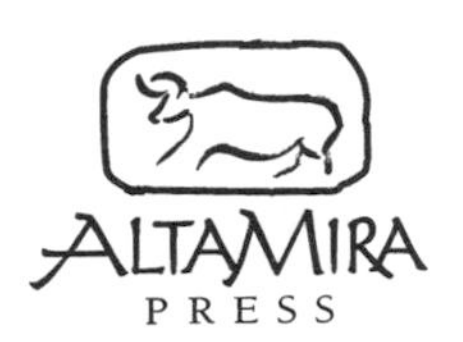

A division of
ROWMAN & LITTLEFIELD PUBLISHERS, INC.
Lanham • New York • Toronto • Plymouth, UK

AltaMira Press
A division of Rowman & Littlefield Publishers, Inc.
A wholly owned subsidiary of The Rowman & Littlefield Publishing Group, Inc.
4501 Forbes Boulevard, Suite 200, Lanham, MD 20706
www.altamirapress.com

Estover Road, Plymouth PL6 7PY, United Kingdom

British Library Cataloguing in Publication Information Available

Library of Congress Cataloging-in-Publication Data

Killer commodities : public health and the corporate production of harm / edited by Merrill Singer and Hans Baer.
p. ; cm.
Includes bibliographical references.
ISBN-13: 978-0-7591-0978-0 (cloth : alk. paper)
ISBN-10: 0-7591-0978-8 (cloth : alk. paper)
ISBN-13: 978-0-7591-0979-7 (pbk. : alk. paper)
ISBN-10: 0-7591-0979-6 (pbk. : alk. paper)
ISBN-13: 978-0-7591-1240-7 (electronic)
ISBN-10: 0-7591-1240-1 (electronic)
1. Health risk assessment. 2. Consumer goods—Health aspects. 3. Consumer goods—Safety measures. 4. Consumer goods—Social aspects. 5. Consumer protection. I. Singer, Merrill. II. Baer, Hans A., 1944–
[DNLM: 1. Consumer Product Safety. 2. Consumer Participation. 3. Economic Competition. 4. Public Policy. WA 288 K48 2009]
RA427.3.K45 2009
362.1028'9—dc22

2008009561

Printed in the United States of America

∞™ The paper used in this publication meets the minimum requirements of American National Standard for Information Sciences—Permanence of Paper for Printed Library Materials, ANSI/NISO Z39.48-1992.

Dedicated to Frances Kathleen Oldham Kelsey, PhD, MD
Because, in the struggle against killer commodities,
there is an enormous need for heroes.

CONTENTS

PREFACE

As various scholars, pundits, and social critics have emphasized, we live in an increasingly commodified world; a world populated by goods, services, and other items that are produced for sale rather than for immediate consumption by the producer. Moreover, we live in a globalized world in which commodities flow quickly from one place to another and travel many miles from the hands of the people who produce them to those of the people who consume them. Additionally, as corporations have become transnational, they have become more powerful and harder to regulate. The result has been growing evidence of dangerous commodities reaching consumers, sometimes with deadly consequences. Such commodities, their health and social impact, and the processes and forces leading to their availability in the market are examined in this book.

This is the second book in an ongoing series initiated by members of the Critical Anthropology of Health Caucus of the Society for Medical Anthropology to turn the bright light of critical theory on global health issues. The first volume, *Unhealthy Health Policy: A Critical Anthropological Examination* (2004), edited by Arachu Castro and Merrill Singer, examined the ways in which health policies can produce illness rather than health because of corporate interest and social inequality. While each of the authors who contributed to this volume—not all of whom are anthropologists—has his or her own perspectives, one of the goals of this book is to contribute to building a critical, socially conscious, and anthropologically informed understanding of killer commodities, while extending awareness of their nature and their health consequences. Beyond contributing to theory building, this book is intended as an aid in the broader social struggle for a safer, healthier world for all people.

INTRODUCTION
HIDDEN HARM
The Complex World of Killer Commodities
Merrill Singer and Hans Baer

On the morning of May 16, 2006, readers of the *New York Times* opened their newspapers to find a full-page, front-section advertisement (cost: approximately $182,000) headlined: "An Important Message from Bausch and Lomb Company." The ad followed an earlier announcement from Bausch and Lomb warning customers about the company's ReNu With Moistureloc soft contact lens cleaner and instructing them to immediately cease and desist using the product. The ad informed readers that the company was recalling the popular cleaning solution worldwide, at a cost of about $50 to $70 million, with a possible additional $100 million in lost sales per year (New York Times 2006). The cause of this dramatic move—not the usual reason a for-profit company wants to take out an expensive advertisement—was a growing body of evidence that use of the cleaning solution could lead to a potentially blinding fungal infection.

What Bausch and Lomb did not explain in its *New York Times* ad was that with over 100 infection cases in Hong Kong and Singapore, the product was withdrawn from those markets, but nothing was reported about it to the U.S. Food and Drug Administration (FDA), as required by law, nor was the product pulled from the U.S. market. Only when infection cases showed up in the United States did the company stop selling Moistureloc in the United States as well. Investigation by the FDA following the recall found 20 additional potential violations of the law at Bausch and

Lomb's factories in South Carolina (Feder 2006). Other company products have been linked with infection by the Centers for Disease Control and Prevention (New York Times 2006). While in its *New York Times* ad, the company affirmed that its number-one priority was the safety of its customers, its sincerity was thrown open to question by its actions (and eventually the company was sold because its failed reputation ruined business). Of course, Bausch and Lomb is not alone.

During the same period that Bausch and Lomb was pulling its contact lens cleaner off of store shelves, the Guidant Corporation, a producer of heart implant devices, like defibrillators, was sanctioned by the FDA for selling thousands of devices after the company became aware that they were flawed and could fail after implantation. The FDA linked seven deaths to faulty Guidant products (Meier 2006a). One of the patients who died was a 21-year-old student named Joshua Oukrop. The company admitted that his Model 186 defibrillator malfunctioned, causing his death.

Three physicians who served on a panel to review safety procedures at Guidant reported, "voluntary independent review [of products] . . . is a notion both foreign and frightening to most corporations, whose perceived need is to protect business interests. . . . But corporate culture fosters loyalty to corporate goals that may create unintended bias and distorted perceptions about product performance" (Meier 2006a:C3). One of the largest makers of medical devices, Guidant recorded $3.8 billion in sales in 2004 (Meier 2005).

These "hidden harm" cases are but the tip of the dangerous products iceberg. We label such products "killer commodities," a term we define as goods that are sold for a profit that result, either directly during use, indirectly through their impact on the environment, or during manufacture on workers, in a notable burden of injuries and death. As the cases presented above suggest, the dangers of killer commodities often are known to their producers and sellers although little effort has been made to assess their inherent risks before they are produced and sold on the open market.

Having glimpsed the tip of the iceberg, the question is raised: what lies beneath the waterline in the deadly arena of unsafe commodities? Over 40 years ago, consumer activist Ralph Nader (1965), published his classic book, *Unsafe at Any Speed: The Designed-In Dangers of the American Automobile*, which detailed the staunch resistance among car manufacturers to the introduction of automobile safety features like seat belts, as well as the fact that many cars were intrinsically unsafe, such as those built with tires that could not bear the weight of a fully-loaded vehicle. Because Nader focused a lot of attention on General Motors' Corvair, the company launched a "dirty tricks" campaign to harass and intimidate Nader into silence, an effort that the president of the company, James Roche, later had to admit and for which he had to apologize to Nader in front of a Senate subcommittee and for which Nader successfully sued General Motors.

Importantly, the issue addressed in this book is not that commodities are inherently bad—a lack of access to needed commodities can be life threatening too—but rather, how commodities are presented to (or withheld from) the public in spite of known risks or because risks were not assessed or only minimally attended to prior to the product going to market. Whether the issue is corporate plotting—which it certainly sometimes is—a corporate culture that, despite numerous assertions to the contrary, puts stockholders' profits far above customer well-being and pushes companies to fight like pit bulls to limit government regulation; the failure of government to protect the public from harmful products while looking out for corporate prosperity; or even consumer willingness to buy items known to be lethal or their failure to fully investigate the products they consume, killer commodities continue to appear and the toll in terms of human life and well-being is painfully high. Three examples of killer commodities with particularly noteworthy consequences are described below.

The Tobacco Industry and the Manufacture of Deadly Addiction

Tobacco, if used as directed by its manufacturers, is guaranteed to cause illness and death. As a result, it constitutes the poster child of killer commodities: a product that kills its users on a scale unmatched by other commodities (Baer, Singer, and Susser 2003). Cigarette smoking, in fact, is the single most preventable cause of premature death in the United States. More than 400,000 Americans die from tobacco-related causes yearly, accounting for one in every five deaths (Centers for Disease Control and Prevention 1993). Internationally, it is estimated that there are one billion smokers. Almost five million people died from smoking worldwide in 2000, about half in resource-poor nations.

Smoky Images

Although he was best known as the Marlboro Man, his real name was Wayne McLaren, and because of the tobacco industry, he gained fame, twice. A rodeo rider, bit actor, and stuntman, McLaren's first rise to notoriety began in 1975 when he was hired by Philip Morris Corporation to appear in magazine ads and on billboard displays, portraying a self-reliant, experience-hardened, yet ruggedly handsome role model for the American smoker. The embodiment of the idealized "man's man" in American culture, the public McLaren, the one seen repeatedly in frontier-influenced photos on horseback in big-sky, open-country settings, helped to sell cigarettes to the American public and beyond. Off camera, the real McLaren was no less a customer of the cigarette companies than those who were influenced by the advertisements in which he was prominently featured. He smoked heavily for 25 years, and was, ironically, in light of his representation as a freedom-seeking individualist, a self-admitted tobacco addict. This development led to his second rise to public visibility. The Marlboro Man, like so many smokers, was diagnosed with lung cancer. Prior to his death from cancer in 1990 at the age of 51, he became an antismoking advocate.

Addiction: Its Psychopharmacology and Neurobiology

What is addiction? Although the term is old and was long controversial because there was no agreed upon definition, the meaning of the term *addiction* has become more precise in recent years. While the World Health Organization (1969:55) has defined addiction as "a state, psychic and sometimes also physical, resulting [from] the interaction between a living organism and a drug, characterized by behavioral and other responses that always include a compulsion to take the drug on a continuous or periodic basis in order to experience its psychic effects, and sometimes to avoid the discomfort of its absences," it is now realized that addiction has specific physical features involving drug-caused changes in the brain.

This discussion is relevant to the issue of cigarette, cigar, and pipe smoking because of nicotine, one of the 4,000 chemicals found in the smoke emitted by tobacco products. Notably, as succinctly summarized by the report of the UK's Department of Health's Scientific Committee on Tobacco and Health (1998), "over the past decade there has been increasing recognition that underlying smoking behavior and its remarkable intractability to change is addiction to the drug nicotine. Nicotine has been shown to have effects on the brain's dopamine systems similar to those of drugs such as heroin and cocaine." Nicotine also impacts other neurotransmitters, significantly intensifying the drug's pleasurable effects. According to Daniel McGehee, a smoking researcher, "it would be difficult to design a better drug to promote addiction" (Zickler 2003:25).

Most cigarettes found in the United States contain ten or more milligrams of nicotine. The average smoker inhales one to two milligrams of nicotine per cigarette. Cigarette smoking causes a rapid delivery of nicotine to all parts of the body, reaching the brain in as little as ten seconds. It is now clear that most smokers use tobacco on a regular basis because they are addicted to nicotine. Indeed, rates of drug dependence, the percentage of people who use a drug who have trouble quitting, "are higher for nicotine than for marijuana, cocaine, or alcohol" (Zickler 2001:39). Some smokers, like the young, may be more vulnerable to developing dependence than others.

The continued use of tobacco is not caused by a lack of information about the risks of smoking, as most smokers in the United States and elsewhere are aware that smoking is very dangerous, and research shows that many want to stop. Each year, almost 35 million people in the United States attempt to quit smoking. Fewer than 7 percent of those who try to quit on their own, however, achieve more than a year of abstinence; most relapse and begin smoking again within a week of attempting to quit. Moreover, after having surgery for lung cancer, almost half of smokers resume smoking; 38 percent of smokers who have had a heart attack begin smoking again while they are still in the hospital; and, among people who have had their larynx removed because of throat cancer, 40 percent go back to smoking (Kessler 1994). Why? As with other drug addictions, those who are addicted to nicotine begin to suffer withdrawal symptoms, including irritability, craving, cognitive and attention deficits, and sleep disruption, once nicotine is no longer regularly reaching the neurons of their brain.

Mendacity, Cancer, and Nicotine Addiction

One of the points of dispute with reference to killer commodities involves the issue of manufacturer awareness and intent. What did the tobacco industry know about the role of their products in causing cancer and other diseases, and when did they first know this information? There is now an abundant body of evidence, contained in industry memos and other sources brought to light in a series of court cases and available through the University of California, San Francisco, Legacy Tobacco Documents Library (2002), to conclude that certainly by the mid-1950s (and probably many years before that), the tobacco industry was well aware of the link between smoking and cancer, an association they continued to deny publicly for decades afterward (Kessler 2001).

Richard Kluger (1996:165), for example, cites the minutes of a meeting held at the Liggett Tobacco Company on March 29, 1954, in which a company scientist is quoted as saying, "if we can eliminate or reduce the carcinogenic agent in smoke we will have made real progress." Similarly, a Philip Morris company document from the early 1960s states that "carcinogens are found in practically every class of compounds in smoke" (Wakeham 1961).

During this era, while publicly denying that cigarettes were dangerous, tobacco company scientists were busy attempting to develop a safe cigarette. Had the industry been able to do so, however, they knew that introducing the new product would present a significant public relations challenge. As a British-American Tobacco Company (BAT 1962) document notes: "When the health question was first raised we had to start by denying it at the PR level. But by continuing that policy we had got ourselves into a corner and left no room to manoeuvre."

As public awareness of the potential risks of smoking increased over the years, tobacco companies—while still denying cigarettes were dangerous—began manipulating their advertising to suggest their own products were safer than those of others. Noted one industry document: "All work in this area should be directed towards providing consumer reassurance about cigarettes and the smoking habit. This can be provided in different ways, e.g. by claiming low deliveries [of tar], by the perception of low deliveries and by the perception of 'mildness'" (Short 1977). The cigarette filter was one device used by the industry to help calm the nerves of an increasingly informed public, although the industry was aware that the filter on cigarettes did not protect smokers (Pepples 1976).

Even cigarettes from this period that were advertised as being low in tar were known to be no safer than other cigarettes. As a memo from a

British-American Tobacco Company (BAT 1979) scientist revealed, it was known in the industry that "the effect of switching to low tar cigarette may be to increase, not decrease, the risks of smoking." From the industry's perspective, however, effective advertisements could be used to sell people on the idea that low-tar cigarettes were safer. A Brown and Williams (B&W) Tobacco Company (1982) document, for example, notes: "B&W will undertake activities designed to generate statements by public health opinion leaders which will indicate tolerance for smoking and improve the consumer's perception of ultra low 'tar' cigarettes (5 mg or less). The first step will be the identification of attractive scientists not previously involved in the low delivery controversy who would produce studies re-emphasizing the lower delivery, less risk concept." All along, the tobacco industry was concerned that nicotine levels remain adequate to ensure addiction. Indeed, in the perspective within the tobacco industry, as documented in an internal memorandum written by the director of research at Philip Morris in 1972 (Kessler 1994), the cigarette is an ideal nicotine delivery system for addicted users: "Smoke is beyond question the most optimized vehicle of nicotine and the cigarette the most optimized dispenser of smoke."

The general pattern of deception—commonly involving a cover-up by the tobacco industry of what it knew about the risks of smoking—is seen as well in other efforts to keep in-house research findings under wraps. A review of documents produced over the years by the British-American Tobacco Company by Hammond, Collishaw, and Callard (2006:781), for example, found a pattern suggesting "a product strategy intended to exploit the limitations of the testing protocols and to intentionally conceal from consumers and regulators the potential toxicity of BAT products."

Twenty-seven years after its 1954 memo admitting that smoking tobacco causes cancer, Liggett broke ranks with fellow cigarette manufacturers and for the first time publicly admitted that nicotine is addictive and smoking causes cancer. Neither admission led Liggett or any other tobacco company to stop making and selling killer commodities. In response to an avalanche of evidence and several successful court cases, even the Philip Morris company (2006), which has been very aggressive in condemning the American Cancer Society and other antismoking advocates, now states on its website that "Philip Morris USA (PM USA) agrees with the overwhelming medical and scientific consensus that cigarette smoking causes lung cancer, heart disease, emphysema and other serious diseases in smokers. Smokers are far more likely to develop serious diseases, like lung cancer, than non-smokers. There is no safe cigarette." Also, "Philip Morris USA agrees with the medical and scientific consensus that cigarette smoking is addictive." Even these admissions, unimaginable not many years ago, have not resulted in the production of fewer cigarettes.

The Tobacco Lab: Manipulating Nicotine and Smokers

Before World War II, the tobacco industry treated the stems and scraps of cigarette manufacture as waste products and discarded them. In order to reduce costs, by the 1950s, tobacco companies were collecting this "waste" and treating it as reconstituted tobacco used in the making of cigarettes. As Kessler (1994) points out, while this change was initially driven by cost-saving motives, it signaled a far more important change in company control over and manipulation of the nicotine content of cigarettes. This change was marked by a series of patents filed by tobacco companies over the years that reflected their research on regulating the amount of nicotine put into cigarettes. Some of the patents involved new ways to increase the nicotine in tobacco, some involved adding nicotine to cigarette filters, and others increased the nicotine of wrappers.

Observes Kessler (1994), "Today, a cigarette company can add or subtract nicotine from tobacco. It can set nicotine levels. In many cigarettes today, the amount of nicotine present is a result of choice, not chance." This capacity is reflected in the language of tobacco company patent applications. As one company patent application (patent no. 3,280,823 C1:43-48) states, "maintaining the nicotine content at a sufficiently high level to provide the desired physiological activity, taste, and odor . . . can thus be seen to be a significant problem in the tobacco art" (Kessler 1994). Similarly, excerpts from industry patent applications identified by Kessler (1994) affirm the growing ability of company scientists to manipulate nicotine levels. While the tobacco industry did not share information about its increasing power to manipulate nicotine with the public, the capacity was openly acknowledged in industry trade publications (Kessler 1994).

Marketing Mortality: Promoting the Use of Tobacco

The tobacco industry, of course, does not merely produce and sell a highly addictive and life-destroying drug; it aggressively advertises and promotes its products, using up-to-date research on how to reach and convince various market segments to become consumers. Each year vast sums are spent by the tobacco companies and allied industries on advertising (about $8 billion annually prior to the tobacco settlement of 1998), event sponsorship, public relations, political campaign contributions (e.g., more than $2 million in contributions to federal candidates from 2003 to 2004), lobbying, and influence peddling at the local, state, and federal levels of government. The impact of tobacco industry spending on policy making can be seen in discussions during 2004 about granting the Food and Drug Administration authority to regulate tobacco products (something it currently cannot do because tobacco is not classified as a food or a medicine). The effort failed when a House-Senate conference committee killed the proposed legislation. Conference committee members who voted against the legislation—a position strongly supported by the tobacco industry—received on average $27,000 in tobacco industry campaign contributions, almost five times as much as was given to those who voted for the bill (Campaign for Tobacco-Free Kids 2005a). Significantly, tobacco and other advertisers have been able to win constitutional protection, known as "commercial speech," under the free speech and press clauses of the First Amendment, although it is not certain that framers of the Constitution envisioned corporations would be among the chief benefactors.

As alluded to earlier, an especially important market for the tobacco industry is the youth and young-adult sector, given the tendency for those who become lifelong smokers to begin smoking while young. The 2004 National Youth Tobacco Survey (YTS) (Centers for Disease Control and Prevention 2004) found that almost 22 percent of U.S. high school students smoke. Notably, about a million young people a year start smoking in the United States.

Available research "shows that tobacco advertising has both predisposing and reinforcing effects on youth smoking, acting as an inducement to experiment with smoking as well as reinforcing continued progression toward regular smoking" (Wakefield et al. 2002:132). Records of tobacco corporations affirm their keen interest in the youth market.

Indeed, industry has segmented the youth market based on research suggesting that at different stages in the developmental process from childhood to adulthood, as well as in the various steps in the process of becoming an addicted smoker, people have different reasons for smoking. In 1973, R. J. Reynolds marketing strategist Claude Teague (1973), for example, pointed out the marketing importance of these stages, including "the pre-smoker," "the learner," and "the confirmed smoker," and urged that tobacco marketing should target each of these stages. The memo in question begins by noting that there are many smokers below the age of 21 and hence "there is certainly nothing immoral or unethical about our Company attempting to attract these smokers to our products." The memo goes on to note that "if our Company is to survive and prosper . . . we must get our share of the youth market. In my opinion this will require new brands tailored to the youth market. . . . Thus we need new brands designed to be particularly attractive to the young smoker." With reference to the presmoking youth and those who are first learning to smoke, "the physical effects of smoking are largely unknown, unneeded, or actually quite unpleasant or awkward," thus psychosocial motivations are most important in getting people to start smoking. While peer approval and curiosity to try something new are most important for the presmoker and cigarette brands "tailored for the beginning smoker should emphasize the desirable psychological effects of smoking," for older teens, including those moving into young adulthood, stress is a more important marketing and branding "hook."

The importance of using stress as a marketing device is indicated by a later R. J. Reynolds document (Business Information Analysis Corporation 1985):

> For young adults who smoke, the use of cigarettes is seen as a mechanism to help ease the stress of transition from teen years to adulthood. The psychological role smoking plays for these young adults can be compared and contrasted with its use for teens and also for adults.

The industry denies that it ever sought to convince people to start smoking. Advertising, corporate spokespersons assert, is about brand warfare; that is, advertisements are targeted at winning customers from competitors, not at nonsmokers. As these historic internal industry documents suggest, however, public statements about advertising are no more truthful than earlier statements about knowledge of the health risks of smoking.

Settlement of massive lawsuits against the tobacco industry in 1998 included a signed agreement that youth would no longer be the targets of smoking advertising. As Philip Morris (2006) now states on its website, "the tobacco settlement agreements prohibit participating manufacturers from taking any action, directly or indirectly, to target youth within any settling state in the advertising, promotion or marketing of tobacco products. The settlements bar the use of cartoons in advertising, promotion, packaging or labeling of tobacco products. They bar most forms of outdoor advertising, including billboards and stadium signs. They ban transit advertisements such as those on taxis and at bus stops. The settlement agreements also prohibit advertising in the form of the distribution of apparel or merchandise such as caps, shirts and backpacks bearing tobacco brand names and logos." To make sure that people are aware that they have changed their ways, tobacco companies have poured millions of dollars into reimaging advertisements. Has the industry been compliant with the agreements as their advertisements claim, or have they found ways around them?

In the assessment of Arnett (2005), tobacco company "talk is cheap." Arnett conducted two studies with adolescents and adults concerning their perceptions of the ages of the models used in new cigarette ads as well as whether the ads portrayed smoking as essential to sexual attraction or success, issues of concern to youth. Findings indicate that for many of the ads, particularly those for brands that are most popular among younger smokers, a majority of the participants perceived the models to be less than 25 years old and a majority also perceived that many of the ads depicted smoking as fundamental for sexual attraction and life success. Concludes Arnett (2005:419), "despite their public pledge, the tobacco companies routinely violate a variety of aspects of the Cigarette Advertising and Promotion Code." A further indication of this pattern is seen in published research on the amount of money spent on advertising in magazines, including youth-oriented magazines. A study by King and Siegel (2001), for example, reviewed the costs of tobacco advertisement in magazines for "youth brands" of cigarettes, namely those such as Camel, Marlboro, and Newport, that are smoked by more than 5 percent of smokers in the eighth, tenth, and 12th grades. They classified magazines as youth oriented if at least 15 percent of their readers, or at least two million of their readers, were between 12 and 17 years of age. Based on the dollar value in the year 2000, these researchers found that the overall advertising expenditures for 15 brands of cigarettes in 38 magazines were $238.2 million in 1995, $219.3 million in 1998, $291.1 million in 1999, and $216.9 million in 2000. Advertisement expenditures for youth brands of cigarettes in youth-oriented magazines were $56.4 million in 1995, $58.5 million in 1998, $67.4 million in 1999, and $59.6 million in 2000. Moreover, they found that in 2000, magazine advertisements for youth brands of cigarettes reached more than 80 percent of young people in the United States an average of 17 times each. King and Siegel (2001:535) conclude the settlement agreement with the tobacco industry on advertising to youth "appears to have had little effect on cigarette advertising in magazines and on the exposure of young people to these advertisements."

Overall, according to the Federal Trade Commission, since the tobacco settlement, tobacco companies have ratcheted up their cigarette advertising expenditures by 125 percent to a record level of over $15 billion per year. This translates to over $41 million a day (Campaign for Tobacco-Free Kids 2005b). Much of this advertising money is still targeted to children and young adults. The Brown & Williamson Company, for example, began advertising its Kool brand of cigarettes with hip-hop images and music. Additionally, the industry has introduced new products that appear to be designed to attract young users, such as candy-flavored cigarettes and smokeless tobacco products.

Despite Philip Morris's impressive new website, there is growing evidence that the more tobacco companies have "changed," the more they have stayed the same. Since the settlement, Philip Morris has fought against a new generation of effective antitobacco ads in Florida, agreed to fund front groups in several states that oppose indoor smoking bans, developed a so-called youth tobacco prevention program that, in fact, was found to actually raise the odds that youth exposed to the program would begin smoking, blamed parents rather than company promotional efforts for youth having access to tobacco, launched foreign efforts to pass out free cigarettes to children, and sponsored youth concerts where cigarettes are distributed (Campaign for Tobacco-Free Kids 2005b).

Moreover, in a national telephone survey of 507 teens aged 12 to 17 from March 6 to 10, 2002, conducted by International Communications Research, it was found that nearly two-thirds (64 percent) of study participants reported that they had seen advertising for cigarettes or spit tobacco products during the previous two weeks, compared to only 27 percent of adults who said they had seen such ads (Campaign for Tobacco-Free Kids 2002). Philip Morris's Marlboro was the brand best remembered by youth in the study, with 61 percent recalling having seen advertisements for Marlboro, compared to 49 percent among adults.

Barring a sea change in the federal government's tendency to limit restriction and regulation of tobacco sales, the multibillion-dollar tobacco industry will continue to find ways to sell tobacco products. In light of the history of the industry, it is likely that the patterns of duplicity described above will continue. The industry is investing heavily in the development of what it is calling "potentially reduced exposure products" (PREPs), including such brands as Eclipse, Omni, Advance Lights, Accord, and Ariva. These products follow on the heels of so-called lite cigarettes, which were supposed to be less dangerous than regular cigarettes until it was discovered that smokers compensated by inhaling more smoke, inhaling more deeply, and/or smoking a greater number of cigarettes per day, resulting in more exposure to toxins than the advertisements suggested. Preliminary research (Caraballo et al. 2006) shows that individuals who have tried these new PREP brands learned about them through advertising or promotion, as well as from family, friends, and coworkers. Users report that the main reasons for first trying PREPs were that the products were free or inexpensive (as the companies have given them away as a promotion strategy), they wanted to stop smoking (and information on the PREP cigarette packages indicates that these products can help users to stop smoking by lessening the cigarette craving), they believed the product claims of fewer health risks, or they simply were curious. As these findings suggest, cynicism from extensive exposure to previous tobacco company misinformation campaigns can be overwhelmed with effective new advertising and creative promotion.

Bad Medicine: Vioxx et al.

In 2004, a Texas jury found that Merck & Co.—a global pharmaceutical company whose motto is "Where patients come first"—was negligent in the death of Robert Ernst, a 59-year-old triathlete and user of Merck's pain relief medication Vioxx. Ernst's widow was awarded $24 million in actual damages, as well as $229 million in punitive damages, for a total award of over $250 million. The outcome of the suit grabbed news media headlines, not only for its size and its defendant (a Big Pharma giant), but also for the over 11,500 additional personal injury lawsuits that were filed against Merck over Vioxx. By the time that Merck & Co. withdrew Vioxx from the market on September 30, 2004, doctors had written over 100 million prescriptions for the drug in the United States alone. With as many as 20 million people having taken Vioxx in the United States since the drug was introduced in 1999, Merck is at risk for judgments that could total $10 to $15 billion dollars (Consumer Affairs 2005), a startling turnaround for a drug that achieved annual sales in 2003 of approximately $2.5 billion.

As a result of the loss of this profitable product, Merck's drug sales for 2005 decreased by 7 percent. The company began a reorganization process in 2005 designed to decrease costs. On May 5, 2005, on the day congressional investigators released documents describing how the company continued to aggressively market Vioxx even after its dangers were known, Merck's CEO resigned.

The case of Vioxx and related COX-2 (cyclooxygenase) selective inhibitor and nonsteroidal anti-inflammatory drugs (e.g., Celebrex and Bextra) raises a number of important questions. No doubt, an issue on the minds of Merck stockholders was what went wrong with a blockbuster drug that began 2004 as a very profitable painkiller and ended the year as a denigrated killer commodity. Some researchers believe that while it was being sold, Vioxx may have contributed to 25,000 heart attacks and strokes (Bazerman and Chugh 2006). Even more startling, David Graham, associate director for science in the Office of Drug Safety at the FDA, told a Senate Finance Committee hearing that a "more realistic and likely range of estimates for the number of excess [heart attack and sudden cardiac death] cases would be from 88,000 to 138,000." To put the death toll in context, Graham reported that it was "the rough equivalent of 500 to 900 aircraft dropping from the sky" (Graham 2004). In this light, two additional questions are: How did Vioxx get FDA approval as a drug, and how did the drug survive for five years on the market?

Significantly, the first evidence of the drug's considerable risk potential began to appear years before it was withdrawn and possibly even before it was put on the market. Consequently, a parallel question on the minds of former users, doctors who prescribed the medication for their patients, and consumer advocates is: Why was the drug still on the market years after major problems were known and why were doctors who were aware of the negative findings on Vioxx still writing prescriptions for it? An additional question about Vioxx, one that may begin to point to an answer to all of the other questions is this: Why was Vioxx (and related drugs) so expensive? While chemically Vioxx ($C_9H_8O_4$) is related to aspirin ($C_{17}H_{14}O_4S$), Vioxx is sold in the United States for about 100 times the cost of aspirin. Was this price justifiable in terms of Merck's research and development costs? Or did the price, as Halpern (2005:319) argues, reflect a greed-driven maneuver "to fleece . . . patients"; the same greed that allowed a dangerous drug to wreak havoc in the lives of its users for years?

Celebrate, Celebrate with Celebrex

When they were first introduced to the market, the COX-2 blockers (all of which were eventually taken off the market) were touted by their respective manufacturers as highly selective, laserlike weapons that, unlike other medications, such as ibuprofen and aspirin, would be very easy on the user's stomach and intestines, reflecting a consistent problem in the long-term use of conventional painkillers. In that they had something powerful to offer—seemingly problem-free relief from the agony of chronic pain—it was not a stretch to use celebratory language in marketing the COX-2 drugs. As the sales volume of these drugs began to be realized globally, there can be no doubt that they produced considerable celebration among pharmaceutical company shareholders as well.

To get to the point of reaching the market and producing profit, new drugs are required to go through a supposedly rigorous process of monitored testing for safety and effectiveness. The gold standard for such testing is the double-blind clinical trial in which neither the researchers nor the study participants know whether they are getting the experimental drug or a placebo. Trials are designed to assess both whether a drug has unacceptable side effects (that is, is it safe for humans to use) and if it achieves its intended purpose (in this case, stopping pain) significantly more than a placebo or an existing drug used for the same purpose. Vioxx successfully passed through the multistage clinical trial process; outcomes showed that Vioxx did not have the adverse stomach effects of conventional nonsteroidal antiinflammatory drugs (such as aspirin) while exhibiting the same painkilling and anti-inflammatory properties. These findings were published in prestigious medical journals and the drug soon won FDA approval. The approved drug was heavily promoted to doctors, who in turn began writing prescriptions for patients. Many patients, anxious to be relieved of pain without suffering damage to their gastrointestinal system, reported they were pleased with Vioxx (many continued to want the drug, in fact, after its significant risks were well known). Later trials would be initiated to ascertain the effectiveness of Vioxx with other health problems, such as cancer.

That is the official story of how Vioxx came to be on the market. Glimpsing behind the scenes at Merck & Co., however, it is clear that the real story is much more complicated. Part of this backstage story has to do with the fact that at the time Merck was preparing Vioxx for clinical trials, the company was facing a loss of highly profitable patent protections on several of its big-earning drug products. The company was badly in need of a new superstar income generator. Consequently, Merck was highly motivated to ensure Vioxx was a success. The other part of the hidden story has to do with early warning signs that Vioxx had major problems, details that finally came to light when, on November 1, 2004, two months after Vioxx had been pulled from the market, the front page of the eastern edition of the *Wall Street Journal* featured an article by Anna Wilde Mathews and Barbara Martinez (2004) titled "Warning Signs: E-Mails Suggest Merck Knew Vioxx's Dangers at Early Stage." The article informed readers that

> when Merck & Co. pulled its big-selling painkiller Vioxx off the market in September, Chief Executive Raymond Gilmartin said the company was "really putting patient safety first." He said the study findings prompting the withdrawal, which tied Vioxx to heart-attack and stroke risk, were "unexpected." But internal Merck e-mails and marketing materials as well as interviews with outside scientists show that the company fought forcefully for years to keep safety concerns from destroying the drug's commercial prospects.

In fact, as it turns out, Merck first recognized there were serious problems with Vioxx in the mid-to-late 1990s. When clinical trials were being organized, Merck officials and scientists began discussing how to shape the trials so that they would minimize the higher level of heart problems that they feared among subjects given Vioxx compared to people on conventional pain medications. Note Mathews and Martinez (2004):

> A Nov. 21, 1996, memo by a Merck official shows the company wrestling with this issue. It wanted to conduct a trial to prove Vioxx was gentler on the stomach than older painkillers. But to show the difference most clearly, the Vioxx patients couldn't take any aspirin. In such a trial, "there is a substantial chance that significantly higher rates" of cardiovascular problems would be seen in the Vioxx group, the memo said. . . . A similar view was expressed in a Feb. 25, 1997 e-mail by a Merck official, Briggs Morrison. He argued that unless patients in the Vioxx group also got aspirin, "you will get more thrombotic events"—that is, blood clots—"and kill [the] drug."

By 2000, it appears fairly certain that Merck not only recognized that Vioxx lacked the protective features of conventional painkillers but also that the drug was linked to an increased rate of heart and other cardiovascular problems (Mathews and Martinez 2004). For four and half years, as the drug was being prescribed to millions of people, Merck nonetheless fought a tough rearguard action hoping to find evidence it could marshal in defense of the drug's safety. Meanwhile, company employees whose job it was to promote Vioxx were trained to dodge direct questions, including those from physicians, about its safety. An internal marketing document for field staff involved in promoting the drug to doctors instructed: "If a doctor said he was worried that Vioxx might raise the risk of a heart attack, he was to be told that the drug 'would not be expected to demonstrate reductions' in heart attacks or other cardiovascular problems and that it was 'not a substitute for aspirin.' This wasn't a direct answer" (Mathews and Martinez 2004).

In addition, the company went on the attack against several academic researchers who questioned the drug's safety. One of those who felt this pressure from the company was a respected Spanish researcher named Joan-Ramon Laporte of the Catalan Institute of Pharmacology in Barcelona. During the summer of 2002, Laporte edited a publication put out by the institute that included criticisms of Merck's handling of Vioxx that had previously been published in the British medical journal *Lancet*. Laporte soon received a correction statement from Merck that they wanted him to publish. He responded that he did not see a problem with the original publication and did not intend to publish a correction. Merck filed suit in a Spanish court against Laporte and the institute, demanding a public correction of inaccuracies in the institute publication. In January 2004, the judge hearing the case ruled in favor of Laporte, saying that the institute publication accurately reflected debate within the medical community about Vioxx and ordered Merck to pay court costs. Company efforts did not stop there. In March 2004, Laporte was a keynote speaker at an annual pharmaceutical conference for Spanish family practitioners and other physicians. In previous years, as is common in the medical world, Merck had helped to pay for the gathering. Prior to the conference, a Merck representative informed the organizer that the company preferred that Laporte be dropped from the program. When this was rejected, Merck withdrew its funding. Later, a corporate lawyer for Merck would assert that the company "is committed to open and vigorous scientific debate" and "never has had a policy of retaliating against scientists" but "has a right to defend its medicines against false claims" (Mathews and Martinez 2004).

Early in 1999, Merck initiated an 8,000-person clinical trial named VIGOR, which stood for the Vioxx Gastrointestinal Outcomes Research study, intended to show that the drug did not tend to cause problems with the gastrointestinal system. In the trial, people given a high dose of Vioxx were compared with those taking a conventional painkiller. Notably, the study excluded patients who were known to be at high risk for heart problems. No patients were allowed to take aspirin. The findings of the study, which were ready in March 2000, showed that Vioxx patients experienced fewer stomach problems than the comparison group; however, they suffered significantly more blood-clot-related health problems, affirming earlier concerns within Merck about Vioxx's safety. The heart attack rate in the Vioxx group ultimately was found to be five times greater than in the comparison group (20 cases versus four cases), not the kind of finding that would support widespread use of the drug. On March 9, 2000, the chief of research at Merck sent an e-mail in which he said the results showed that the cardiovascular problems "are clearly there," adding, "it is a shame but it is a low incidence and it is mechanism based as we worried it was." Alluding to other highly profitable drugs that had adverse effects, he concluded, "We have a great drug and like angioedema with vasotec and seizures with primaxin and myopathy with mevacor there is always a hazard. The class will do well and so will we" (Mathews and Martinez 2004).

With the results of the VIGOR study in hand, Merck issued a media release. The company's statement did not mention the apparent problem. A subsequent release was headlined "Merck confirms favorable cardiovascular safety profile of Vioxx." While acknowledging the VIGOR results, Merck maintained that other trials it had run showed "no difference in the incidence of cardiovascular events" between Vioxx and a placebo or between Vioxx and conventional painkillers (Mathews and Martinez 2004). Toward the end of 2000, paid scientific consultants of Merck and Merck's own scientists, including Alise Reicin, the company's vice president for clinical research, jointly published the findings of the VIGOR study in the prestigious *New England Journal of Medicine.* The article, while noting study findings suggesting the drug would be safe for people who were not at high risk for heart attacks, failed to provide known information about other serious cardiovascular complications, including strokes and blood clots associated with Vioxx use.

Subsequently, a review of the findings from the VIGOR trial by Harvard Medical School instructor John Abramson (2004) was discussed in his book *Overdosed America: The Broken Promise of American Medicine*, including his conclusion that even those patients who did not have a history of heart problems doubled their risk of developing a cardiovascular problem as a result of taking Vioxx instead of a conventional painkiller. The Vioxx case, according to Abramson (Heslam 2005), reflects a common pattern in the pharmaceutical industry: "American health care may not be the best at improving health most effectively and efficiently but it is certainly the best in the world at generating profits for the drug industry. . . . There's very little money to be made by the medical industry by pushing a healthy lifestyle."

The pharmaceutical industry, according to Abramson (2004), regularly engages in sleight-of-hand manipulation of information. Abramson is not alone in his response to the way Merck presented its data on Vioxx to the medical world. In a damning editorial in the *New England Journal of Medicine* published in 2005, written by the journal's editor-in-chief, Jeffrey

Frazen; executive editor, Gregory Curfman; and managing editor, Stephen Morrissey, the authors asserted that in their article on Vioxx published in the year 2000, Merck consultants and scientists failed to disclose three additional heart attack deaths among those taking Merck's drug as well as other relevant data from the VIGOR clinical trial. According to these physicians and medical editors (Johnson 2005:E1), "taken together these inaccuracies and deletions call into question the integrity of the data on adverse cardiovascular events in this article." Added Curfman, "the health of the public, of many, many thousands of people was at stake here" (Johnson 2005:E10).

In an effort to increase the windfall profits produced by Vioxx, Merck initiated a new clinical trial, ironically called Approve, to test the drug's effectiveness in preventing colon polyps, a significant risk for colon cancer. The trial, however, was cut short by a safety monitoring board whose job in a health study is to determine whether a trial should be halted prior to completion, either because the findings are so overwhelmingly positive that no further study participants should be subjected to the less effective comparison drug or a placebo, or because adverse effects are mounting for the experimental drug. In the case of Vioxx's cancer clinical trial, the latter was the case. The safety monitoring board found that among patients taking Vioxx for more than 18 months, there were 15 heart attacks or strokes for every 1,000 patients compared with 7.5 per 1,000 among those on the placebo. This finding was the death knell for Vioxx. Merck pulled it from the market. Consistent with the pattern of previous years, when Merck and consulting scientists submitted a paper to the *New England Journal of Medicine* on the findings from the Approve study, peer reviewers assigned to assess the manuscript had reservations. One commented: "The 'hand' of the study sponsor [i.e., Merck] seems too evident throughout the manuscript, which is written consistently in a fashion designed to support the company's public positions," while another reviewer noted that the paper "aggressively promotes the safety of up to 18 months of use of rofecoxib [i.e., Vioxx]. This goes beyond the data of the study" (Pollack and Abelson 2006).

In retrospect, Richard Horton (2004:1995–1996), editor of *Lancet*, concluded:

> The licensing of Vioxx and its continued use in the face of unambiguous evidence of harm have been public-health catastrophes. . . . The most important legacy of this episode is the continued erosion of trust that

> public-health institutions will suffer. . . . For with Vioxx, Merck and the FDA acted out of ruthless, short-sighted, and irresponsible self-interest.

Pulling the FDA into the Fray

When called before a U.S. Senate committee to testify about Vioxx, FDA whistle-blower David Graham (2004) began with a chilling assessment of the FDA's track record in approving pharmaceutical drugs for sale to the public that later turn out to be as dangerous as Vioxx.

> My research and efforts within FDA led to the withdrawal from the U.S. market of Omniflox, an antibiotic that caused hemolytic anemia; Rezulin, a diabetes drug that caused acute liver failure; Fen-Phen and Redux, weight loss drugs that caused heart valve injury; and PPA (phenylpropanolamine), an over-the-counter decongestant and weight loss product that caused hemorrhagic stroke in young women. My research also led to the withdrawal from outpatient use of Trovan, an antibiotic that caused acute liver failure and death.

Graham lends support to the assessment by *Lancet* chief editor Horton (2004:1995) that

> The public expects national drug regulators to complete research . . . in their ongoing efforts to protect patients from undue harm. But, too often, the FDA saw and continues to see the pharmaceutical industry as its customer—a vital source of funding for its activities—and not as a sector of society in need of strong regulation.

Indeed, as Graham suggests, part of the mission of the FDA, through its Center for Drug Evaluation and Research (CDER), is to ensure that medicines and vaccines for humans (as well as animals) are safe and effective. CDER, which traces its roots to the 1902 meeting of the American Pharmaceutical Association and passage a few years later of the federal Pure Food and Drugs Act, asserts that its mission is to provide "rigorous review" of new drugs to ensure that they meet "the highest scientific standards and are demonstrated to be safe and effective."

After detailing the case against Vioxx, in his Senate testimony, Graham (2004) reported the response at the FDA to findings that Vioxx was causing heart attacks, and lots of them. When Graham (2004) presented his findings to the FDA's Office of New Drugs, it triggered "an explosive response." Graham testified that he was pressured to change his conclusions about Vioxx and his recommendations about banning the drug. Unless findings were changed, Graham was told, he could not present his findings, as planned, at the International Conference on Pharmacoepidemiology. Meanwhile, the director of the Office of New Drugs e-mailed Graham to say that the FDA was not contemplating putting a warning label on Vioxx. Even within a few weeks of when Merck stopped producing and selling Vioxx, no one at the FDA besides Graham was expressing safety concerns about the drug. In Graham's assessment, the problem is the "corporate culture" within the FDA, a case of the fox guarding the henhouse.

Support for Graham's scornful assessment of the FDA was not long in coming. A study of the individuals who serve on the 50 advisory boards that are supposed to provide objective and detached advice on awarding FDA approval for drugs and other medical products (e.g., silicone breast implants) found that almost 30 percent of panel members had financial connections to companies whose products need FDA approval but that members rarely excuse themselves for conflict of interest. Dr. Steven Nissen, a well-known cardiologist at the Cleveland Clinic and an FDA adviser, affirmed during a panel discussion organized by the Center for Science in the Public Interest that

> the American people no longer trust the FDA to protect their health. The entire FDA budget for drug regulation is only about $500 million and relies extensively on user fees. As a consequence, the FDA is financially indebted to the companies it must regulate. This is a fundamental conflict of interest. (Alonso-Zaldivar 2006)

Moreover, as concluded in the aftermath of Vioxx in the report of the Subcommittee on Science and Technology (2007:2), "science at the FDA is in a precarious position: the Agency suffers from serious scientific deficiencies and is not positioned to meet current or emerging regulatory responsibilities."

Did Merck fold because of the Vioxx catastrophe? While the company suffered losses and lawsuits are pending, by the second quarter of

2006, Merck reported a net income of $1.5 billion, up from $750 million for the same quarter the year before (Associated Press 2006). Based on the strength of two of its products, Fosamax (for osteoporosis) and Singulair (for asthma), the company's stock was doing well, its stock value was rising, and Vioxx had disappeared from the headlines.

Asbestos Still

While asbestos has often been touted, at least until recent decades, as one of the marvels of the industrial era, its use is quite old. Indeed, the word *asbestos* comes from the Greek for "inextinguishable" or "indestructible." A number of epidemiological studies conducted in Britain and the United States during the 1930s and 1940s brought attention to various complications, including cancer and pulmonary ones, associated with asbestosis. Exposure to asbestos endangers workers involved in the mining and processing of asbestos and the manufacture of asbestos-containing products as well as people exposed to asbestos already in place. The public health impact of the latter was made visible in the aftermath of the two attacks on the World Trade Center in 2001, with the release of in-place asbestos into the surrounding environment.

Despite an early recognition of the health hazards associated with asbestos, it is a substance that is utilized in a wide range of products, including insulation. In recent decades, as public health officials have made people aware of the health hazards associated with asbestos, numerous asbestos abatement projects have been implemented, particularly in developed societies.

For anyone familiar with books like Michael Bowker's *Fatal Deception* (2003), one is never sure whether such assurances on the part of the powers-that-be are trustworthy. His account focuses upon the activities of W. R. Grace and Company, a well-known chemical and oil conglomerate based in Columbia, Maryland, with operations in far-flung locations such as France, Germany, Japan, Australia, and New Zealand. In 1963, the company purchased a mining facility in Libby, Montana, in order to extract a rare and versatile ore called vermiculite, which is used in insulation, animal feed, potting soil, gypsum plaster, fertilizer, brake pads, fireproof safes, paints, fireplaces, and other products. The vermiculite deposit at Libby is situated on the top of a mountain about six miles north of town. Montana state health officials had discovered that vermiculite dust contains high levels of tremoli asbestos, a substance that is used in more than 3,000 products (Bowker 2003).

In Australia, James Hardie Industries Ltd., which moved its headquarters to the Netherlands in 2001 in order to avoid compensating asbestos victims, has been a major producer of asbestos products (Haigh 2006). The company dominated the Australian asbestos cement products market for decades, with a market share of nearly 90 percent. It also produced insulation products, pipes, brakes, and clutch linings that contained asbestos. James Hardie asbestos products contributed to numerous instances of people developing asbestosis and mesothelioma; however, it was not until the late 1980s that James Hardie admitted that asbestos products are killer commodities. Ironically, as far back as 1935, a factory inspector reported on the health hazards of asbestos workers at a James Hardie factory in Perth (Pearce 2004). As a result of pressure from labor unions, the company was forced to set up the Medical Research and Compensation Foundation to provide financial compensation for victims of its products. Fortunately, Australia and the Netherlands have a treaty that allows the company's Australian victims to sue for compensation in Dutch courts.

Indeed, more than 250,000 tons of asbestos reportedly were imported and used in U.S. products between 1991 and 2001 alone. The asbestos industry maintains that asbestos is safe as long as it remains sealed in place, such as in cements and tiles, but virtually all asbestos products become friable as they age, which means that fibers can easily flake off. Asbestos reportedly results in the death of over 100,000 workers worldwide per annum (Bowker 2003). The most prominent victims of asbestos-related diseases include U.S. Navy admiral Elmo Zumwalt, movie actor Steve McQueen, natural scientist Stephen Jay Gould, and Democratic Minnesota congressman Bruce Vento. The United Nations has estimated that some three million people in developing countries will die from asbestos-related diseases by 2030 (Bowker 2003:244). Asbestos-related diseases generally require from ten to 50 years to manifest themselves in the form of serious symptoms. Over 600,000 U.S. asbestos victims have filed lawsuits and claims (Bowker 2003). The Environmental Protection Agency (EPA), the Occupational Safety and Health Administration (OSHA), and various other federal and state regulatory agencies each have their own rules dictating the number of asbestos fibers that are permissible and considered safe in dwelling units and/or worksites. While OSHA requires warning labels on raw asbestos materials in worksites, it rarely requires such warnings on consumer products and conducts little monitoring in the manufacturing processes involving asbestos-containing products, with the exception of a worker filing a complaint about a possible hazardous procedure. Conversely, the EPA website (www.epa.gov) admits that "there is no known safe exposure level for asbestos." By the mid-1980s, the EPA conceded that about 20 percent of public buildings in the United States included some form of asbestos-containing friable material and that asbestos removals often expose both workers and building occupants to fibers.

In 1989, the EPA implemented a phaseout program that was intended to completely ban the manufacture, importation, processing, and distribution of asbestos and the sale of certain products containing asbestos. Lobbying by the U.S. and Canadian asbestos industries contributed to a decision on the part of the fifth court of appeals in 1991 rejecting most of the EPA's guidelines (Darcey and Alleman 2004:18). EPA rules to phase out asbestos were overturned in a court decision in 2004. Most asbestos is used in cement sheets and pipes, despite warnings that this is especially dangerous because many people are exposed to the substance in airborne ducts.

In contrast to the United States, over 35 countries, including most European ones and Australia, have banned asbestos (Bowker 2003). Indeed, Collaegium Ramazzini, an international nongovernmental organization that focuses on occupational and health policy matters, has proposed a global ban on asbestos use (Darcey and Alleman 2004:18). Although Canada prohibits use of asbestos products within its borders, it exports an estimated 680 million pounds per annum of chrysotile asbestos. Indeed, it and Russia continue to be world's leading asbestos exporters. A new asbestos factory opened in India in 2004. Although the use of asbestos in the United States has declined, it continues to be imported into the country.

Theorizing Killer Commodities: Conspiracies, Systematics, and Hegemonies

This review of several killer commodity cases, and the chapters that follow, raise critical questions about theoretical models for understanding what drives the killer commodities market. Several alternative theories present themselves. One points to the issue of conspiracies within corporations to hide known information about the risks of their products so as not to threaten the bottom line (i.e., making money), as well as a pattern of collusion with governmental regulatory bodies that seem at times more concerned with protecting corporate profits than public health. As the cases presented thus far suggest, there is evidence of both conspiracy and collusion. Given patterns of appointment to regulatory bodies, however, it seems fair to ask whether collusion is even the right designation, in that those doing the appointing, those being appointed, and those appointed to monitor are all members of the same social class with similar values and commitments.

As suggested by other information presented in this book, the prevalence of killer commodities goes beyond overt conspiracy and backroom complicity. It suggests built-in, systemic structures and widely diffused and extensively reinforced cultural constructions. To some degree, we all participate in the culture of consumerism that helps to fuel the toxification of commodities: we buy products known to be environmentally harmful, we allow ourselves to be nagged by our (advertisement-coaxed) children into buying questionable foods or playthings, we seek instant chemical relief from all pains and upsets, we fail to demand a high standard of corporate responsibility, and we reelect politicians who have been shown to be in bed with corporations that demand welfare for the rich in the form of single-bidder contracts, tax cuts, government services, and toothless regulatory agencies. Some might ask: are we all to blame for killer commodities? Is the best model for understanding them a systems theory like the kind developed half a century ago by thinkers like Ludwig von Bertalanffy and William Ross Ashby, and more recently within cybernetics, catastrophe theory, and chaos theory, that directs analysis away from a "corporation good" versus "public good" way of thinking and toward an understanding of the connections among circular and interlocking components that comprise a complex societal whole? Certainly there are those who would embrace such a model of killer commodities.

Alternately, there is the theoretical concept of hegemony developed by Antonio Gramsci, an Italian political activist and political theorist, who sought to elaborate the observation of Marx and Engels that ruling ideas in society in every era are the ideas of (and that benefit) the ruling class. In the modern era of the capitalist world system, critical hegemony theorists seek to understand the processes by which capitalist assumptions, concepts, and values come to permeate the core institutions of society, including government bodies and agencies, churches, the schools, the media, and families. From this perspective, the ruling class—namely the wealthiest and most powerful sector of society, those who populate corporate boards of directors and who control much of the wealth in society—is understood to exert direct domination through the coercive vehicles of the state apparatus (e.g., the government, courts, military, police, and prisons) as well as the ability to use wealth to buy and enforce influence. Additionally, and equally if not more important in the view of hegemony theorists, the dominant class exerts control of the cognitive and intellectual life of society by structural means as opposed to coercive ones. Hegemony is achieved through the diffusion and constant reinforcement throughout the key institutions of society of certain values, attitudes, beliefs, social norms, and legal precepts. Hegemony theorists, in other words, recognize that in the same way that prisoners participate in their own imprisonment (by not constantly rebelling, by giving incriminating information to guards about fellow prisoners, by physically enforcing social control among inmates) so too consumers participate in the acceptance of killer commodities and the structural relationships that support their gaining access to the market. In this sense, producer/consumer relations in the market constitute an arena of hegemonic interaction. Studies of these interactions (e.g., Baer, Singer, and Susser 2003; Castro and Singer 2004) show that they reinforce corporate hegemony by: 1) generating needs and desires while defining product consumption as the route to fulfillment, success, pleasure, and a sense of self-worth; 2) stressing the need for the consumer to comply with a social superior's or expert's judgment (a common argument made for corporate self-regulation as well as the common use of "experts" to affirm product safety); and 3) directing consumer attention to the immediate causes of product-related injury or death (e.g., lack of parental supervision) and away from structural factors (e.g., corporate influence over product regulation, cooptation of academicians and academies that play a role in commodity production and evaluation) that underlie the flow to market of killer commodities.

We will return to the issue of killer commodity theory in the final chapter. The chapters in between this introduction and the conclusion offer ample material to assess alternative theories. Based on original contributions from 16 authors, this volume provides a theoretically grounded introduction to the analysis of killer commodities and their impact on contemporary society and public health. Given the number of dangerous products on the market, in some ways this book only scratches the surface. Many known killer commodities are not examined. Still, there is sufficient coverage here to affirm the discomforting sense that something is terribly wrong and the public is in harm's way from a host of products of a quite diverse sort, in their homes, in their communities, on the job, and in the wider environment. The government regulatory systems—however limited—that were erected to protect the public from earlier waves of deadly commodities, have been, in many ways, disempowered. The fox, in the form of industry representatives, now guards the henhouse (e.g., the FDA, the CPSC), and, to use Shakespeare's apt phrase from *Henry IV*, "stony-hearted villains" have an increasingly free hand to peddle dangerous wares at the public's expense.

References

Abramson, John
2004 Overdosed America: The Broken Promise of American Medicine. New York: HarperCollins.
Alonso-Zaldivar, Ricardo
2006 FDA Pledges Conflict Reforms. Los Angeles Times, July 25: A12.
Arnett, J.
2005 Talk Is Cheap: The Tobacco Companies' Violations of Their Own Cigarette Advertising Code. Journal of Health Communications 10(5):419–431.
Associated Press
2006 Merck Reports Major Gains. July 26.
B&W (Brown and Williamson Tobacco Company)
1982 What Are the Obstacles/Enemies of a Swing to Low "Tar" and What Action Should We Take? Minnesota Trial Exhibit #26. July 2: 185.

Baer, Hans, Merrill Singer, and Ida Susser
2003 Medical Anthropology and the World System. Westport, CT: Praeger.
BAT (British-American Tobacco Company)
1959 BAT Research & Development, Complexity of the P.A.5.A. Machine and Variables Pool. Minnesota Trial Exhibit #10,392. August 26.
1962 A. McCormick, Smoking and Health: Policy on Research, Minutes of Southampton Meeting. Document #1102.01.
1979 P. Lee, Note on Tar Reduction for Hunter, Tobacco Advisory Council. July 19 (L&D UK Ind 33).
Bazerman, M., and D. Chugh
2006 Decisions without Blinders. Harvard Business Review 84(1):88–97.
Bowker, Michael
2003 Fatal Deception: The Untold Story of Asbestos—Why It Is Still Legal and Still Killing Us. Emmaus, PA: Rodale.
Business Information Analysis Corporation.
1985 RJR Young Adult Motivational Research. R. J. Reynolds Tobacco Company. January 10, http://www.rjrtdocs.com/rjrtdocs/index.wmt?tab=home.
Campaign for Tobacco-Free Kids
2002 New Poll Shows Kids Still Bombarded with Tobacco Advertising. Electronic document, www.tobaccofreekids.org/Script/DisplayPressRelease.php3?Display=472.
2005a Campaign Contributions by Tobacco Interests. Electronic document, http://tobaccofreeaction.org/contributions.
2005b Special Report; Big Tobacco Still Targeting Kids. Electronic document, www.tobaccofreekids.org/reports/targeting.
Caraballo, R., L. Pederson, and N. Gupta
2006 New Tobacco Products: Do Smokers Like Them? Tobacco Control 15:39–44.
Castro, Arachu, and Merrill Singer, eds.
2004 Unhealthy Health Policy: A Critical Anthropological Examination. Lanham, MD: AltaMira Press.
Centers for Disease Control and Prevention
1993 Smoking-Attributable Mortality and Years of Potential Life Lost—United States, 1990. Morbidity and Mortality Weekly Report 1993 42(33):645–648.
2004 National Youth Tobacco Survey Atlanta.
Consumer Affairs
2005 Class Action Could Cost Merck Billions. Electronic document, www.consumeraffairs.com/news04/2005/vioxx_class_action02.html.

Darcey, Dennis J., and Tony Alleman
2004 Occupational and Environmental Exposure to Asbestos. *In* Pathology of Asbestos-Associated Diseases. Victor L. Roggli, Tim D. Oury, and Thomas A. Sporn, eds. Pp. 17–33. New York: Springer.
Feder, Barnaby
2006 Lens Cleaner Is Recalled Worldwide. New York Times, May 16: C1, C8.
Graham, David
2004 Testimony to Congress. Electronic document, http://finance.senate.gov/hearings/testimony/2004test/111804dgtest.pdf.
Haigh, Gideon
2006 Asbestos House: The Secret History of James Hardie Industries. Melbourne: Scribe.
Halpern, Georges
2005 COX-2 Inhibitors: A Story of Greed, Deception and Death. Inflammopharmacology 13(4):419–425.
Hammond, D., N. Collishaw, and C. Callard
2006 Secret Science: Tobacco Industry Research on Smoking Behaviour and Cigarette Toxicity. Lancet 367(9512):781–787.
Heslam, Jessica
2005 Harvard Doc: You May Not Need that Lipitor. Boston Herald, June 19: 4.
Horton, Richard
2004 Vioxx, the Implosion of Merck, and Aftershocks at the FDA. Lancet 364:1995–1996.
Johnson, Linda
2005 Journal Assails Vioxx Study. Hartford Courant, December 9: E1, E10.
Kessler, David
1994 Statement on Nicotine-Containing Cigarettes to the House Subcommittee on Health and the Environment by the Commissioner of the Food and Drug Administration. Electronic document, www.fda.gov/bbs/topics/SPEECH/SPE00052.htm.
2001 A Question of Intent: A Great American Battle with a Deadly Industry. New York: PublicAffairs.
King, C., and Michael Siegel
2001 The Master Settlement Agreement with the Tobacco Industry and Cigarette Advertising in Magazines. New England Journal of Medicine 345(7):535–537.
Kluger, Richard
1996 Ashes to Ashes: America's Hundred-Year Cigarette War, the Public Health, and the Unabashed Triumph of Philip Morris. New York: Vintage Books.

Mathews, Anna Wilde, and Barbara Martinez
2004 Warning Signs: E-Mails Suggest Merck Knew Vioxx's Dangers at Early Stage. Wall Street Journal, November 1: A1.

Meier, Barry
2005 Heart Device Sold Despite Flaw, Data Shows. New York Times, June 2: C1.
2006a Heart Device Makers Plan Enhanced Safety Review. New York Times, May 16: C3.
2006b Study Finds High Rate of Recalls of Heart Devices Used in Emergencies. New York Times, May 16: C1.

Nader, Ralph
1965 Unsafe at Any Speed: The Designed-In Dangers of the American Automobile. New York: Grossman.

National Institute on Drug Abuse
1998 NIDA Research Report—Nicotine Addiction: NIH Publication no. 01–4342.

New York Times
2006 F.D.A. Report Faults Maker of Contact Lens Solution. New York Times, May 17: C6.

Pearce, Rohan
2004 James Hardie: Murder by Any Other Name. Green Left Weekly, September 15.

Pepples, E.
1976 Industry Response to the Cigarette/Health Controversy, 1976. Internal memo #2205.01.

Philip Morris
2006 Smoking and Health Issues. Electronic document, www.philipmorrisusa.com/en/health_issues/cigarette_smoking_and_disease.as.

Pollack, Andrew, and Reed Abelson
2006 Why the Data Diverge on the Dangers of Vioxx. New York Times, May 22. Electronic document, www.nytimes.com/2006/05/22/business/22drug.html?pagewanted=1.

Short, P.
1977 Smoking and Health Item 7: The Effect on Marketing. Minnesota Trial Exhibit #10,585. April 14.

Subcommittee on Science and Technology
2007 FDA Science and Mission at Risk. Electronic document, www.fda.gov/ohrms/dockets/ac/07/briefing/2007-4329b_02_01_FDA%20Report%20on%20Science%20and%20Technology.pdf.

Teague, Claude
1973 Some Thoughts about New Brands of Cigarettes for the Youth Market. R. J. Reynolds. Electronic document, www.rjrtdocs.com/

rjrtdocs/image_downloader.wmt?MODE=PDF&SEARCH=4&ROW=2&DOC_RANGE=502987407+-7418&CAMEFROM=2.

UK Department of Health

1998 Report of the Scientific Committee on Tobacco and Health. Electronic document, www.archive.official-documents.co.uk/document/doh/tobacco/part-1.htm#1.30.

University of California, San Francisco

2002 Legacy Tobacco Documents Library. Electronic document, http://legacy.library.ucsf.edu.

Wakefield, Melanie, Yvonne Terry-McElrath, Frank Chaloupka, Dianne Barker, Sandy Slater, Pamela Clark, and Gary Giovino

2002 Tobacco Industry Marketing at Point of Purchase after the 1998 MSA Billboard Advertising Ban. American Journal of Public Health 92(6):131–133.

Wakeham, H.

1961 Tobacco and Health—R&D Approach. Cipollone 608. Minnesota Trial Exhibit #10,300. November 15.

World Health Organization

1969 WHO Technical Report Series, no. 407. Geneva.

Zickler, Patrick

2001 Adolescents, Women and Whites More Vulnerable Than Others to Becoming Nicotine Dependent. NIDA Notes 16(2):39–40.

2003 Nicotine's Multiple Effects on the Brain's Reward System Drive Addiction. NIDA Notes 17(6):24–25.

Part One
HOME COMMODITIES

CHAPTER ONE

STEALTHY KILLERS AND GOVERNING MENTALITIES

Chemicals in Consumer Products

Edward J. Woodhouse and Jeff Howard

Rachel Carson's *Silent Spring* (1962) is credited with revolutionizing public understanding of the hazards posed by industrial chemicals. On reflection, however, one must wonder how thoroughly technological society has grasped the landmark book's implications. For, despite the environmental movement's success in reducing some specific hazards, such as those from persistent pesticides, chemical toxicity generally reaches more deeply and more broadly into the fabric of daily life in our era than it did in Carson's.

This has occurred despite the fact that scientific and public knowledge of health and environmental effects has improved enormously over the past half century. Even casual observers have encountered a steady stream of news stories documenting that industrial chemicals emitted during the manufacture, use, and disposal of consumer products cause cancer and birth defects; impair the respiratory, nervous, and immune systems; and disrupt the body's hormonal balance and reproductive capacities. Why, then, have such chemical hazards been allowed to proliferate?

Anyone who tries to think about this subject is immediately confronted with its scientific complexity: more than a million different consumer products containing diverse combinations of some one hundred thousand commercial chemicals—and additional substances generated during production, use, disposal, or degradation of the original constituents. Most of these chemicals have never been assessed toxicologically, and understanding the combined effects of even a few hundred synthetic organic chemicals within a living organism is beyond scientific capacities (see Montague 2004). Nor have governments or businesses yet systematically mapped the flow of chemicals in and around consumer products: Wal-Mart alone carries a hundred thousand items (Frontline 2004), and even that giant retailer with its virtually unlimited resources has only recently begun to trace some of the environmental implications of the raw materials that go into its products, the production of those goods, and their packaging, transport, and retail distribution (Gunther et al. 2006).

Readily available information is damning, however, and we begin by briefly examining a representative set of everyday toxic products. These include PVC (polyvinyl chloride), plastic household items containing phthalates, dandruff shampoos, an agricultural fumigant that leaves toxic residues on food, a chemical for decaffeinating coffee, flame retardants, and Teflon-coated cookware. Some of these are toxic during use, whereas others are problematic during manufacture or disposal. We provide just enough technical information to demonstrate the basics of this fascinating and disturbing—but, thus far, mostly latent—controversy. In the process, and in the remainder of this chapter, we address a question that in an increasingly technological society is of considerable importance: What social norms and arrangements have contributed to this "toxification"?

As a modest contribution to the growing literature on sustainable consumption (Cohen and Murphy 2001), we propose that toxic commodities exist in the numbers and varieties they do less because of technological necessity than because a substantial majority of people in most Western nations tacitly share a set of political assumptions that inadvertently have enabled this toxification. Our aim is both to document the ubiquity of toxic threats associated with households and to derive insights concerning the *governing mentalities* at work in this domain.

Examples of Toxic Household Products

Polyvinyl chloride (PVC), commonly known as vinyl, is a plastic now ubiquitous in homes, schools, and businesses across the planet. Approximately 30 million tons are produced annually. "Quite simply, PVC is now one of the most common synthetic materials in the world. There are few if any major economic activities that it does not touch in one way or another" (McGinn 2000:47). Because PVC has the advantages of being cheap, not rusting like metal, and not decaying like wood, most drinking water now moves through PVC pipes and the plastic is used for everything from food wrap to patio furniture. Vinyl pipe, siding, doors, and window frames have made substantial inroads at the expense of iron, aluminum, and wood (Greenpeace n.d.).

Manufacturing PVC involves a number of toxicologically nasty chemicals, including ethylene dichloride, a known carcinogen and suspected neurotoxin that ranks among the most environmentally harmful synthetic chemicals (Scorecard 2006). In addition to routine chemical releases during the manufacturing process, there are industrial accidents and fires, the largest of which to date burned 400 tons of PVC. Several million fires occur annually in homes, restaurants, and other businesses around the world, and many people deliberately burn meat wrappers on barbeque grills. Chemical constituents of PVC can leach into one's body from medical plastics (Lakshmi and Jayakrishnan 2003) and from water pipes (Baue 2001). Disposal of PVC trimmings and discarded PVC products via incineration generates dioxins and other chlorinated by-products (McGinn 2000:55ff; Costner 2000). Highly toxic chlorinated dioxin formed as a by-product during manufacture is an unintentional contaminant in PVC cling film and other consumer products. More than 120,000 tons of lead, a potent neurotoxin, are used annually to improve the plastic's durability, some of which is released into the household as window blinds and other PVC products age (Thornton 2000:313).

The flexibility of many PVC products comes from additives known as "plasticizers." *Phthalates* are added to PVC to enhance the flexibility of nipples for baby bottles, chewable baby toys (see chapter 2), and an array of other items from raincoats and vinyl flooring to garden hoses and electrical wiring (CDC 2006). These substances often do not entirely remain within the plastic, because they

> are not chemically bonded to the PVC polymer but are merely mixed into the plastic during its formulation. Over time, they leach out of vinyl products, entering the air, water, or other liquids with which the product

> comes into contact. Phthalates . . . are especially likely to evaporate, creating the familiar smell we associate with a new vinyl shower curtain. . . . Some 42,000 tons of phthalates are emitted into the air from PVC products in the world each year. (Thornton 2000:313)

Phthalates also are used as ingredients in cosmetics and toiletries, including aftershaves, deodorants, skin creams, hair preparations, nail polishes, and fragrances and in household floor polishes, adhesives, caulks, and paints (NIH 2006).

Phthalates are suspected carcinogens, disrupt the endocrine (hormonal) system, and are believed to interfere with mammalian reproductive systems over several generations (CREDO n.d.). Approximately five million tons of phthalates are produced annually, most of which goes into PVC (McGinn 2000:52). Phthalates have come to be nearly ubiquitous in the household, the global environment, and human body fluids, with especially high levels in the blood of children using PVC pacifiers and teething rings (Costner et al. 2005). According to a public health advocacy organization, "aggregate phthalate exposures, from multiple sources, raise a significant public health concern" (DiGangi et al. 2002:5).

What ought one make of the fact that many parents who would not let children eat food off the floor allow them to chew on toxic toys? Why do many pediatricians fail to communicate effectively with parents regarding such chronic risks? Of course the manufacturers are primarily to blame for creating the risks, but to stop there is to fail to probe large questions regarding the human system of inquiry—and lack of inquiry.

Unlike PVC and phthalates, which have received considerable attention from environmental scientists and activists, *dandruff shampoos* are so ordinary as to be almost beneath notice. Yet they contain fungicides that are intended *not* to be innocuous. Approximately ten million pounds of zinc pyrithione are used annually in dandruff shampoos. While this chemical has human health consequences, including the potential for rapid and irreversible eye damage, its main risks may be elsewhere. Shampoo washed down shower drains ends up in wastewater treatment plants that use bacteria to help decompose sewage and other waste. Because zinc pyrithione is toxic to microorganisms—the reason it is used in shampoos—the chemical kills or inhibits the bacteria that are being used to treat wastes (SSNC 2004). The useful bacteria in these systems grow slowly, so they are not easy to regenerate. To the extent that natural bacterial processing of wastes fails to work, there are indirect and potentially serious consequences for human health, especially in parts of the world where waste and water treatment is already problematic. Additional treatments such as chlorination of water supplies can partially compensate, but these bring their own risks, including higher levels of hazardous chlorine by-products. Boat-hull paint containing zinc pyrithione "poses a significant risk to nontarget aquatic organisms," according to the New York State Department of Environmental Conservation (2003).

It is fair to ask why any ordinary user of dandruff shampoos or marine paint would think about their environmental side effects. The answer is that these substances are simply lightweight versions of the chemicals that troubled Rachel Carson: pesticides. Any chemical designed to kill something annoying may be dangerous to other living organisms, and members of an advanced technological civilization ought to be attuned to that reality. Opinions of course will differ about how far to go in worrying about such matters, but there is a case to be made, as we said earlier, that Carson's story has not been fully grasped. Most users evidently are incurious about the effects of dandruff fungicides and zinc-containing pesticidal paint on nontarget organisms, and the lack of curiosity assists manufacturers who want to sell such products.

Some chemicals that show up in homes are more commonly used in industrial applications. These include the chemical solvent *methylene chloride*, which was introduced into commerce in the mid–20th century as a replacement for more flammable solvents. Approximately 200 million pounds of methylene chloride are used annually in the United States, principally in paint removers and industrial adhesives, in manufacturing of pharmaceuticals and urethane foam, and as a cleaning agent for fabricated metal parts (HSIA 2003).

One connection to consumer commodities is the chemical's use as a solvent for extracting caffeine from coffee. The fine print on some bags of Starbucks coffee beans reads: "If this bag contains decaffeinated coffee other than Decaf Komodo Dragon Blend, it was decaffeinated with methylene chloride." The U.S. Food and Drug Administration long ago banned methylene chloride in hairspray and cosmetics but allows its use in treating coffee. Tested samples of coffee have residual methylene chloride far below the maximum allowed level of ten parts per million. Given that no lower limit has been demonstrated for carcinogenic potential, however, as Michael F. Jacobson, of the Center for Science in the Public Interest, puts it, "it's an insane policy to allow the use of an unnecessary and acknowledged carcinogen" (Molotsky 1985).

Other ways to decaffeinate coffee, although sometimes more expensive, do not rely on a toxic solvent: Folgers uses ethyl acetate, a chemical naturally occurring in apples, and Nestlé's Nescafé Taster's Choice uses a water-based process. An alternative of particular interest is supercritical carbon dioxide, one of a family of "green solvents" that are a centerpiece of green chemistry. Rather than merely trying to keep toxic levels low enough to pass governmental scrutiny, green chemists design chemicals and production processes to be benign from the start. Supercriticality is fairly simple: put a gas under the right pressure and temperature, and it becomes a fluid with very different chemical properties. Carbon dioxide becomes a powerful solvent that can replace benzene and toluene in many applications, such as cleaning circuit boards for electronics. Of course CO_2 evaporates when returned to room temperature and pressure and is generally regarded as nontoxic (done properly, the process does not contribute to climate change). Its usefulness in decaffeinating coffee has been clear for many years (Katz 1987), yet the use of methylene chloride persists.

One of the sources quoted above was published in the *New York Times* more than two decades ago, and Starbucks bags are handled, if not read, by many, many highly educated persons. Is it reasonable to expect ordinary people to know about the many alternative, nontoxic technologies such as supercritical CO_2? When handed a bag of coffee with what is in effect a warning label, how would members of an intelligent civilization respond? And what stands between most people's present inquiry skills or interests and the probing capacities that might be desirable?

Questions arise as well about relationships between ordinary people and the experts to whom crucial tasks are delegated in a technological civilization's complex division of labor. Supercriticality has been understood for about a century, yet industrial chemists and chemical engineers barely used it until recently and failed to publicize the potentials. Who ought to have asked what, when? What responsibilities do nonchemists have to inquire into the structuring of chemistry curricula and the governmental institutions that oversee academic and industrial chemistry?

Another toxics issue involving food is that of the pesticide *methyl bromide*. The Montreal Protocol of 1991 listed the chemical as contributing to depletion of the ozone layer, and the U.S. Environmental Protection Agency (EPA) shortly thereafter initiated action under the Clean Air Act "to phase out use and production of methyl bromide by January 1, 2001" (USDA 1995). Various exceptions and delays have pushed the date back again and again. The odorless, colorless gas is used to fumigate soil prior to planting tomatoes, peppers, and strawberries, and the food-processing industry uses methyl bromide to keep rodents and insects from contaminating cookies, crackers, pasta, chips, spices, herbs, cocoa, powdered milk, and coffee beans (NIH 2006). Not surprisingly, residual amounts remain on the food. Toxicologists consider the chemical especially dangerous to children; the state of California has labeled it as a developmental toxicant on the basis of animal experiments showing birth defects (Hallier et al. 1993; Hodgson and Rose 2005).

A U.S. ban on methyl bromide formally took effect in 2005, but growers remain able to use the fumigant on a limited basis if granted a "critical-use exemption" by the EPA. In fact, more of the chemical was used in the United States in 2006 than a year earlier, although the long-term trend is downward. There are said to be "no technically feasible alternatives that can be used without incurring significant economic losses" (USEPA 2004:2), but the definition of "loss" turns out to be squishy. Alternative fumigants take longer to kill target pests, so production lines have to be slowed; yet if every competitor were required to take the same care, none would necessarily suffer economically. There also are nonchemical alternatives to methyl bromide, including "controlled atmospheres, cold and carbon dioxide under pressure," technologies that the EPA claims would require "major investments for appropriate treatment units and/or major retrofits of existing warehouses" (USEPA 2004:7). Alternatively, such investments could be construed simply as a cost of doing business in an environmentally responsible manner, so one needs to ask: What accounts for the high priority given to cost relative to health?

As methyl bromide is phased out, the chemical replacing it is metam-sodium, which "decomposes rapidly to methyl isothiocyanate, a highly toxic compound capable of killing a wide spectrum of soil-borne pests" (Li et al. 2006). This same chemical was involved in the Bhopal disaster of 1986, which may illustrate the difficulty of learning from experience in the chemicals business. Without a broad shift in public consciousness favoring detoxification of economic activities, industry executives have the latitude to substitute one kind of hazard for another, a form of socially delegated authority discussed further in the next section.

Flame retardants are chemicals that suppress or inhibit the combustibility of textiles and upholstered furniture, construction materials, electronic circuit-board resins, and the plastic casings for coffeemakers, fax machines, computers, and vacuum cleaners (BSEF 2000). For example, polyurethane foam—itself toxic in some formulations—is too flammable to be used safely in upholstered furniture unless treated with a flame retardant. And many electronic devices constitute inherent fire hazards unless treated. Several environmental organizations have pushed for safer flame retardants, and a number of U.S. states and other nations have partially responded; but there is little public awareness of the issue despite numerous stories in the mass media as well as fictional accounts depicting death by asphyxiation from "thick, acrid smoke—the sort of smoke produced by synthetic stuffing in cheap furniture" (Barnard 1990:98). Given that fire is so cognitively vivid, one might expect people to be more concerned about the subject; that they are not raises questions: Does this constitute an implicit trust in manufacturers and in government regulators, trust at odds with the widespread skepticism toward these institutions reflected in opinion surveys? Or a kind of resignation? Or obliviousness?

Another way to think about it is to consider the learning environment in which consumers operate. It is easy for people to observe that the products of technological innovation often work fairly well for their intended purposes, and it is much more difficult to learn about the products' unintended (but inevitable) secondary and tertiary consequences. Thus, many cooks have direct positive experience of *Teflon-coated cookware*, for example; they can easily recognize that it is easier to clean than old-fashioned cast iron, copper, or aluminum. To purchase and use such a product is much easier than learning that the manufacture of Teflon involves PFOA, a perfluorinated chemical that "is broadly toxic. It does not break down in the environment, and is considered to be persistent over geologic time scales. It nearly universally pollutes human blood" (EWG 2004).

Similar perfluorinated compounds are created from decomposition of stain-resistant coatings for carpeting and couches, microwave-popcorn bags, fast-food wrappers, polishes, and paints. PFOA and related chemicals, after being transported by global air currents, are found in increasing concentrations in Arctic wildlife. Levels of these chemicals inside North American homes actually are about 100 times higher than are found outdoors, volatilizing from carpeting and other household products (Shoeib et al. 2004). Manufacturers began learning of potential health effects in 1961, but workers exposed to PFOA were not ordered to wear respirators until 1980. Executives of 3M became sufficiently concerned about health effects to cease production of PFOA in 2000, whereas eight other manufacturers began a phaseout only in 2006, after pressure from the EPA. Accumulating scientific evidence helped drive the change, as did lawsuits forcing DuPont to reveal internal documents showing that the company had violated the law by failing to disclose what it knew about the chemical's risks. The company was assessed more than $100 million in damages in 2005 and faces additional liabilities (PSKPP n.d.).

The chemicals discussed above are a small sample, of course, but in combination they make the point that Western households are low-level chemical waste dumps and are intimately linked to an even broader range of toxic emissions during manufacturing and waste disposal. The ubiquity of toxic products raises troubling questions about the political roots of the toxification of consumer culture. To probe these questions, we now undertake what might be considered a *political toxicology of consumption.*

Acquiescence to Toxification

What ought one make of the fact that most of these problematic chemical products—and many others—came into widespread use *after* Rachel Carson's widely publicized warning in 1962? Is toxification simply the price of progress, as some people say with a macabre shrug, or a matter-of-fact willingness to make tradeoffs? If large-scale toxification were technologically essential to meet consumer needs/wants, or economically unavoidable, then many people might be prepared to make a Faustian bargain. However, there is little reason to believe that this sort of deal with the devil is necessary.

Advocates for green chemicals generally admit that some contemporary activities might prove impossible without toxic side effects (e.g., Thornton 2000:chs. 9–10). Just as tradeoffs occur when people take blood pressure medications and run a risk of complications, it is conceivable, say, that leather tanning or solar panels or computer screens might have to involve something toxic. However, chemists have demonstrated remarkable ingenuity in figuring out how to get the lead out of paint, create "natural" flavors and fragrances, synthesize plastics from corn, trick the body into not recognizing sugar molecules (yielding sweetness without calories), and get pharmaceuticals to break down quickly in the body. These developments must be considered only a foretaste of the kinds of detoxification that are feasible, because so far such ingenuity is being applied to the goal of across-the-board detoxification by only a relative handful of chemists and chemical engineers.

The low level of effort to date is striking. Most universities do not offer even a single course in green chemistry. Most PhD programs in chemistry still do not require students to pass exams in toxicology. The vast majority of the world's chemists do not trouble themselves to assess direct and indirect toxicities of products and production processes, catalogue available alternatives, or research nontoxic approaches. Such is the extraordinary inertia of conventional chemistry, which green chemistry proponents call "brown chemistry." Despite this inertia, a diversity of nontoxic or substantially less toxic alternative products gradually has become available, some derived from natural sources, such as cleaning products made from citrus derivatives, and others highly industrialized but designed to be benign, such as supercritical solvents. According to a small but thoughtful minority of chemists and environmentally oriented industry executives, many more such detoxifications would become possible with concerted efforts (Collins 2001; Matlack 2001; Poliakoff et al. 2002; see U.S. House of Representatives, Committee on Science 2004; Woodhouse and Breyman 2005).

Business concerns about profit margins also have played an important role in the limited adoption of low-toxicity approaches, of course, but precisely because Dow and DuPont have oligopoly power, chemical industry executives could have chosen different approaches to toxicity long ago. Under regulatory pressure, chemical firms worldwide have cut certain air and water emissions from manufacturing by more than 90 percent, while making roughly the same level of profit as in the high-pollution era. When chlorofluorocarbons were found to endanger the ozone layer, chemical firms led by DuPont adapted without long-term damage to the bottom line.

In more than a few cases, the less toxic way of doing business actually has proven less expensive: water is a cheaper raw material than benzene, for example, and is now being used along with other safer solvents in a growing number of industrial applications. This also is occurring, in a limited way, in the domain of consumer products, where, for example, water-based paints and polishes with low VOCs (volatile organic compounds) in many applications are functionally indistinguishable from the more toxic oil-based paints of yesteryear and significantly easier to use. When chemical processes are changed in ways that reduce the production of hazardous byproducts, moreover, disposal costs are reduced along with the complex (and expensive) paperwork required for cradle-to-grave tracking of chemical wastes. If it can be as profitable to detoxify as not, continuing toxicity is all the more puzzling.

Relatively few people know the green chemical story, of course, but it is nevertheless worth asking why several billion consumers are as willing as they are to bring toxic products into their homes without making more of a fuss. Even if they were in some sense impelled by a lack of reasonable alternatives, many could be expected to express anguish, participate in boycotts, or otherwise demonstrate visible frustration with their predicament. Europeans have successfully resisted most genetically modified agricultural products, so why is there no equivalent movement challenging toxic consumer products? Why have most environmental organizations tended to oppose primarily a handful of especially egregious toxicities, such as those involving the "dirty dozen" persistent pesticides? Why no campus protests of "brown" research and curricula in chemistry and chemical engineering departments? From the shortage of such opposition, one must infer that a great many citizens/consumers somehow take widespread chemical toxicity for granted or at least are resigned to it.

At the moment, no one can say just what the average person's perspective on all of this is. Social scientists have not studied public attitudes and behaviors toward toxics at the level we are trying to probe, with the partial exception of Werner (2003). In fact, unable to locate surveys or other empirical work on consumers' understanding of the chemical content of products, we checked with a social psychologist who specializes in consumer studies and with a prominent proponent of nontoxic living. Both confirmed our sense that public thinking on this question remains almost entirely unstudied, the latter suggesting: "I think the apathy on this subject is so deep that studies haven't yet been done." Her own reading of prevailing attitudes is "that the general public is not very interested [in product toxicity]. The people who *are* interested generally have had some experience with a chemical injury or cancer. Most people don't want to confront this as a problem" (personal communication with Debra Lynn Dadd, 2006).

Activists sometimes speak as if social problems require each person to better think through issues and make more conscious choices, whereas our assumption is that broad patterns of acceptance, toleration, and acquiescence are socially constructed in ways that often keep underlying issues from getting onto individual and collective agendas for direct examination and assessment. We see two main social patterns that help keep the brown-versus-green chemicals issue off the public agenda. Each imposes—and is reinforced by—a *governing mentality*: a tacit and often ill-considered pattern of assumptions that fundamentally shapes political relationships, interactions, and dialogue, often in ways that conflict with democratic ideals (see Campbell 2000:ch. 2). Thus the patterns we identify here are structural/institutional/behavioral but intimately linked to patterns that are mental/attitudinal.

First, the social construction of everyday toxicity is constituted in part by the *delegation of authority to business executives* (Lindblom 1977). That entrepreneurs should enjoy substantial latitude in deciding what to bring to market may seem entirely natural; yet, on reflection, it clearly is a cultural and legal convention that could be otherwise. Although there are good reasons to let executives of manufacturing firms exercise almost sole discretion about what and how to produce, there also are good reasons not to let them do so. One of the best counterreasons is that executives tend to choose what is convenient and profitable for their firms even if it is not what informed customers and an engaged citizenry actually would or should want.

Illustrations of the problem can be found in many domains of consumption, not just in chemicals. In the automotive domain, for example, hybrid vehicles were successfully demonstrated as early as 1898, yet executives decided not to manufacture and sell such vehicles until Toyota led the way a century later. Executives may or may not have been correct to believe the market too small and potential profits too thin; but it was they who made the choice, and everyone else deferred to their judgment. A few observers groused, to be sure, but hardly anyone goes around thinking that major decisions about automobiles are too important to be left to automotive executives. On reflection, everyone knows that automobile design, manufacturing, and marketing choices have significant implications for energy usage, air quality, global climate, labor, and geopolitics. In effect, however, humanity has removed large chunks of those matters from democratic decision and delegated them to a small number of unelected, largely unaccountable corporate executives. We propose that the same kind of mistake, on a larger scale, has been made in delegating chemical innovation so completely to industry executives and their technical employees.

A different way of proceeding would require executives to share authority for public facets of chemical design. A small downpayment on such a scheme is a modest reform effort catalyzed by the GreenBlue Institute, which was founded by visionary environmental architect William McDonough and former Greenpeace chemist Michael Braungart. Together with participants from industry and from the not-for-profit sector, GreenBlue has developed a CleanGredients website showing which chemicals used in cleaning compounds are relatively benign (GreenBlue 2006). The site is being actively used by industrial companies that purchase raw materials from chemical manufacturers to formulate and sell cleaning products. Schools, hospitals, nursing homes, and other end users also consult the site as a guide to ordering the large quantities of cleaning supplies used in institutional settings. The project has cost less than a million dollars, which for the chemical industry is a pittance; but it took until 2006 to make the information available, because no one had a strong incentive to do it. Hundreds of different companies are represented in the database, and none of them will make enough money from it in the near term to justify the time and effort required to get the database up and running—a classic problem of market failure, in which markets leave an important public need unmet (Lindblom 2001). In this case, environmental organizations eventually stepped in, but other aspects of chemical greening await even such a modest move.

From the perspective of democratic theory, this state of affairs reflects a defect in the design of technological governance. Public choices are being made without representative deliberation and without full consent of the governed. It might be going too far to call it laissez-faire, but businesses have been left relatively free to design, produce, and market chemicals as their executives and technologists deem appropriate. Limited exceptions, such as prohibition on lead in most paint and gasoline, were generally enacted only *after* health and environmental problems arose, the delay due at least in part to lack of institutionalized mechanisms for "civic science" (Fortun and Fortun 2005) and for engagement of public interest advocates in "upstream" decisions about chemical design and production (Thornton 2000; Commoner 1992; O'Connor 1993). This is not the place to delve into organizational arrangements for melding public and private considerations in chemical design, but one simple example would be laws mandating best available technology—leaving it to lawsuits and threats thereof to work out what that would mean at any given time for a particular class of chemicals or chemically intensive consumer products.

A second set of institutional arrangements and mentalities supporting toxification involves *granting scientists, engineers, and their institutions a privileged position* in inquiry and decision making about technology. Everyone knows not to let the plumber decide how many bathrooms to have in one's house: the expert knows *how* to do the task, but it is the homeowner who chooses *what* is to be done. When science and engineering rather than plumbing are involved, however, this simple distinction often becomes obscured. Tasks that appropriately belong to citizen-consumers and government officials are delegated, instead, to experts.

The privileged position of science interpenetrates with the privileged position of business, especially for chemistry, which historically has been one of the scientific fields most closely associated with industry. But scientific privilege emanates from different assumptions and social processes than does deference to business.

Crucially, the privileged position of science involves a careless definition of what activities ought to be protected by "academic freedom" in universities. For example, it becomes unthinkable to consider removing the accreditation of chemistry and chemical engineering departments that operate environmentally destructive curricula or that align their research agendas too closely with those of corporations practicing brown chemistry (Woodhouse 2006). Although critical scholarly writing about the new corporate university has been developing steadily over the past decade, the focus to date has been on ordinary conflicts of interest more than on failing to rethink outdated curricula and accountability mechanisms (Slaughter and Leslie 1997; Twitchell 2004; cf. Vanderburg 2006).

Support for what we consider excessive academic freedom for scientists is rooted in a naive, idealized view of science as selfless, independent truth seeking that more or less automatically improves the human condition (Sarewitz 1996). Social studies of science have established that scientists and their institutions behave pretty much like other humans and organizations. Scientists pursue research they think will win funding, build their careers, and be interesting to themselves and their closest colleagues. They try to persuade each other and reach negotiated understandings of what is to be considered forefront knowledge. "Science" may thereby be improved in some sense, but the only certain beneficiaries of most scientific projects are the scientists and technicians employed to conduct those projects and, in an increasing proportion of cases, the projects' corporate funders.

Meanwhile, curricula are designed to train future scientists more than to serve the liberal arts and management students who become the majority of future government officials, business executives, and college-educated citizens. Reformers have criticized science textbooks and teaching for generations, and every issue of the *Journal of Chemical Education* contains useful ideas regarding how to make classrooms relevant to everyday life (e.g., acid rain, recycling tires). However, especially in the United States, schools of education offer little training for teaching high-school chemistry, and chemistry courses are still dominated by formulas and by memorization of minutiae. The criticism applies doubly to organic chemistry, which is overwhelming even to many chemistry majors; and yet this is precisely where students should be learning about the environmental consequences of synthetic chemicals. Chemistry for nonmajors courses are more user-friendly, but they are taken by only a small minority of college students and rarely teach anything about green chemistry.

Overall, chemistry teaching does not prepare most students for participation in a chemically intensive civilization, and few university chemistry professors are making that problem a high priority. A study of public opinion about science a quarter-century ago concluded: "The most striking aspect of public attitudes toward science, and scientists . . . is that they appear to be based on nebulous and distorted conceptions" (Pion and

Lipsey 1981:303). That public preparation for participation in chemical governance has not improved substantially in the intervening decades is suggested by surveys showing that public attitudes toward nanoscience and nanotechnology tend to parrot media stories emphasizing speculative economic benefits and gee-whiz capabilities (Scheufele and Lowenstein, 2005).

At the same time that university chemistry curricula fail to adequately educate the average college graduate, they, along with chemical engineering curricula, play a pivotal role in maintaining the "brown" status quo within the professions. In many environmental arenas, gradual change has taken place as new cohorts of recent graduates enter the workplace, bringing assumptions different from those of their forebears. This arguably is not nearly as true in industrial chemistry, where new cohorts continue to be trained in the toxifying culture of 20th-century chemistry and chemical engineering. One carpet industry executive committed to nontoxic and biodegradable carpeting reports that when graduates come to work for him they are flummoxed by the mandate to apply green-chemistry design principles. He has to take them by the shoulders, look them in the eye, and say, "yes, you *can* make it that way, go back and try again." With a few such exceptions, the new generation of industrial chemists and chemical engineers learns during schooling and then in the workplace not to treat toxicity as being of primary significance for most chemical products. To the extent that they focus on toxicity problems at all (as opposed to shunting the problem off to toxicologists, government regulators, or hazardous waste managers), the fledgling chemical experts learn to think of toxics control as a matter of careful containment and disposal (e.g., via high-temperature combustion). They do not learn in school or on the job to elegantly redesign molecules and chemical production processes to avoid producing toxicity, and they generally seem to have little trouble accommodating their new bosses' expectation that the toxic approaches of the 20th century are to be extended more than reshaped.

The privileged position of scientists and engineers in technological decision making is also protected by the simple fact that forefront research occurs largely within institutions substantially removed from public scrutiny. Even when state legislatures cut the budgets or otherwise "interfere" with state universities, legislators usually prove unable or unwilling to actually change much that happens in classrooms or laboratories. And private universities obviously are even further removed from public scrutiny and accountability by not-for-profit legal structures, historically high prestige, and an assumption that they are either unimportant to everyday consumer life or else adequately self-governing.

Organizations that might be expected to facilitate oversight of science rarely do. Government bureaucrats in environmental agencies sometimes are quite adept at interacting with scientific advisory committees and other technoscientists and could, conceivably, serve as a check on excessive deference to science. But regulatory agencies in the United States and many other nations are hamstrung by legal dictates and political environments favorable to business. They also are bureaucratic organizations difficult for most outsiders to understand or greatly influence. When scientific jargon is added to the mix, science in government becomes opaque much of the time to all but the most expert and most persistent outsiders (Laird 1990). Chemistry's arcane subject matter completes the protective screen.

Professional organizations such as the American Chemical Society and the American Institute of Chemical Engineers have the expertise to monitor university, governmental, and even corporate science and technology (Coeckelbergh 2006). Instead, however, professional organizations' executives usually focus primarily on building membership, lobbying for more research funds, planning conferences, and performing other functions peripheral to public policy. Partly because professional organizations have not generally been involved in public controversies, they are not recognized by government officials, journalists, or the public as potential resources for monitoring science; hence there is little pressure on them to do so. Professional scientific organizations of all kinds "easily degenerate into self-serving trade associations" (Pellegrino and Relman 1999), thereby adding to the problem of excessive deference to scientists, rather than being a resource for counteracting it.

Thus, just as corporate executive discretion is deployed in ways that typically serve the aims of corporate executives better than public values, scientific discretion is deployed disproportionately to serve the interests of scientists and their clients (often commercial enterprises). In the absence of systematic efforts to publicly reorganize science funding, incentive systems, and the enculturation of scientists, chemistry and other sciences have little systematic motivation to assist with tasks that would directly benefit the majority of humanity. For example, very few chemists lend their expertise to not-for-profit environmental organizations to understand and combat toxic pollution, because doing so is not perceived as a viable way to build a chemistry career. Green chemistry thereby remains unrecognized even by many environmental activists, and it has low status within the discipline of chemistry. And even a relatively well-known green chemist such as Terrence Collins of Carnegie Mellon University is considered a maverick for daring to suggest that graduates of chemistry departments need courses in ethics and a working knowledge of toxicology—a subject most chemists now consider a foreign discipline that is someone else's responsibility.

These issues obviously raise a deep and complex set of questions concerning how scientific research, teaching, and consulting can be shaped to serve public ends. For our purposes, it is sufficient to point out that cultural norms and organizational practices delegate substantial autonomy to research chemists, which has made it easy for them to avoid intense grappling with how to rearrange chemical structures to achieve detoxification.

One of the world's few activist chemists asks: "Why are manufacturers putting toxic chemicals in . . . the products they sell for household and personal use when, sooner or later, those chemicals become household contaminants that threaten the health of their customers?" (Costner et al. 2005:7) The same could be asked about products whose toxicity is most pronounced outside the home, during production or disposal. Our answer thus far has been that social conventions and institutions—and corresponding governing mentalities—delegate primary authority for chemical innovation to technoscientists and business executives. Because research chemists have found it interesting and convenient to pursue "brown" rather than green chemistry, and because corporate executives (and industry chemists and engineers) have found it legal, profitable, and otherwise acceptable to manufacture and distribute synthetic organic chemicals without designing to eliminate toxicity, this delegation of authority has amounted to a structural predisposition to toxification. Although the chemical industry has faced significant regulation, neither scientist nor business executive has yet been impelled by regulation, market forces, or public pressure to fundamentally revamp the approach to toxic chemicals developed in the early and mid–20th century.

Interwoven with the first two governing mentalitics is a third mentality, to which we have already implicitly alluded: the *fundamental assumption that high levels of toxicity are unavoidable in an affluent consumer society*. Most citizen-consumers, government officials, business executives, and chemists alike have made this key assumption, which has made good public policy about chemicals almost impossible. Despite the paucity of effort so far devoted to systematic detoxification and despite the seemingly great promise of green chemistry, public discussion, negotiation, and (usually) acquiescence to toxicity has occurred along the unidimensional spectrum depicted in figure 1.1: more toxicity with a better/cheaper consumer lifestyle versus less toxicity with a lower-consumption, more expensive, and/or less interesting lifestyle.

Where to locate on this continuum has been determined more by business executives and technoscientists than by government officials or citizen-consumers. Government officials in environmental and health agencies have interacted extensively with business and with environmental organizations concerned about chemical pollution, of course; but except in a relative handful of high-profile cases such as those involving DDT and PCBs, the result has generally been merely a minor tweaking of industry practice. The overall situation is more complex than simply elites taking authority, manipulating citizens, and deceiving consumers, however. Citizen-consumers have ceded authority, purchasing the items put on store shelves with little objection. Of course most of us know very little about the particulars, such as whether the plastic parts of the coffeemaker will contaminate the coffee or emit toxic gases in the kitchen. Given the number and variety of news stories about toxicity over the past generation, however, no one can credibly claim to have no inkling of the general risks.

How can one make sense of this striking and patently dangerous acquiescence to toxification? Social scientists have developed a cluster of concepts that are helpful in understanding the phenomenon.

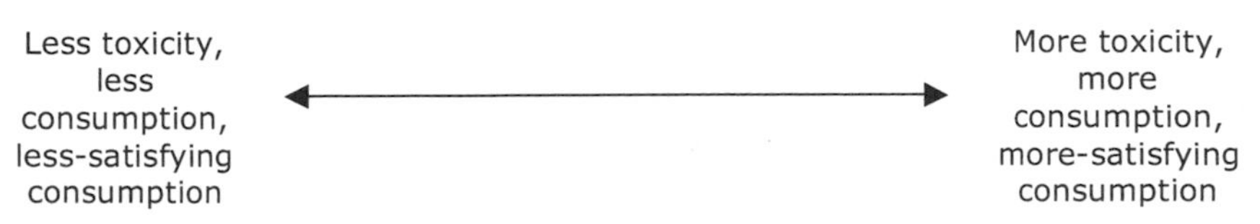

Figure 1.1. A Third Governing Mentality

One is Gramsci's notion of *hegemony*, wherein the ruling class dominates through the very institutions of civil society—churches, schools, and fraternal organizations—that might be imagined to serve as countervailing forces (Gramsci 1971). Today we could reasonably add the chemistry and chemical engineering professions to that list. As usually employed, the term "refers to the process by which one class exerts control of the cognitive and intellectual life of society by structural means as opposed to coercive ones. Hegemony is achieved through the diffusion and reinforcement of certain values, attitudes, beliefs, social norms, and legal precepts that . . . come to permeate civil society" (Baer et al. 2003:15). In the case of consumer products, the legal and political arrangements that enforce (or at least reinforce) the delegation of authority to business executives, scientists, and engineers have served to diffuse these elites' values, norms, and perceptions, including those supporting the acceptability and inevitability of toxification.

A second approach is provided by political theorist Murray Edelman, who notes that dominant groups typically are able to use symbolic benefits to distract and purchase the allegiance of dominated groups, producing in the latter a strange *quiescence*, or passivity. "Far from representing an obstacle to [dominant groups]," he argues, the dominated "become defenders of the very system of law which permits the [dominant] to pursue their interests effectively" (Edelman 1995:31). Weak chemical laws enable toxic consumption, and plastics and other toxic consumer products clearly have served to enroll mass publics into consumer culture. Moreover, the symbolic benefits of freedom to purchase are as important to many people as the tangible benefits actually accruing from possessing what has been purchased. These symbolic benefits probably have distracted the public from subtle toxification of everyday life, and the combination of tangible and symbolic benefits certainly has helped promote acquiescence.

Third, Peter Bachrach and Morton Baratz point to the *mobilization of bias*, in which "a set of predominant values, beliefs, rituals, and institutional procedures ('rules of the game') . . . operate systematically and consistently to the benefit of certain persons and groups at the expense of others" (Bachrach and Baratz 1962:43). Steven Lukes (2005) extends the idea, noting that this mobilization operates so systematically that it need not be intentional or even conscious and that one of its principal consequences is invisibly preempting challenges to the status quo. Charles

Lindblom (1977) refines the insight by showing how policy making comes to exhibit a peculiar *circularity*: most citizens learn to ask for no more than political and economic elites are prepared to give. Industries reliant on synthetic organic chemicals (e.g., the toy, kitchenware, and furniture industries) almost effortlessly avoid most challenges to the toxic status quo. There is a kind of "nondecision making" in which only the most controversial chemicals make it onto priority agendas for actual debate, and many of those debates result in little or no regulation. Far-reaching alternatives including green chemicals are rarely considered seriously, because even ostensible opponents of the status quo tend to share fundamental assumptions—rarely made explicit, much less debated—that bend both production and consumption toward toxification. Even most environmental organizations ask for not much more than elites can give without undermining profitability or chemical business as usual.

Discussion

The toxification of everyday life that is evident from a casual reading of the daily news becomes more striking as one ponders the specific toxicities associated with PVC, phthalates, dandruff shampoos, methylene chloride, methyl bromide, flame retardants, and Teflon. From the ubiquity of toxicity coupled with the rarity of direct challenges to it, we have inferred that there is widespread acquiescence to toxic consumption. We have identified three governing mentalities that seem to be at work in shaping public acceptance of toxic consumer products: the assumption that business executives (and staff chemists and engineers) should enjoy broad authority to decide what innovations will be researched, which will be marketed, and how chemicals and chemical products will be formulated and manufactured; the assumption that academic scientists and engineers should have nearly complete freedom to pursue research trajectories substantially of their own (or their corporate patrons') choosing; and the assumption that extensive toxicity is the price that must be paid for participation in Western consumer culture.

The three mentalities are thoroughly intertwined, of course. If a customer at Kroger or even at an upscale grocery such as Whole Foods cannot choose between deli cheese wrapped in plastic containing phthalates and deli cheese wrapped in a material containing no phthalates, it is most proximately because store executives and deli managers set policy dictating how their workers wrap cheese. In turn, the grocery managers' choices are constrained by what executives in companies supplying the food industry choose to provide, which for many years has meant plastic cling film containing an endocrine-disrupting chemical that readily dissolves in fatty foods such as cheese and is subsequently deposited in the fat tissue of the consumer.

If the deli manager takes phthalate-laden cling wrap for granted, it is partly because public-interest groups have not courted journalists and otherwise mounted public education campaigns. This relatively weak nongovernmental organization (NGO) activism can itself be traced to the fact that few environmental groups have chemists on staff and that the overwhelming majority of academic and corporate chemists avoid civic engagement of just about any kind. The apolitical tendencies of chemical experts contrast with the greater activism of wildlife biologists, toxicologists (Fortun and Fortun 2005), and those who study environmental mutagenesis (Frickel 2004). These researchers study environmental problems, are less closely tied to chemical manufacturing, and generally come closer than the industrial chemists to behaving as civic scientists willing to participate in public conversation about chemical problems and prospects.

The intertwining of the three governing mentalities also can be seen through the lens of another mundane component of consumer culture: cotton. As conventionally grown, the fiber requires enormous quantities of pesticides and water, and mechanically drying wet cotton clothing uses considerably more energy than drying synthetic fibers. Setting aside the issue of whether overall cotton production ought to be reduced, consider just the issue of organically grown cotton versus cotton grown with pesticides. "Organic cotton has been embraced enthusiastically by environmental activists but not by consumers," a World Bank study finds, and hence "the scope for expanding organic cotton appears to be limited" (Baffes 2004:263).

Organic production on a large scale might add only a few cents to the cost of a pound of cotton, but to a textile manufacturer purchasing millions of pounds, that adds up to a substantial investment. Buyers for retail chains ordering clothing from textile manufacturers think in terms of what will sell; they are not out to change agriculture. Retail customers, in turn, are thinking about style, color, fit, and price more than about the kind of fiber in their shirts and skirts. And whereas customers at many grocery stores come face to face with organic produce, clothing shoppers rarely receive such prompting to consider buying organic. In the absence of consumer demand, growers, manufacturers, and retailers lack motivation to change their practices.

This case illustrates several factors at work in the social construction of the toxic products phenomenon: 1) the shortage of civic science devoted to the matter, with scientists and engineers devoting less effort to assisting organic growers or catalyzing public discussion than to helping develop genetically modified cotton tolerant of high levels of pesticides and herbicides; 2) market failure: lack of consumer demand coupled with business executives' choice to mostly stick with pesticide-grown cotton; and 3) the lack of systematic attention to the problem by governments, where, for example, departments of agriculture tend to be captured by major agricultural interests. We do not mean to say that most people who wear cotton clothing are consciously deciding in favor of increased toxicity, but it also would be a mistake to miss the fact of consumer cooperation or acquiescence. Much the same can be said of thousands of other products entailing toxicity during one or more parts of their life cycles.

The idea that the public plays a fundamental role in this cycle is not incompatible with findings that mass publics in most nations have long been broadly supportive of enhanced environmental protection (Kempton et al. 1996). A substantial majority in opinion surveys report that they do not believe government protects adequately against chemical hazards, and green consumerism clearly is on the rise (Adler 2006). Yet public support for the environment, like support for most good causes, is accompanied by a considerable gap between attitudes and actions (Johnson and Scicchitano 2000; Barr 2006). In a recent poll, 81 percent of U.S. Catholics indicated that lifestyle change is necessary to protect the environment, but only 32 percent reported considering the impact of products they buy regularly (LeMoyne College/Zogby International 2005). And cognitive psychologists long have understood that learning tends to be context specific, so it is unsurprising that public attitudes toward some environmental concerns (e.g., climate change) might not carry over to concerns about subtle toxicities of consumer goods in the home.

The discrepancy between general concern and individual inaction also can be partially reconciled by placing opinions about everyday toxics in the context of larger social processes that catalyze or suppress people's knowledge, thinking, caring, and action. Just as interest in political matters rises and falls depending on whether candidates for office and their political parties engage and activate voters, so also with toxic household products. Consumer-citizens rarely get a realistic chance to vote on the matter either with dollars or at the ballot box, and therefore are rarely prompted to learn about the issues and to deliberate concerning tradeoffs—except perhaps individually as a retail purchaser considering a display of upscale organic cotton bedding or pesticide-free grapes.

Ironically, a kind of public information campaign could be on the horizon from the corporation most associated with mindless proliferation of plastic household products, Wal-Mart. The world's largest business is promising to lead the way toward sustainable retailing (Kabel 2005). Although reduced energy use is the chain's primary near-term objective, Wal-Mart already has become the world's largest buyer of organic cotton. CEO Lee Scott says that "there can't be anything good about putting all these chemicals in the air. . . . There can't be anything good about putting chemicals in these rivers in Third World countries so that somebody can buy an item for less money in a developed country. Those things are just inherently wrong" (quoted in Gunther et al. 2006:42).

One environmental organization executive observing the process suggests that "the potential here is to democratize the whole sustainability idea—not make it something that just the elites on the coasts do but something that small-town and middle America also embrace" (quoted in Gunther et al. 2006:57). This probably overstates the likely outcome, but Environmental Defense takes the initiative seriously enough to have established a branch office in Benton, Arkansas, near Wal-Mart's headquarters. At Wal-Mart's expense, the management consulting firm Sky-Blue devoted a year to studying every product the retailer sells to determine some limited aspects of its environmental impact, and fourteen different networks now bring buyers, suppliers, and relevant environmental experts together to reassess various facets of the corporation's operations. One of these networks is devoted specifically to chemicals, and the company's huge grocery store operation is becoming one of the biggest sellers of organic produce and coffee. These actions seem to go well beyond the public-relations moves typically associated with "greenwashing" (Tokar 1997), although placating customers concerned about the chain's treatment of workers and the environment certainly is part of the motivation.

The giant retailer is in a position to bring the issue of household toxicity to the attention of tens of millions of people. Just as agenda setting is hugely important in politics, so it is at the individual level. There is too much to pay attention to, and ideas without a persuasive spokesperson in one's reference group tend to be ideas to which one gives little attention. It is too early to know whether Wal-Mart actually will follow through or how customers will react. But the effort provides a telling contrast with conventional retailing, where executives and managers rarely apply public values to systematically assess the items on a store's shelves. The most likely outcome is that Wal-Mart executives and suppliers will simply act to reduce some of the worst toxicities. We hope, though, that they will also facilitate the public's own deliberation by supplying information that will assist customers in reconsidering the types of toxicities they are buying for their homes. Given the privileged position of business, that choice, too, rests with Wal-Mart executives.

Conclusion

In our teaching and in conversations with friends and interviewees, we rarely encounter anyone who signals a belief that it is inappropriate for corporate executives to have primary authority to decide how products are designed and manufactured. Many of these same people probably would hesitate to say that business executives have a right to decide how much toxicity will enter homes and bodies; but by delegating most aspects of product design to so-called private enterprise, even many politically progressive people in effect do just that.

We also find that most people implicitly endorse laissez-faire and corporate-oriented science. Even highly educated, liberal alumnae of elite academic institutions generally fail to question how chemistry is taught or how forefront research is prioritized and overseen. Of course hardly anyone except chemists and chemical engineers really *thinks* about chemistry at all, and that is exactly our point. Failing to think is implicitly to delegate choices about research and teaching of chemistry and chemical engineering to the very faculty who have facilitated the creation of a toxic planet.

There are, of course, limited efforts to challenge the toxification of everyday life. It is impossible to miss the efforts of Greenpeace and the Environmental Working Group, for example, and even mainstream environmental organizations such as Sierra Club selectively work for toxics reform. An organization as staid as the U.S. Senate Committee on Labor and Resources held hearings in 2006 aimed at revision of the outdated Toxic Substances Control Act of 1976. Bill Moyers and other journalists periodically attack aspects of the chemical industry. The Sustainable Cotton Project in the past dozen years has helped organic cotton come out of nowhere to make it into several lines of clothing that achieve reasonably broad distribution. International treaties have reduced production of the dozen or so very worst chemicals. And a handful of activist organizations are beginning to promote green chemistry.

Although important and encouraging, all of this nibbles at the problem of toxics rather than going to the heart of the phenomenon. More fundamental changes in the toxicity of everyday consumption are improbable unless three ideas are adopted into mainstream public thought:

1. In most cases it probably is not necessary to choose between high toxicity and low affluence, for green chemistry seems capable of moving most products well along the path to "benign by design";
2. It is inappropriate to leave choices about chemical innovation primarily to business executives and their staff chemists and engineers, because toxification and detoxification are public issues; and
3. Chemistry teaching and research are too important to be shaped entirely by chemists and chemical engineers, for humanity relies on chemical experts and we need them to behave as "civic scientists" conversing and negotiating with the rest of us.

Most generally, perhaps, the case of toxic consumer products suggests that intelligent democratic governance of a technological civilization requires democratizing decision making about technology (see Sclove 1995). Many of the changes in mentalities and institutions required to evolve a partially synthetic planet safe for humans and other living organisms also would be conducive to fairer, wiser governance of technological civilization more generally.

References

Adler, Jerry
2006 Going Green. Newsweek, July 17. Electronic document, www.msnbc.msn.com/id/13768213/site/newsweek, accessed June 22, 2007.

Bachrach, Peter, and Morton Baratz
1962 The Two Faces of Power. American Political Science Review 56:947–952.

Baer, Hans A., Merrill Singer, and Ida Susser
2003 Medical Anthropology and the World System, 2nd ed. London: Praeger.

Baffes, John
2004 Cotton: Market Setting, Trade Policies, and Issues. *In* Global Agricultural Trade and Developing Countries. M. Aksoy Ataman and John C. Beghin, eds. Pp. 259–273. Washington, DC: World Bank Publications.

Barnard, Robert
1990 A City of Strangers. New York: Charles Scribner's Sons.

Barr, Stewart
2006 Environmental Action in the Home: Investigating the "Value-Action" Gap. Geography 91(Spring):43–54.

Baue, Bill
2001 Safe Pipes Mean Safe Water. Children's Health Environmental Coalition. Electronic document, www.checnet.org/healtheHouse/education/articles-detail.asp?Main_ID=148, accessed June 22, 2007.

BSEF (Bromine Science and Environmental Forum)
2000 An Introduction to Brominated Flame Retardants. October 19. Electronic document, www.ebfrip.org/download/weeeqa.pdf, accessed June 22, 2007.

Campbell, Nancy D.
2000 Using Women: Gender, Drug Policy, and Social Justice. New York: Routledge.

Carson, Rachel
1962 Silent Spring. Greenwich, CT: Fawcett Publications.

CDC (Centers for Disease Control and Prevention)
2006 Background and Environmental Exposures to Di(2-Ethylhexyl)-Phthalate in the United States. Electronic document, www.atsdr.cdc.gov/toxprofiles/tp9-c2.pdf, accessed June 22, 2007.

Coeckelbergh, Mark
2006 Regulation or Responsibility? Autonomy, Moral Imagination, and Engineering. Science, Technology & Human Values 31(3):237–260.
Cohen, Maurie J., and Joseph Murphy, eds.
2001 Exploring Sustainable Consumption: Environmental Policy and the Social Sciences. New York: Pergamon.
Collins, Terry
2001 Toward Sustainable Chemistry. Science 291(5501):48–49.
Commoner, Barry
1992 The Failure of the Environmental Effort. Current History 91(564):176–181.
Costner, Pat
2000 Dioxin Elimination: A Global Imperative. Amsterdam: Greenpeace International.
Costner, Pat, Beverly Thorpe, and Alexandra McPherson
2005 Sick of Dust: Chemicals in Common Products—A Needless Health Risk in Our Homes. Spring Brook, NY: Safer Products Project, Clean Production Action.
CREDO (Cluster of Research into Endocrine Disruption in Europe)
N.d. Information on European Research Projects into Endocrine Disruption. Electronic document, www.credocluster.info, accessed June 22, 2007.
DiGangi, Joseph, Ted Schettler, Madeleine Cobbing, and Mark Rossi
2002 Aggregate Exposures to Phthalates in Humans. Washington, DC: Health Care Without Harm. Electronic document, www.noharm.org/details.cfm?type=document&id=662, accessed June 22, 2007.
Edelman, Murray J.
1995 Symbols and Political Quiescence. *In* Public Policy: The Essential Readings. S. Z. Theodoulou and M. A. Cahn, eds. Pp. 26–33. Englewood Cliffs, NJ: Prentice-Hall.
EWG (Environmental Working Group)
2004 Dupont Suppresses Teflon Blood Study. November 17. Electronic document, www.ewg.org/node/8738, accessed June 22, 2007.
Fortun, Kim, and Mike Fortun
2005 Scientific Imaginaries and Ethical Plateaus in Contemporary U.S. Toxicology. American Anthropologist 107(1):43–54.
Frickel, Scott
2004 Chemical Consequences: Environmental Mutagens, Scientist Activism, and the Rise of Genetic Toxicology. New Brunswick, NJ: Rutgers University Press.
Frontline
2004 Is Wal-Mart Good for America? Boston: WGBH.

Gramsci, Antonio
1971 State of Civil Society: Problem of the "Collective Man" or of "Social Conformism." *In* Selections from the Prison Notebooks. New York: International Publishers.
GreenBlue
2006 Online database of institutional and industrial cleaning product ingredient chemicals, www.cleangredients.org, accessed June 22, 2007.
Greenpeace
N.d. PVC: The Poison Plastic. Electronic document, http://archive.greenpeace.org/toxics/html/content/pvc1.html, accessed June 22, 2007.
Gunther, Marc, Doris Burke, and Jia Lynn Yang
2006 The Green Machine. Fortune 154(3):42–57.
Hallier, Ernst, Thomas Langhof, Doris Dannappel, Monika Leutbecher, Klaus Schröder, Hans Werner Goergens, Andreas Müller, and Hermann M. Bolt
1993 Polymorphism of Glutathione Conjugation of Methyl Bromide, Ethylene Oxide and Dichloromethane in Human Blood: Influence on the Induction of Sister Chromatid Exchanges (SCE) in Lymphocytes. Archives of Toxicology 67(3):173–178.
Hodgson, Ernest, and Randy L. Rose
2005 Toxicology of AHS Implant Chemicals. Journal of Biochemical and Molecular Toxicology 19(3):180–181.
HSIA (Halogenated Solvents Industry Alliance)
2003 White Paper on Methylene Chloride. Electronic document, www.hsia.org/white_papers/dcm%20wp.htm, accessed June 22, 2007.
Johnson, Renee J., and Michael J. Scicchitano
2000 Uncertainty, Risk, Trust, and Information: Public Perceptions of Environmental Issues and Willingness to Take Action. Policy Studies Journal 28(3):633–647.
Kabel, Marcus
2005 Wal-Mart Nudges Foreign Suppliers: Retailer to Demand Environmental and Social Responsibility. Washington Post, October 21: D02.
Katz, S. N.
1987 Decaffeination of Coffee. *In* Coffee: Technology. R. J. Clarke and R. Macrae, eds. New York: Elsevier Applied Science.
Kempton, Willett, James Boster, and Jennifer A. Hartley
1996 Environmental Values in American Culture. Cambridge: MIT.
Laird, Frank N.
1990 Technocracy Revisited: Knowledge, Power and the Crisis in Energy Decision Making. Organization & Environment 4(1):49–61.

Lakshmi, S., and A. Jayakrishnan
2003 Properties and Performance of Sulfide-Substituted Plasticized Poly(Vinyl Chloride) as a Biomaterial. Journal of Biomedical Materials Research 65B:204–210.
LeMoyne College/Zogby International
2005 Survey data, October 14–23, as summarized by Polling the Nations. Electronic document, www.orspub.com, accessed August 4, 2006.
Li, Lin Ying, Terrell Barry, Kevin Mongar, and Pamela Wofford
2006 Modeling Methyl Isothiocyanate Soil Flux and Emission Ratio from a Field Following a Chemigation of Metam-Sodium. Journal of Environmental Quality 35:707–713.
Lindblom, Charles E.
1977 Politics and Markets: The World's Political-Economic Systems. New York: Basic Books.
2001 The Market System: What It Is, How It Works, and What to Make of It. New Haven, CT: Yale University Press.
Lukes, Steven
2005 Power: A Radical View, 2nd ed. New York: Palgrave Macmillan.
Matlack, Albert S.
2001 Introduction to Green Chemistry. New York: Marcel Dekker.
McGinn, Anne Platt
2000 Why Poison Ourselves? A Precautionary Approach to Synthetic Chemicals—Worldwatch Paper 153. Washington, DC: Worldwatch Institute.
Molotsky, Irvin
1985 Agency Says Solvent Is Safe for Processing Coffee. New York Times, December 21: A3.
Montague, Peter
2004 The Chemical Wars. New Solutions 14(1):19–42.
New York State Department of Environmental Conservation
2003 Zinc Pyrithione NYS DEC Letter—Denial of Registration Application 9/03. Electronic document, http://pmep.cce.cornell.edu/profiles/miscpesticides/methylchloride-xanthangum/zinc_pyrithione/zinc_pyr_let_903.html, accessed June 22, 2007.
NIH (National Institutes of Health)
2006 Household Products Database. Electronic document, http://householdproducts.nlm.nih.gov, accessed June 22, 2007.
O'Connor, John
1993 The Promise of Environmental Democracy. *In* Toxic Struggles: The Theory and Practice of Environmental Justice. R. Hofrichter, ed. Pp. 47–57. Philadelphia, PA: New Society.

Pellegrino, E. D., and A. S. Relman
1999 Professional Medical Associations: Ethical and Practical Guidelines. JAMA 282:984–986, quoted at 985.
Pion, Georgine M., and Mark W. Lipsey
1981 Public Attitudes Toward Science and Technology: What Have the Surveys Told Us? Public Opinion Quarterly 45(3):303–316.
Poliakoff, Martyn, J. Michael Fitzpatrick, Trevor R. Farren, and Paul T. Anastas
2002 Green Chemistry: Science and Politics of Change. Science 297(August 2):807–810.
PSKPP (Project on Scientific Knowledge and Public Policy)
N.d. Perfluorooctanic Acid. Electronic document, www.defending-science.org/case_studies/perfluorooctanoic-acid.cfm, accessed June 25, 2007.
Sarewitz, Daniel
1996 Frontiers of Illusion: Science, Technology, and the Politics of Progress. Philadelphia, PA: Temple University.
Scheufele, Dietrich A., and Bruce V. Lowenstein
2005 The Public and Nanotechnology: How Citizens Make Sense of Emerging Technologies. Journal of Nanoparticle Research 7(6):659–667.
Sclove, Richard E.
1995 Democracy and Technology. New York: Guilford.
Scorecard: The Pollution Information Site
2006 Chemical Profiles. Electronic document, www.scorecard.org/chemical-profiles, accessed June 22, 2007.
Shoeib, Mahiba, Tom Harner, Michael Ikonomou, and Kurunthachalam Kannan
2004 Indoor and Outdoor Air Concentrations and Phase Partitioning of Perfluoroalkyl Sulfonamides and Polybrominated Diphenyl Ethers. Environmental Science and Technology 38(5):1313–1320.
Slaughter, Sheila A., and Larry L. Leslie
1997 Academic Capitalism: Politics, Policies, and the Entrepreneurial University. Baltimore, MD: Johns Hopkins University Press.
SSNC (Swedish Society for Nature Conservation)
2004 The Investigation of Zinc Pyrithione in Dandruff Shampoo: A Presentation of the Facts. Gothenburg: Svenska Naturskyddsföreningen.
Thornton, Joe
2000 Pandora's Poison: Organochlorines and Health. Cambridge: MIT.
Tokar, Brian
1997 Earth for Sale: Reclaiming Ecology in the Age of Corporate Greenwash. Boston: South End.

Twitchell, James B.
2004 Higher Ed, Inc. Wilson Quarterly 18(Summer):46–59.
USDA (U.S. Department of Agriculture), Agricultural Research Service
1995 Methyl Bromide Alternatives. Newsletter. October.
USEPA (U.S. Environmental Protection Agency)
2004 Methyl Bromide Critical Use Nomination for Post Harvest Use by NPMA for Facilities and Commodities. Electronic document, www.epa.gov/Ozone/mbr/2004_USPostHarvest_Commodities_Facilities_%20NPMA.pdf, accessed June 22, 2007.
U.S. House of Representatives, Committee on Science
2004 Hearing on Proposed Legislation for Green Chemistry Research and Development, March 17. Electronic document, www.house.gov/science/hearings/full04/mar17/charter.pdf, accessed March 28, 2004.
Vanderburg, Willem H.
2006 Can the University Escape from the Labyrinth of Technology? Part 1: Rethinking the Intellectual and Professional Division of Labor and Its Knowledge Infrastructure. Bulletin of Science, Technology & Society 26(3):171–177.
Werner, Carol M.
2003 Changing Homeowners' Use of Toxic Household Products: A Transactional Approach. Journal of Environmental Psychology 23(1):33–45.
Woodhouse, Edward J.
2006 Nanoscience, Green Chemistry, and the Privileged Position of Science. *In* The New Political Sociology of Science. Scott Frickel and Kelly Moore, eds. University of Wisconsin Press.
Woodhouse, Edward J., and Steve Breyman
2005 Green Chemistry as Social Movement? Science, Technology & Human Values 30(2):199–222.

CHAPTER TWO

NOTHING TO PLAY AROUND WITH

Dangerous Toys for Girls and Boys

Merrill Singer and Pamela I. Erickson

In the days before he was rushed to a Minneapolis hospital, four-year-old Jarnell Brown had been acting strangely and was clearly under increasing distress. Always an active, bubbly child, he became cranky and out of sorts and then began vomiting. According to his mother, Jarnell was unable to tell her what was wrong: "He [began] hollering and screaming all the time. He just did not know what was causing it" (Hawley 2006:1). At the hospital, doctors initially thought the boy was suffering from viral gastroenteritis. He was administered medications to prevent nausea and vomiting and released from the emergency room only to return two days later. The vomiting had become worse and he was listless. Doctors found that he was dehydrated and had elevated blood urea nitrogen levels (suggesting his kidneys were not operating normally, a common feature of dehydration). He was admitted to the hospital and put on intravenous fluids.

Ten hours after admission, Jarnell became highly agitated and combative. He was sent to radiology for X-rays but on the way he suffered a seizure and stopped breathing. Successfully resuscitated, Jarnell was placed on mechanical ventilation and underwent a CT scan of his head and chest and his stomach was X-rayed. Review of the X-ray revealed that a foreign object was in his stomach, and doctors ordered a blood test for heavy metal levels. The test found that Jarnell had a blood lead level (BLL) of 180 μg/dL (the Centers for Disease Control and Prevention views levels of

≥10 μg/dL as cause for medical concern and levels over 60 μg/dL to be an extreme medical emergency). By this point, a cerebral blood flow check showed that blood was no longer reaching Jarnell's brain. On the fourth day after his admission, Jarnell was removed from life support and soon declared dead (Berg et al. 2006).

Subsequent autopsy produced a heart-shaped metal charm imprinted with the word "Reebok" lodged in the child's stomach. Jarnell's mother recognized the charm, which she said came with a pair of sneakers belonging to one of Jarnell's friends. Examination of the shoes showed that they were manufactured by Reebok International, Ltd. Acid-digesting tests on the charm removed from Jarnell's stomach showed that it was 99.1 percent lead. The Minneapolis Department of Regulatory Services then acquired a similar charm from a local shoe store and found that it was 67% lead by weight. When she learned the cause of Jarnell's death, his mother addressed manufacturers saying, "Think about kids when you're making stuff. . . . It's not about money, because my son will never come back—and for the price of a shoe" (Hawley 2006).

The discovery of high lead levels in imported jewelry, like the Reebok charm, is not unusual. The year Jarnell died, the Consumer Product Safety Commission (CPSC) recalled 150 million pieces of imported metallic toy jewelry that were being sold through vending machines, like those often found at the exits of supermarkets. In March 2006, the CPSC recalled almost 600,000 necklace and ring sets packaged under various labels, such as "Mood Necklace," "Mood Ring," "Glow in the Dark Necklace," "Glow in the Dark Ring," "UV Necklace," or "UV Ring," that had been sold for several years at various discount stores including Dollar Tree, Dollar Bills, Dollar Express, Greenbacks, and Only $1.

As these examples suggest, there are millions of dangerous toys and other play items sold every day by toy stores, supermarkets, department stores, novelty stores, and vending machines, as well as by street-corner vendors, over the Internet, and at many other venues.

While people generally like to talk about toys and to reminisce about the favorite toys of their childhood, the topic of dangerous toys is a highly emotional one, both because children's vulnerability is widely recognized (although this certainly was not always the case) and because of the place toys now hold in our cultural imagination: they are defined generally as a source of unregulated fun, not of fear and suffering. How people have thought about toys, of course, and what items have been considered toys have changed over time and place, reflecting wider patterns in the cultural landscape. The term *toy* is believed to be over 600 years old and to be etymologically related to *tool*, implying that children's play with toys helps prepare them for adult work with tools, a theme expressed in many toys including toy jewelry, but also dolls, weapons, vehicles, miniature kitchens, and construction toys. Large toy companies began to appear in the late 1800s and early 1900s, and mass marketing of toys soon followed. The late 20th century introduced ever more complex and costly electronic toys, but also the global production (at factories in numerous countries) and international distribution of both cheap and expensive toys of diverse kinds (Hampshire Museums Service 2006). Along with dolls that looked quite real, that could talk, move limbs, or perform other bodily functions, there also came ever more fanciful toys, including beings of imaginative origin. Contemporary toys are often influenced by television programs and movies that are advertised directly and heavily to children as consumers (a promotional strategy that began with the Barbie doll), suggesting a basic tension in the Western attitude between expecting toys to teach children about things of real-world, practical value versus wanting them to assist the childlike imagination to run wild.

Reflecting some of this tension, toy design may be pulled in opposing directions. Increasingly, for example, toys have taken on a serious role in society, especially in the public arena where debates about healthy child development are aired, while at the same time becoming a quite lucrative source of profit among producers and distributors. Marianne Szymanski (Brockenbrough 2006:1), head of an independent company that provides Web-based advice to parents on toy purchases, captures an important element in the contemporary Western view of toys as educational and developmental aids, noting, "through play, children use sensory and developmental skills that prepare them for real life." That real life is dangerous, of course, is not one of the things most parents think about when making choices about toy purchases, and it is certainly not something they want to associate with toys or children. At the same time, how children play with toys and which toys they choose to play with now are interpreted as informative markers of important developmental milestones (e.g., using toys in make-believe dramas is seen as a marker of the emergence of imagination). Moreover, toys have come to be defined as providing opportunities for children to learn (Brockenbrough 2006).

Even when they take the form of deadly implements (e.g., rubber knives, plastic machine guns, murderous video games, toy soldiers) or promote homicidal activities, play items often are defended as being "just toys," and hence nothing to worry about. Nonetheless, the sometimes blurry boundaries between toys and implements of harm, and perhaps societal ambiguities about how we view children, as well (i.e., simultaneously seeing them as having great potential for cruelty while celebrating their innocence), have become fodder for comedians and other societal commentators. Of growing concern among some parent groups has been the ever-stronger emphasis on violence in real toys and video games, another sign of the hand of the capitalist market on toy design. As O'Keefe (1998:1) emphasizes:

> Critics accuse the media and the toy companies of pushing violence because it sells, even if it might endanger children's minds. The industry offers the usual market defense—they're only giving the audience what it wants. "These kids have seen it all," said one industry spokesperson. "They don't relate to feel-good shows filled with sweetness and innocence. It's not our job to tell kids what is or isn't good for them. And it's not our job to change the world."

In sum, in contemporary Western culture, toys have come to be seen as simultaneously wondrous, liberating, educational, fun, and necessary for normal development, which can also give vent to troublesome emotions. In fact, as Jarnell's sad case underlines, however, there is a particularly dark cloud that envelops our most romantic ideas about playthings: because of the push for profits, toys themselves, and not just the emotions they may give expression to, are often injurious and occasionally lethal. The purpose of this chapter is to examine this upsetting connection, socially, economically, and politically.

The Political Economy of Playthings: The Multibillion-Dollar Global Toy Industry

From the perspective of producers and distributors, toys are anything but child's play; rather they are very big business. Moreover, they are a business that is rapidly being concentrated in fewer and fewer hands. Like the fashion or automobile industries, toys are very fad and trend driven. This year's popular toys are rapidly replaced by next year's, as highly coveted toys at one point in time—the kind parents fight over in toy store aisles—can quickly become ugly ducklings without much customer appeal. Stoking the toy trend engine is the American International Toy Fair (AITG), an annual event in New York City at which toy companies, old and new, showcase their products and vie for buyers. The annual four-day event began over 100 years ago and has debuted many of the toys that went on to be industry leaders, including Barbie, Monopoly, Slinky, the Mighty Morphin Power Rangers, and Trivial Pursuit.

The trend-driven nature of the toy market is important because it pushes toy manufacturers to constantly turn out new products, and further, to rush them to market as fast as possible, especially during the holiday season. A survey by the NPD Group, for example, found that toys that had been introduced during the preceding three-year period accounted for 55 percent of sales in the United States in 2003 (Hong Kong Trade Development Council 2006). The dog-eat-dog competition and accelerated pace of the toy industry, driven always by the hunger for ever-greater bottom-line returns, as well as the cultural pressure parents feel to make sure their children have the most trendy playthings (as if not doing so is a sign of failed parenting in our highly achievement-conscious culture) are significant contributors to the hasty tempo with which harmful toys come to be in the hands of small children.

In 1997, in the United States alone, the toy industry had retail sales of $22 billion. Three years later, the toy sales figure had jumped to $29 billion, which translates to $400 a year for every child 14 years of age and younger (although the industry slipped back to 1997 levels in subsequent years, with educational and building-set toys countering the general decline in overall toy sales in the U.S. market) (NPD Group 2006). Toys, however, are a global product, and thus sales worldwide are far higher ($55 billion by 2002), with producers from Canada, France, Germany, Hong Kong, Italy, Japan, the UK, and the United States aligned in the promotion of the world toy market through the International Council of Toy Industries. Cross and Smits (2005:873) note that a "complex dynamic of globalization of children's culture . . . has been developing for several decades." One consequence of this trend is that toys produced in countries with limited safety enforcement during manufacture may be readily exported to other countries, while toys that do not pass safety checks in one country may be marketed in others where inspection is inadequate.

Beyond changing designs and the globalization of toy production and sales, various additional factors impact the toy market, a number of which have implications for the availability of dangerous toys. While U.S. toy company executives "like to say the industry is 'recession proof' because parents will always find a way to buy toys for their children, analysts [of the toy market] do not fully agree" (Maestri 2005:1). According to a spokesperson of the NDP Group, "while it is our view that 'Christmas always happens for kids,' we think fewer dollars are available for gifts and moms/dads will seek bargains" (Maestri 2005:1). A bargain-hunting mentality among parents increases the appeal of discount outlets that specialize in cheaper playthings like the toy jewelry discussed above.

Availability also affects parent toy purchase decisions. The U.S. toy market is characterized by what has been called "the Toy Wars" (Miller 1995), namely commitment to driving the competition out of business both at the manufacturing and retail levels. As O'Keefe (1998:1) observed a number of years ago: "The toy business—which once consisted of scores of manufacturers, hundreds of wholesalers and tens of thousands of 'mom-and-pop' toy stores—has compressed itself down into a thin layer of giant producers and a small cadre of superstores, led by Toys"R"Us and Wal-Mart, which together account for almost two-thirds of all the toys sold in America." On the retail side, there are two primary types of outlets that sell toys: the toy specialty stores that feature a wide variety of toys and the toy discounters, multidepartment stores that carry a diverse array of consumer goods from clothes to televisions as well as a limited inventory of toys carrying a comparatively low price tag. Toys"R"Us is the leader in toy specialty stores and the second largest toy seller overall; Wal-Mart ranks number one in the toy discounter market by volume and is also the number-one overall toy seller (Oligopoly Watch 2004). By 2005, specialty toy stores controlled only about 20 percent of the toy market share, compared to 54 percent at general discount outlets like Wal-Mart. Online purchase of toys, which significantly limits the ability of parents to inspect items prior to payment, also has been growing and now constitutes about 6 percent of the toy market in the United States (NPD Group 2006). Toys sold over the Internet are not required to carry safety messages.

In recent years, a growing number of second-tier specialty toy stores have been pushed out of the market or been forced to restrict their scale of operation. In December 2003, for example, the celebrated high-end FAO Schwarz company (which was referred to in the industry as the Rolls-Royce of toy stores) filed for bankruptcy and sold off all of its stores.

One consequence of what might be called the "Wal-Mart effect" (in toys and other product lines) is that by destroying its "big-box" (i.e., large store) retail competition, Wal-Mart has inadvertently created space for super-discount stores (e.g., so-called dollar stores) to gain a foothold in the toy market. The number of super-discount chain outlets has surged, with sales reaching $265 billion in the United States by the year 2000. Super-discount stores especially target two market niches: rural areas and low-income neighborhoods—to the degree that the push to find extremely cheap toys to sell results in super-discount stores stocking more dangerous toys, and rural and low-income shoppers are most likely to suffer the consequences.

Where do those who seek rapid profits from toys find cheap toys to sell? One important source is countries with expanding production capacity and comparatively low labor costs. STK International Inc., of Los Angeles, for example, has been cited multiple times for importing dangerous toys that break easily, producing small parts that pose a choking hazard (CPSC 2002). Similarly, several toys imported from China by California International Trading of Los Angeles were recalled because they break easily, producing swallowable parts. The toys were selling for $1 to $2, primarily at swap meets and flea markets (CPSC 2005a). Many other companies also have been caught attempting to bring dangerous toys into the country. Consequently, there have been repeated exposures to dangerous imported toys in recent years.

One final factor driving the sale of toys is advertising. Advertisers spend over $12 billion a year to reach the child market, most of it on fanciful and often overglamorized television commercials, the dominant medium of toy advertising (Lauro 1999; Rice 2001). With the emergence of cable and satellite television and specialty channels like Nickelodeon, the availability of children's programming has expanded enormously throughout the day and evening hours. As a result, it is estimated that the average child in the United States now views more than 40,000 television commercials each year, many of them for toys or toy-related products, such as cereals that contain a small toy prize in the box (Kunkel 2001). Advertisers have learned key lessons in how to create demand for particular toys among children, such as using a widely known celebrity endorser in advertising campaigns. Studies comparing the same ad with and without a popular idol show that such figures significantly improve the appeal of the featured product to children (Ross et al. 1984). Children from ethnic minority families have been found to have heavier exposure to television than children from white families, and they view a higher number of commercials as a result (Huston and Wright 1998).

Scope of the Dangerous Toy Quandary

On October 13, 2005, Russel Roeger, then the executive director of the U.S. Consumer Products Safety Commission (CPSC 2005b), an independent federal agency established in 1973 to protect the public from killer (and injurious) commodities, issued a memorandum on toy-related deaths and injuries that had been reported to and investigated by the commission during the year 2004. During the year, 16 children, nine years of age and under, died as a result of play with various kinds of toys. Four of the children choked to death on toy balls or balloons, game dice, or toy premiums (like cereal-box inserts). Several other children died from asphyxia after becoming entangled in toy parts, while others died from accidents while riding on toy vehicles (not including motorized scooters or other vehicles marketed to children). For the 15-year period between 1990 and 2004, U.S. PIRG (Cassady 2005) reported that there were a total of 272 known toy-related child deaths in the United States, 58 percent of which were due to choking.

In addition to fatalities, the CPSC reported that there were over 210,000 toy-related injuries in the year 2004 that were treated in U.S. hospital emergency rooms, down somewhat from the 255,100 injuries reported in 2001. The total annual cost of toy-related injuries treated in emergency rooms nationwide among children four years of age and younger was approximately $385 million in 2001. Inclusion of injuries that never involved the ER, which very likely far outnumbered those that resulted in emergency intervention, would drive these numbers up significantly. In short, as these statistics suggest, far more children are injured while playing with toys than are killed (a fact that has been significantly influenced by improved emergency response and intervention capability).

One of the duties of the CPSC is to issue product recalls when it determines that a commodity is dangerous to consumers and to publicize recalls issued by toy companies. The number of children's product recalls, the vast majority of which are voluntary recalls, issued by the CPSC rose 32 percent, to 87 between 2003 and 2004, but this still represents a drop of 26 percent from the number of recalls issued in 2001. In 2000 and 2001, recalls of children's products accounted for over half of all consumer product recalls; in 2003 and 2004 they only comprised 31 percent of total product recalls. Some parents and consumer product safety groups have begun to wonder whether the CPSC can keep up or is, so to speak, dropping the ball on toy safety.

The toy industry strongly favors voluntary standards, claiming that "too much regulation takes away parental choices and amounts to the government's taking over the parent's job . . . [while parents] innocently assume . . . that the necessary regulations are in place to minimize hazards from toys and maximize toy safety" (Stern and Schoenhaus 1990:213). Moreover, industry spokespersons often emphasize the importance of parental supervision while children are playing, "conveniently ignoring the fact that one of the primary uses of toys is to amuse children when adults are not playing with them" (Stern and Schoenhaus 1990:213).

Critics have charged that the CPSC has taken a narrow legalistic and technocratic approach to regulation, reflective of its sitting members, all of whom are lawyers, one with a background in corporate law. The current chairman of the CPSC is Hal Stratton. He was nominated by President George W. Bush and confirmed by the U.S. Senate for that position on July 25, 2002. Born in Muskogee, Oklahoma, he is an enrolled member of the Cherokee Nation. He holds degrees in geology and law from the University of Oklahoma. Prior to joining the CPSC, he was a member of the New Mexico House of Representatives from 1979 to 1986 and the attorney general of New Mexico from 1987 to 1990. The person Bush had at first wanted to head the CPSC (for which he could not get congressional support) was Mary Sheila Gall, who, as a CPSC member (appointed by President George H. W. Bush), did not support choke-hazard warnings on small toys; opposed setting federal standards for baby walkers (1994), baby bath seats (1994), and bunk beds (1999) on the grounds that voluntary standards were sufficient to ensure child safety; and supported the elimination of fire-safety standards for children's pajamas. Gall's nomination was strongly opposed by various consumer groups, including Consumers' Union, publisher of *Consumer Reports*, because of her record of voting against setting safety standards and her tendency to publicly blame parents for product-related child injuries.

The character and approach of the CPSC have changed several times since the agency was established. The agency was considered on its deathbed during the Reagan presidency because of drastic budget and staff cuts. Under Ronald Reagan, the commission was chaired by Terrence Scalon. Scalon, a former vice president for corporate relations of the Heritage Foundation, is president and chairman of the Capital Research Center, a conservative Washington, D.C., think tank concerned with monitoring the activities and funding of progressive advocacy organizations. Additionally, Scalon is affiliated with Consumer Alert, a national, nonprofit membership organization concerned with what it feels is excessive growth of government regulation. Consumer Alert's funding comes primarily from major corporations with an interest in limiting regulation, including Chevron, Eli Lilly, and Philip Morris. By 1997, the General Accounting Office criticized the CPSC for inadequate information gathering, among other problems. When President Bill Clinton appointed Ann Winkleman Brown, a child-safety advocate, to the commission, she publicly stated that the CPSC was a waste of money, labeling it a "bun without beef," an idiom of the era. The activist approach she brought to the commission disappeared when she resigned in 2001, and the Bush administration began to appoint commissioners who thought the agency should have a narrower focus and a more collaborative relationship with industry. The standard procedure is for the CPSC to negotiate with the manufacturer (or importer or seller) to reach a mutually agreed upon approach (Felcher 2001).

Among the toys that were recalled by the CPSC in 2004, those that caused the most injuries prior to recall are listed in table 2.1. Two companies, Graco Children's Products, Inc., and Hasbro, Inc., each had two of their products recalled during 2004 because of child injuries. The injuries caused by these children's products ranged from contusions and fractures to strangulation and included several fatalities.

While manufacturers often comply with voluntary recalls issued by the CPSC and retail outlets remove the toy from their sales shelves, in the case of Magnetix this was not the case. RoseArt Industries, the producer, announced that it would offer replacement toys suitable for children under six

Table 2.1. Injuries and Toy Recalls in 2004

Manufacturer	*Product*	*Number of Injuries*	*Type of Injuries*
Graco Children's Products, Inc.	Travel Lite Swing	128	Bloodied lips, bumps, bruises
Mattel, Inc.	Batman Batmobile	14	Lacerations, punctures, scratches
Hasbro, Inc.	Nerf Big Play Football	9	Facial injuries, cuts requiring stitches
Hasbro, Inc.	Super Soaker Monster Rocket	6	Concussions, cuts
Backyard Products	Backyard Products Swing	6	Sore back, cuts, bruises
Graco Children's Products, Inc.	Bumblebee toys with blue antennae	6	Choking, scratched throat
Kids II, Inc.	Vinyl Mirror Books	6	Cuts, pinched fingers

Source: Hazards of Child's Play: Children's Product Recalls in 2004. 2005. Chicago: Kids in Danger.

years of age to parents who wanted a substitution, but it would not recall Magnetix building sets that were already in toy stores or other outlets. A company spokesperson, Jennifer Zerczy, maintained that the toy's package was labeled for children age six and over and there was a small-parts warning on the package. In fact, a check by journalists found that the warning label states that the toy is not intended for children younger than age three. Zerczy responded to reporters' questions about this discrepancy by saying that it is the responsibility of parents to buy age-appropriate toys and to supervise their children when at play (Mayer 2006). In Kenny Sweet's case, the toy was purchased for his ten-year-old brother and Kenny's mother specifically instructed him not to play with it in front of Kenny. About ten days later, however, Kenny became sick. When his symptoms did not subside, he was taken to the hospital, but he died several hours later. Eight small magnets from the Magnetix building set were found at autopsy, bonded to each other in two groups through the walls of his intestines.

Table 2.2 presents the most common toy-related injuries based on a review of consumer reports, injury case studies, CPSC data, and media accounts.

Suffocation and Strangulation

The colorful advertisement announces that you can throw it, catch it, squeeze it, and bounce it. Parents who have watched it wrap suddenly

Table 2.2. Most Common Toy-Related Injuries

Injury	*Cause*
Suffocation and strangulation	Swallowing small toy parts, becoming entangled in ropes or cords, mouth and nose covered by plush or other toys
Poisoning	Swallowing or touching noxious substances in or on toys
Loss of hearing or ear perforations	Sirens and other loud toys
Trauma	Toys breaking, falls, crashes, and being struck
Burns	Toys overheating or causing fires
Musculoskeletal injury	Repetitive use of video game controls
Drowning	Riding toy vehicles into pools, using water toys
Eye impairment	Being struck by a toy projectile

around their child's neck and begin strangling him or her have another idea about what to do with the toy: they want to ban it. The toy in question, called the Flashing Yo-Yo Waterball, is a liquid-filled gel ball that, according to promotional material, has "the preferred long yo-yo 'string' which stretches from 8 inches to several feet." Produced in China by the Shenzhen Dingsinfa Industrial Co. Ltd., the Yo-Yo Waterball has been the object of intense controversy. One parent, Lisa Lipin, was pulled into the fray when her seven-year-old-son, Andrew, ran to her for help when he was unable to remove the rubber string trailing from the ball that had wrapped around his neck. Recalls Lisa:

> I just worked the thing up over his head. I wasn't able to break it because I couldn't rip it apart. He was left with strangulation marks and [his] eyes were bulging, the color from his face was gone. (Hope 2005:1)

Lisa Lipin's frightening experience was not unique. In 2006, Wisconsin state senator Julie Lassa and Representative Amy Sue Vruwink issued a press release that reported on an even more traumatic experience with the toy.

> According to Autumn Deedon, of Pittsville, her 7-year old son was playing with the yo-yo waterball when the toy wrapped around his neck, cutting off his blood supply. As a result, he passed out and fell head first to the ground. Ms. Deedon rushed her son to the emergency room and found that he suffered from a concussion. (Lassa and Vruwink 2006)

Alerted by the media and hundreds of consumer complaints, the CPSC (2003a) reported that in the cases it investigated "there were no lasting injuries, [although] seven cases reported broken blood vessels affecting eyes, eyelids, cheeks, neck, scalp or the area behind the ears." Based on these findings, the CPSC (2003a) concluded that the toy "does not meet congressionally mandated standards for product recall." While some retail stores have responded to consumer complaints and taken it off their shelves, the toy is still legally sold in most parts of the United States and can be readily acquired from several different sites on the Internet.

With regard to strangulation and choking risk in toys, the Yo-Yo Waterball is but the tip of the iceberg. Over 25 years ago, the CPSC banned the sale of toys that contained small parts if they were intended for use by children under three years of age because of the recognized risk of choking. Because it has led to a number of court cases resulting in testimony under oath, the issue of children choking on toys has produced some insights about the views of toy companies about toy safety (aside from public relations pronouncements with expectable messages). One such case, reported by Edward Swartz in his book *Toys That Kill* (1986), was the lawsuit brought by Ronald and Margaret Cunningham against the Quaker Oats Company, producer of the Fisher-Price brand Little People Play Family figurines, after their son almost choked to death and suffered enduring injuries after swallowing one of the toy figures. During the trial, it was revealed that parents had been writing to the company since the toy hit the market complaining about the risks of swallowing and choking on the small toy figures. When Henry Coords, the company president, testified, he admitted that the company ran no tests to see if children could swallow and choke on the figures. The company's former director of research and development claimed, however, that two medical doctors had been consulted about the toy's safety. When called to testify, both doctors denied ever meeting with company representatives about the safety of the toy. Why didn't the company redesign the toy after letters of complaint began pouring in? A company executive told a reporter that the reason is that it would cost too much money. Although the company's motto was "safety first," the company's behavior showed that profit was a higher priority. Although the jury found the company negligent for manufacturing and marketing the dangerous toy, the well-selling and highly profitable product remained on the market without significant redesign. In 1991, under continued pressure from parents and product safety advocates, the original Little People became what toy collectors came to call the

"Chunky People," because the figures were redesigned to be much wider and harder to swallow.

Poisoning

One of the most common materials used to construct toys is plastic. It is comparatively cheap, easy to clean, and remarkably flexible. Especially malleable plastics like vinyl find their way into many toys, from dolls to teething toys for babies. The reason vinyl is so bendable is the injection of a plasticizing substance during production. Plasticizers do not bond with plastic molecules but rather slip between them. The most commonly used plasticizer in vinyl toys is called diisononyl phthalate (DINP). There has been tremendous international debate about whether DINP is poisonous to humans. Research has shown that laboratory animals fed high doses of DINP for long periods develop liver and kidney tumors. Moreover, New York PIRG (2002) reported that testing has shown that phthalates leach out of plastic over time. Convinced of the seriousness of the threat to small children posed by plasticizers, in 2005 the European Parliament voted to ban DINP and five other phthalate softeners in toys and other products that can be placed in a child's mouth.

By contrast to the European stance, in the United States the CPSC (2003b) released its review of the risks of DINP in children's products in 1998 which concluded that "few if any children are at risk from the chemical because the amount that they ingest does not reach a level that would be harmful. Generally, the amount ingested does not even come close to a harmful level." Nonetheless, the CPSC requested toy makers not to use phthalates in soft rattles and teething toys as a precautionary measure. Subsequently, the CPSC convened a committee of experts called the Chronic Hazard Advisory Panel (CHAP), to review existing research on the health effects of DINP. The CHAP report, published in 2001, found "minimal to non-existent risk of injury" for most children, but also noted that there might be a risk for children who mouth plastic toys containing DINP for 75 minutes a day or more for an extended period of time. In 2002 the CPSC staff issued another report which again concluded that children who mouth toys containing DINP face "no demonstrated health risk" and recommended denial of public petitions that called for a ban on the use of vinyl in toys, a recommendation that was accepted by CPSC commissioners (CPSC 2003b). In 2003, however, the government of Japan imposed a ban on the use of phthalates in toys intended for small children, and the debate continues.

Hearing Loss

The unit of sound measurement is the decibel. Each increase of ten decibels represents a doubling of loudness (e.g., 60 decibels is twice as loud as 50 decibels). According to Deafness Research UK (2004), the average conversation between two people is usually about 60 decibels, while a busy street tends to range between 80 and 90 decibels. When decibel levels range above 120 decibels, some ear damage may result. Ear damage is not caused by sound levels alone; rather, damage is a result of loudness combined with duration of the sound. Thus, while very loud sounds above 140 decibels can cause damage in a short period of time (even instantly), most ear damage is a product of continuous exposure to a loud noise over time. At 105 decibels, for example, the period before damage begins is only about 15 minutes. Standards for decibel ceilings on toys have been implemented for a number of years. In the UK, toys that tend to be held close to a child's ear are not allowed to exceed 80 decibels. Reviews of studies on toy noise (e.g., Fleischer et al. 1998) by Luxon (1998) and Deafness Research UK (2004) have found that: 1) children's hearing may be particularly vulnerable to noise-related damage; 2) toy pistols fired close to the ear can be much louder than military rifles; and 3) regulations in some countries allow toys to be much louder than workplace noise levels for adults. A study by Yaremchuk et al. (1997) of 25 toys that were purchased at a national toy chain store, for example, found noise levels ranging from 81 decibels to 125 decibels measured at 2.5 centimeters distance and 80 decibels to 115 decibels measured at 25 centimeters (equal to the average length of a child's arm). When the Department of Trade and Industry in the UK tested toys at 25 centimeters distance it found the decibel levels reported in table 2.3.

Retrospective research by Siegal et al. (2003) demonstrates the effects of exposure to higher-decibel toys. In a study with 53 children under the age of 14 who had been exposed to noise from toy guns and firecrackers, they found that 39 of the children had suffered unilateral hearing loss while 14 showed loss in both ears. Most of the loss (over 70 percent) was

Table 2.3. Noise Levels (in decibels) Produced by Various Toys

Toy	Decibels
Gun with sound effect	96.9
Talking soft toy	97.1
Musical top	100.6
Toy airplane	106.0
Squeeze toy	108.9
Teething rattle	109.9
Electronic pinball	118.8
Drum	125.1
Electronic megaphone	132.6
Cap gun	150.5

Source: Deafness Research UK.

in the high-frequency range, although nine children also suffered mid-frequency damage. Twenty of the children complained of dizziness or tinnitus and seven were found to have eardrum perforation.

Because of the appeal of loud sounds to children (which is part of the reason fireworks, video games, squeeze toys, toy guns, and toys with sirens are popular), manufacturers seek to improve toy sales by ensuring their products have a high-sound volume. The damage done to children's hearing as a result only becomes evident over time, often, because young children do not know how to report such problems, after considerable hearing loss has occurred.

Trauma

A review of toys recalled by CPSC over the years shows that a common shortcoming of such toys is that they have a high potential to break in some way, causing traumatic injury to the children using them. In 2005, for example, Fisher-Price agreed to recall over 150,000 Grow-to-Pro Pogo Sticks following a growing number of accidents, including reports of teeth being knocked out and of cuts requiring stitches. The toy had an internal metal pin that tended to wear down with use, causing the pogo stick to become stuck in the down position and then release suddenly, knocking children to the ground (CPSC 2005c).

Some items marketed to children cause injury because of the nature of the product and the age of the consumers it targets. The baby walker is an example of this type, even if some would argue that it is not a toy per se (although the line between toy, vehicle, and furniture is not always clear in children's products). Nonetheless, it is responsible for many childhood trauma injuries. In a Swedish study (Emanuelson 2003) of mild brain injuries (concussions) due to a fall, an accident, or a blow to the head among children (zero to four years of age) between 1998 and 1999, it was found that the single product most associated with these wounds was the baby walker, followed by playground equipment (another frequent source of child injuries).

Nonmotorized scooters also fall into the category of toys that are marketed to children who are too young to use them safely. To determine how significant, Gaines, Shultz, and Ford (2004) examined the records of 27 children admitted to one hospital during the two-year period between January 1, 2000, and December 31, 2001, because of a scooter-related injury. The average age of the patients was about nine years and most (63 percent) were boys. The most common immediate cause of injury was a fall, although about a fourth of the cases involved a collision with another vehicle. The most frequent injury was to children's heads.

Burns

Electrical toys are a common source of burn injuries among children, as well as fires that cause additional injuries as well as property damage. While many electric toys are labeled as UL-approved, burns and shocks can occur when wires become frayed over time. Additionally, chemistry sets and other kinds of hobby kits sometimes contain flammable substances that can explode or catch fire, causing skin and eye injuries. In the case of the battery-powered riding vehicle (sold under several different names), the Peg Perego USA company received almost 200 consumer reports of the vehicle's electrical components overheating, causing smoking, melting, and fire between April 1994 and March 1997. These incidents resulted in several burn injuries as well as approximately $55,000 in property damage to three houses and garages. The company was aware of at least 20 other incidents in which the toy failed to stop, resulting in injuries.

Beyond these direct causes of burns to children, toys, and the way they are presented to children, can contribute to burn injuries in indirect ways as well. While most children are taught not to play with fire, each year thousands of children, mostly boys, are burned while doing so. Might toys contribute to this dangerous behavior? Noting that fire imagery often appears on toy packaging, and that this may send a message to children about how much fun fire can be, Curri et al. (2003) examined all the toys on display in a national toy store to identify those that had clear, unambiguous images of fire on their packaging. The researchers found 404 toys with fire imagery, 97 percent of which were targeted to boys. Video games constituted the toy type that was most likely to exhibit fire on its cover, accounting for 51 percent of the toys on the fire imagery list, followed by toy cars and trucks (21 percent). In toys targeted to girls, fire images usually were contained and safe (e.g., images of food cooking on stove tops on toy stove packages), while on boys' toys, fire tended to be shown in wild and exciting settings. The researchers conclude that boys are receiving a "powerful, consistent [and dangerous] message from [the] images of fire on toy packaging" (Curri et al. 2003:163).

Musculoskeletal Injury

The most common complaints leveled at video games are that they promote aggressive behavior and sedentary lifestyles, and they are addictive. Research has shown that about one-third of U.S. children in their early teens play video games daily, and that about 7 percent play for at least 30 hours a week. Some researchers have expressed concern that a fundamental cultural shift is taking place characterized by the rise of what has been called "videophilia," defined as "the new human tendency to focus on sedentary activities involving electronic media" (Pergams and Zaradic 2006). Excessive video and computer game playing also has been linked to a form of tendonitis that has been called both "Nintendinitis" and "PlayStation thumb," a repetitive strain disease characterized by severe pain in the extensor tendon of the thumb as a result of repeated pressing on the video controls during play (Brasington 1990).

Various studies have assessed the development of repetitive strain disorders among video game players. Burke and Peper (2002) interviewed a convenience sample of 211 students in grades one through 12 and their parents to assess frequency and duration of video and computer game use, type of products, and input devices (e.g., joysticks) being used, experience of physical discomfort, and parental concerns about their child's computer use. They found that many of the children reported pain in the wrist (30 percent) and the back (15 percent) that they associated with game playing. Almost half of the parents (46 percent) complained that they had difficulty convincing their children to get off of the computer or video player, and about a third (35 percent) expressed concern that their children were spending less time outdoors. Similar findings on video game playing and neck pain have been reported for parochial school students in New York studied by Ramos, James, and Bear-Lehman (2005), while Ma and Jones (2003) found an association between wrist and forearm fractures and the number of hours spent playing video games among Australian youth. While these studies are suggestive, thus far, they are limited and are not supported by other research. Zapata et al. (2006), for example, conducted a cross-section study of 833 adolescents enrolled in a private school in São Paulo, Brazil, and found that the majority (58 percent) played video games. Just under 40 percent reported suffering from pain while about 16 percent were diagnosed as having a musculoskeletal pain syndrome.

Drowning

In 2002, over 850 children under the age of 14 died of drowning in the United States; the majority (60 percent) were under age four. Drowning accounts for 16 percent of accidental injury-related death in the United States among children 14 years of age and younger. Additionally, about 15 percent of children admitted to hospitals for near-drowning incidents suffer severe or permanent brain injury. Typical medical costs for a near drowning of a child 14 and under ranges from more than $8,000 for the initial hospital treatment to more than $250,000 a year for long-term care. The cost of a single near drowning that causes brain damage can be more than $5.5 million (Safe Kids Worldwide 2004).

Toys are involved in cases of drowning or near-drowning incidents in three primary ways. The first involves rubberized toy pools. The second toy-related drowning risk for children involves the use of water toys in pools or other swimming locations. In the state of Washington, for example, 80 children died of drowning between 1999 and 2001. A view of these cases by the state department of health (Washington Department of

Health 2002) found that 42 percent were playing in the water or on a rubber raft or inner tube just prior to drowning. The third way toys are involved in drownings occurs when children ride their tricycles or other small vehicles into bodies of water. Of the 16 children who suffered toy-related deaths in the United States in 2004, for example, two, a boy of two years and a girl of four, drowned when they apparently rode their respective tricycles into in-ground family pools (CPSC 2005b).

Loss of Sight

The poster child of injurious projectile toys, those that are thrown or fired and capable of causing eye damage as well as other bodily injuries, was Yard Darts (or Lawn Darts). These 12-inch, heavy darts, which were intended for outdoor play, had full metal tips (although some types had plastic tips) and were capable of causing serious injury. While the "intended" use of the toy, as prescribed by the manufacturer, was to employ an underhand toss in hopes of sticking the dart into the ground inside a plastic hoop, bored and creative children quickly invented other uses.

Injuries caused by the toy were not unusual. While the CPSC at first maintained that it had received very few complaints about the toy, the death of a seven-year-old girl who was impaled in the top of the head by a yard dart resulted in further investigation. This led to the discovery of three yard dart–related deaths and over 6,000 injuries. As a result, in 1988 Yard Darts were outlawed for sale or import in both the United States and Canada (although at least one child was killed even after the ban was implemented).

Sometimes, however, the dangers of such toys do not lead to their removal from the market. In an online advertisement (Your Web Store 2006), the Supremo Slingshot produced by Prime Time Toys, Ltd., is described as being "designed to launch only soft foam balls for worry free fun." In 2003, however, the Boston-based consumer watchdog group WATCH included the Supremo Slingshot on its annual Worst-Toy List. According to WATCH, which is headed by product-liability lawyer Ed Swartz, the Supremo Slingshot is capable of "forcefully firing the balls with which it is sold and has the potential to cause serious eye injuries" (Bhatnagar 2003). WATCH contacted Massachusetts's attorney general Tom Reilly about the toy. He concurred with their assessment that the toy is covered by the state's prohibited weapons statute. Reilly, in turn, then contacted Toys"R"Us, the primary retail outlet selling the slingshot in the state, which removed the toy from its shelves and agreed to refund customers who returned the items to a company store. CPSC, however, did not ban the slingshot. According to WATCH, "some hazardous toys remain in toy boxes because purchasers have not received notice of a recall. Others remain available because they were never tagged for recall by the CPSC despite proven hazards" (Bhatnagar 2003).

One type of projectile toy that has regularly been associated with injuries is the nonpowder gun (including BB guns, pellet guns, air rifles, and paintball guns). The muzzle velocity on some of these "toy guns" can range from 150 feet per second to 1,200 feet per second, compared to 750 feet per second to 1,450 feet per second for many types of "real" or powder guns (Laraque 2004). A retrospective pediatric hospital medical chart review of children who suffered air-gun injuries during the years 1991 to 2002 by Keller et al. (2004) found 35 cases with children averaging ten years old. Of these, 21 required admission to the hospital, 19 needed surgery, and five experienced long-term disability. Because the wounds caused by these guns are small and there is limited injury to surrounding tissue, the extent of the damage is often overlooked.

The considerable popularity of paintball guns has accelerated the pace of eye and other injuries caused by projectile toys. Vassilev and Marcus (2004), for example, reviewed the computerized database of the New Jersey Poison Information and Education System for the years 2000 to 2003 and identified 79 cases of paintball-related injuries, 75 percent of which were in children five years of age and younger. Listman (2004) conducted a review of unpublished CPSC data to determine the frequency of eye injuries in children and reviewed English-language research literature on such injuries. He found that the incidence of paintball-related eye injuries treated in emergency rooms jumped from an estimated 545 in 1998 to over 1,200 in 2000, with 40 percent occurring among children under 15 years of age.

Each year manufacturers introduce a new crop of projectile toys, including crossbows, dart guns, bow and arrow sets, and related items, many with labels warning of their potential dangers. These manufacturers seem to be unmindful, however, of the fact that children do not tend to read warning labels, that parents cannot monitor their children's behavior around the clock, that the toys of older children are coveted by their younger siblings, and that children commonly find new ways to play with their toys that were not "intended" by the manufacturer. Without doubt, there is strong appeal for these kinds of toys, especially among young boys who are exposed to uncounted messages about the social value, sense of empowerment, and adventure associated with the use of weaponry and violence generally. Do toy manufacturers and distributors help to create a "culture of combat" as a means of enhancing profit or are they merely giving children what they want? Very likely, both are probably true.

Conclusion: Who Is Minding the Store?

As the American Academy of Pediatrics (2000) notes, "what seems to be harmless fun could result in a serious injury. . . . Thousands of children suffer toy-related injuries every year." These injuries are the result of many different types of toys produced and sold by a shrinking array of companies, including major U.S.-based corporations and foreign manufacturers whose products may only be available on the Internet. From the perspective of critical medical anthropology, the starting point for understanding the domain of dangerous toys lies in thoughtful examination of the reasons that: 1) so many hazardous toys reach the market to begin with; 2) some kinds of known toy-related risks, like dangerous levels of lead content or a tendency to break apart under normal use into swallowable multicolored shiny parts, continue to appear year after year with each new wave of toys to hit the market; 3) the dangers of many toys often only are discovered *after* they are widely sold to consumers and causing harm to their children; 4) most recalls of even very dangerous toys are voluntary and fines and punishments for producing or marketing harm in a fancy wrapper are rare; 5) certain types of toys, such as those capable of high-velocity firing of projectiles or emitting deafening levels of noise, continue to appear unimpeded each year; and 6) parents and other consumers select toys with risky features, poorly or problematically labeled packages, or toys that may contribute to behaviors the parents do not condone.

Unfortunately, most of the available data on dangerous toys that can be marshaled in addressing these issues are limited to the United States, the United Kingdom, Australia, and Canadian sources, although toys that cause harm are produced in and exported to countries around the world and the toy business now is a globalized industry. In the United States, the Consumer Product Safety Commission, whose president is appointed by the president of the United States, is charged with protecting the public from harmful commodities. To the degree that manufacturers and retailers are cooperative with CPSC efforts, the commission is in a position to contribute to a drop in toy-related injuries and death and has had successes in this regard. That the CPSC often is slow to act or resistant to label some toys that have caused considerable harm as too dangerous to be sold suggests contradictions in the agency's mission, the commitments of its leaders, and the degree to which government regulation is still valued in society (e.g., the CPSC has gone from almost 1,000 employees in the early 1980s to under 500 today). Certainly, at times, the CPSC has not been slow to criticize consumer groups like WATCH (e.g., on the grounds that it creates needless concern among parents about toys the CPSC deems safe). Moreover, sometimes when companies decide not to voluntarily recall products that have been found to be risky, it is only public outcry and organizing that prompts the CPSC to take protective action.

Without question, it is evident in our modern, fast-paced, rapidly shifting, globalized world that a tense relationship exists between toy profits and toy safety. The general social trend toward reductions in government regulatory powers, promotion of self-monitoring by the corporate community, and the building of cozy collaborative relationships between corporations and government regulatory agencies (and a revolving door of employment between these two sectors) does not point toward greater vigilance in the promotion of toy safety in the immediate future. Only public demand for and organizing around toy safety will protect children from the toy industry and its concern with the bottom line. Dangerous toys, after all, are nothing to play around with.

References

American Academy of Pediatrics

2000 Toy Safety: How Children Are Injured. Electronic document, www.medem.com/medlb/article_detaillb.cfm?article_ID=ZZZ9LYOOQ7C&sub_cat=104.

Bhatnagar, P.

2003 Ten Worst Toys Are Unwrapped: Consumer Group WATCH Raises Red Flag for Supremo Slingshots, Ribbets the Frog and

Rubber Yo-Yos. CNN Money. Electronic document, http://money.cnn.com/2003/11/18/news/companies/dangerous_toys/index.htm.

Berg, K., H. Hull, E. Zabel, P. Staley, M. Brown, and D. Homa
2006 Death of a Child After Ingestion of a Metallic Charm: Minnesota, 2006. Morbidity and Mortality Weekly Review 55(12):340–341.

Brasington, R.
1990 Nintendinitis. New England Journal of Medicine 322:1473–1474.

Brockenbrough, Martha
2006 Grown-ups in Toyland: How to Pick a Good Toy. Electronic document, http://encarta.msn.com/encnet/features/columns/?article=toymain.

Burke, A., and E. Peper
2002 Cumulative Trauma Disorder Risk for Children Using Computer Products: Results of a Pilot Investigation with a Student Convenience Sample. Public Health Reports 117(4):350–357.

Cassady, Alison
2005 Trouble in Toyland: 20th Annual Toy Safety Survey. Washington, DC: U.S. PIRG Educational Fund.

CPSC (Consumer Product Safety Commission)
2002 California Company Pleads Guilty to Importing and Selling Dangerous Children's Toys. Media release. Washington, DC: CPSC.
2003a CPSC Announces Results of Investigation of Yo-Yo Water Ball Toys. Media release. Washington, DC: CPSC.
2003b Letter to Jeffery Beck Wise, National Environmental Trust Fund. Washington, DC., www.cpsc.gov/library/foia/foia03/petition/ageunder.pdf.
2005a CPSC, California International Trading Announce Recall of Pacifiers and Two Electronic Toys. Media release. Washington, DC: CPSC.
2005b Toy-Related Deaths and Injuries, Calendar Year 2004. Washington, DC: CPSC.
2005c CPSC, Fisher-Price Announce Recall of Pogo Sticks. Media release. Washington, DC.

Cross, Gary, and Gregory Smits
2005 Japan, the U.S. and the Globalization of Children's Consumer Culture. Journal of Social History 38(4):873–890.

Curri, T., T. Palmieri, A. Aok, C. Kaulkin, M. Lunn, C. Gregory, and D. Greenhalgh
2003 Playing with Fire: Images of Fire on Toy Packaging. Journal of Burn Care and Rehabilitation 24(2):163–165.

Deafness Research UK
2004 Noise-Induced Hearing Loss: Children and Toys. Electronic document, www.deafnessresearch.org.uk/factsheets/noise-children.pdf.

Emanuelson, Ingrid
2003 How Safe Are Children's Products, Toys and Playground Equipment? A Swedish Analysis of Mild Brain Injuries at Home and During Leisure Time 1998–1999. Injury Control and Safety Promotion 10(3):139–144.

Felcher, E. Marla
2001 It's No Accident: How Corporations Sell Dangerous Baby Products. Monroe, ME: Common Courage Press.

Fleischer, G., E. Hoffmann, R. Muller, and R. Lang
1998 Toy Cap Pistols and Their Effect on Hearing. HNO 46(9):815–820.

Gaines, B., B. Shultz, and H. Ford
2004 Nonmotorized Scooters: A Source of Significant Morbidity in Children. Journal of Trauma 57(1):111–113.

Hampshire Museums Service
2006 A Brief History of Toys. Electronic document, www.hants.gov.uk/museum/toys/history/index.html.

Hawley, David
2006 Reebok Recalls Bracelet After Lead Poisoning Kills Minnesota Boy. Kansas City Star, March 24. Electronic document, www.kansascity.com/mld/kansascity/news/breaking_news/14177452.htm.

Hong Kong Trade Development Council
2006 Hong Kong's Toy Industry. Electronic document, www.tdctrade.com/main/industries/t2_2_39.htm.

Hope, Leah
2005 State to Ban Sale of Yo-Yo Waterball. Electronic document, http://abclocal.go.com/wls/story?section=News&id=3139447.

Huston, A., and J. Wright
1998 Mass Media and Children's Development. *In* Handbook of Child Psychology, vol. 4: Child Psychology in Practice. W. Damon, ed. Pp. 999–1058. New York: Wiley.

Keller, J., J. Hindman, J. Kidd, R. Jackson, S. Smith, and C. Wagner
2004 Air-Gun Injuries: Initial Evaluation and Resultant Morbidity. American Surgeon 70(6):480–490.

Kids in Danger
2005 Hazards of Child's Play: Children's Product Recalls in 2004. Chicago: Kids in Danger.

Kunkel, D.
2001 Children and Television Advertising. *In* The Handbook of Children and Media. D. Singer and J. Singer, eds. Pp. 375–394. Thousand Oaks, CA: Sage Publications.

Laraque, D.
2004 Injury Risk of Nonpowder Guns. Pediatrics 114(5):1357–1361.
Lassa, Julie, and Amy Sue Vruwink
2006 Press Release, April 24. Milwaukee, Wisconsin.
Lauro, P.
1999 Coaxing the Smile That Sells: Baby Wranglers in Demand in Marketing for Children. New York Times, November 1: C1.
Listman, David
2004 Paintball Injuries in Children: More Than Meets the Eye. Pediatrics 113(1):e15–e18.
Luxon, Linda
1998 Toys and Games: Poorly Recognised Hearing Hazards? British Medical Journal 316:1473–1480.
Ma, D., and G. Jones
2003 Television, Computer, and Video Viewing; Physical Activity; and Upper Limb Fracture Risk in Children: A Population-Based Case Control Study. Journal of Bone and Mineral Research 18(11):1970–1977.
Maestri, Nicole
2005 Toy Company Results May Be no Fun and Game. Electronic document, http://today.reuters.com/business/newsArticle.aspx?type=consumerProducts&storyID=nN11699817.
Mayer, Caroline
2006 Firm Won't Pull Magnetic Toy After Child's Death. Seattle Times, April 2: A7.
Miller, G. Wayne
1995 Toy Wars: The Epic Struggle Between G.I. Joe, Barbic, and the Companies That Make Them. New York: Random House.
New York PIRG
2002 Phthalates in Children's Toys. Trouble in Toyland, New York PIRG's Toy Safety Report.
NPD Group
2006 The NPD Group Reports on 2005 U.S. Toy Sales. Press release. Port Washington, NY: NPD Group.
O'Keefe, Terry
1998 "Toy Wars" Reveals Brutally Competitive Industry. Executive Bookshelf, Atlantic Business Chronicle, February 27: 1.
Oligopoly Watch
2004 Toy Industry Turmoil. Electronic document, www.oligopolywatch.com/2004/03/20.html.
Pergams, O., and P. Zaradic
2006 Is Love of Nature in the US Becoming Love of Electronic Media? 16-year Downtrend in National Park Visits Explained by Watching

Movies, Playing Video Games, Internet Use, and Oil Prices. Journal of Environmental Management (in press).

Ramos, E., C. James, and J. Bear-Lehman
1995 Children's Computer Usage: Are They at Risk of Developing Repetitive Strain Injury? Work 25(2):143–154.

Rice, F.
2001 Superstars of Spending: Marketers Clamor for Kids. Advertising Age, February 12: S1.

Ross, R., T. Campbell, J. Wright, A. Huston, M. Rice, and P. Turk
1984 When Celebrities Talk, Children Listen: An Experimental Analysis of Children's Responses to TV Ads with Celebrity Endorsements. Journal of Applied Developmental Psychology 5:185–202.

Safe Kids Worldwide
2004 Facts about Childhood Drowning Fact Sheet. Electronic document, www.usa.safekids.org/content_documents/Drowning_facts.pdf.

Siegal, S., E. Eviatar, J. Lapinsky, N. Shlamkovitch, and A. Kessler
2003 Inner Ear Damage in Children Due to Noise Exposure from Toy Cap Pistols and Firecrackers: A Retrospective Review of 53 Cases. Noise Health 5(18):13–18.

Stern, Sydney Ladensohn, and Ted Schoenhaus
1990 Toyland: The High-Stakes Game of the Toy Industry. Chicago: Contemporary Books.

Swartz, Edward
1986 Toys That Kill. New York: Vintage Books.

VanArsdale, J., B. Horowitz, T. Merritt, D. Peddycord, E. Severson, K. Moore, N. Pusel, R. Leiker, B. Zeal, M. Scott, and M. Kohn
2004 Brief Report: Lead Poisoning from Ingestion of a Toy Necklace—Oregon, 2003. Morbidity and Mortality Weekly Review 53(23):509–511.

Vassilev, Zdravko, and Steven Marcus
2004 Paintball Injuries in Children: The Cases Managed Out of Hospitals. Pediatrics (letter) 113(5):1468.

Washington Department of Health
2002 Circumstances Surrounding Deaths from the Washington Child Death Review Data. Electronic document, www.doh.wa.gov/hsqa/emstrauma/injury/pubs/wscir/WSCIR_Drowning.pdf.

Yaremchuk, K., L. Dickson, K. Burk, and B. Shivapuja
1997 Noise Level Analysis of Commercially Available Toys. International Journal of Pediatric Otorhinolaryngology 41(2):187–197.

Your Web Store
2006 www.camppacs.com/cgi-bin/shopper.cgi?preadd=action&key=PRIM6149.

Zapata, A., A. Moaes, C. Leone, U. Doria-Filho, and C. Silva
2006 Pain and Musculoskeletal Pain Syndromes Related to Computer and Video Game Use in Adolescents. European Journal of Pediatrics 165(6): 408–414.

CHAPTER THREE

THE ENVIRONMENTAL AND HEALTH CONSEQUENCES OF MOTOR VEHICLES

A Case Study in Capitalist Technological Hegemony and Grassroots Responses to It

Hans Baer

Motor vehicles, with their internal combustion engines, perhaps more than any other machine embody the social structural, cultural, and environmental contradictions of the capitalist world system. They have had major impacts upon patterns of consumption, settlement (e.g., urban sprawl), traffic congestion, mass transportation, social relations, public policy, the environment, and health. In essence, they have become a hegemonic force in the 20th century and beyond. As Paul Gilroy observes:

> The twentieth century was the century of the automobile, of automobility and mass motorization. Commerce in motor vehicles still constitutes the overheated core of unchecked and unsustainable consumer capitalism, but the impact of car culture extends far beyond those buoyant commercial processes. . . . Novel and damaging patterns created by motorization have profoundly altered the political economy of everyday life. (Gilroy 2001:81–83)

This chapter discusses the role of motor vehicles, particularly automobiles, within the larger context of capitalist production and the culture of consumption. It particularly focuses upon the environmental and health consequences of motor vehicles. I examine the impact of automobilization upon the ecological body, individual body, and the body politic. Motor vehicles are a major contributor to air and noise pollution and global warming, all of which have significant negative health consequences. Further, they contribute directly to a wide variety of physical and mental health problems, including accidents resulting in deaths and serious injuries, respiratory and cardiovascular diseases, cancer, musculoskeletal disorders, stress, and social isolation. This chapter also examines counterhegemonic movements, particularly ones that have appeared in developed societies, that challenge the technological hegemony that motor vehicles have assumed within the capitalist world system. As a critical anthropologist, in part following in the footsteps of critical sociologists Freund and Martin (1993), I seek to contribute in this chapter to both the political ecology and the political economy of health of motor vehicles.

Motor Vehicles, Capitalist Production, and the Culture of Consumption

James Flink (1988:viii) contends that the rise of the automobile industry and a massive network of roads are "central to the history of the advanced capitalist countries in the twentieth century, and explain an especially large part of the history of the American people." Although Europeans invented the internal combustion engine, the United States assumed the lead in automobile production by the early 20th century. Indeed, the production and consumption of automobiles became a major component of Fordism, a term coined by Antonio Gramsci to designate the 20th-century corporate vision of mechanized production coupled with the mass consumption of standardized products. As Lee (1993:77) observes,

> during the 1920s, mass production in the US was drifting rapidly towards both a crisis of production and a crisis of consumption. The new productive regime pioneered by Henry Ford had succeeded in changing dramatically the quantitative and qualitative output of commodities, but it had not significantly altered the established wage/labour relation. . . . But the arrival of mass production, of course, required mass consumption: a sufficiently sized mass market composed of the wage-earning classes that would be able to absorb the influx of mass-produced commodities.

In addition to having offered his workers the then unheard of five-dollar-eight-hour day incentive one year after the opening of his first plant in 1914, Ford embarked upon a campaign to socialize his workers into core American values that included abstinence from alcohol but also adoption of stable familial patterns and mass consumerism, which included purchase of one of his automobiles at a relatively affordable price. His initial efforts met with some resistance to the notion that automobiles constituted symbols of modernity and prestige affordable to even those workers who toiled on his assembly lines (Lee 1993). As a result of the stock market crash of 1929 and the Depression of the 1930s, more progressive segments of the U.S. capitalist class found a new ally in Roosevelt's New Deal, which utilized the state as a "means of providing enough employment to generate sufficient consumer demand so as to absorb the very worst excesses of overproduction" (Lee 1993:80).

The role of the state in advanced capitalist societies has been to resolve the contradictions that develop in a market economy and to reduce social conflicts that may threaten the stability of the social system. The state must be responsive both to the requirements of the economy and the organized demands of the public. Although the state must cater to the latter to some extent, it never questions the logic of the corporate economy and a stratified social system. Studies by Mills (1956), Domhoff (1990), and others have documented the upper-class origins of many high-echelon members of the U.S. state, particularly those in the executive branch of the federal government. Consequently, when the state promotes changes in public policy, including those related to various aspects of motor vehicle production and highway construction, they tend to be in harmony with the interests of the corporate sector. As Taebel and Cornehls (1977:75) observe,

> corporate administrators and technicians, particularly those of the auto industry, have long moved freely in and out of the federal government, thus blurring the line between governmental interests and those of private business concerns. Nowhere is this mutuality of interests more clearly understood or more staunchly promoted than among the leaders of the auto corporations themselves.

Roosevelt's vision of economic stability and democratic welfarism did not come to full fruition until after World War II—an event that did much to overcome the Depression and to propel the United States into the position of the foremost capitalist nation and the leading culture of consumption in the world. A key component of the new corporate-state alliance was the "concentration of industrial activity into a few key sectors, most notably those of automobile production, building and construction, shipping and other transportation equipment, petro-chemicals, steel, rubber" and the production of a wide array of household appliances and goods (Lee 1993:84). The automobile became a link between the suburban home and the workplace, shopping centers, movie theaters, sports stadiums and arenas, and tourist sights and vacation resorts. Furthermore, the automobile served to "bypass the threatened social alienation which was said to result from the geographical dispersal of localized communities and the physical rupture of traditional kinship bonds that followed from the ease of modern spatial mobility" (Lee 1993:130). Automobile advertisements, which in the United States alone come to $40 billion a year (Kay 1997:17), frequently have promised and continue to promise their target populations that they will achieve power, prestige, freedom, sexual desirability, and prowess if they choose to become the proud owners of a highly individualized form of transportation.

The reality that North Americans, encouraged by corporate advertising, have come to love their cars is well captured in Flink's book *The Car Culture*. He observes: "during the 1920s automobility became the backbone of a new consumer-goods-oriented society and economy that has persisted into the present" (Flink 1973:140). By this time, as Barnet and Cavanaugh (1994:262) so aptly note, "the car became a primary locus of recreation, a badge of affluence, a power fantasy on wheels, a gleaming sex symbol," all images that have been heavily promoted by the automobile industry through intensive advertising. In their classic community study of Middletown (Muncie, Indiana) during the 1920s, the Lynds (1929:950) reported that "the make of one's car is rivaling the looks of one's place as an evidence of one's belonging" among members of the "business class." Despite the Depression, they reported that by the mid-1930s, the automobile had become an essential object of ownership for the Middletown worker for whom "it gives the status which his job increasingly denies, and, more than any other facility to which he has access, it symbolizes living, having a good time, that thing that keeps you working" (Lynd and Lynd 1937:245). Particularly following World War II, the automobile symbolized the affluence that many young working-class Americans now enjoyed compared to the socioeconomic circumstances of either their parents or themselves in earlier times (Moorhouse 1983).

Aside of the fact that the U.S. military relies upon a diversity of motor vehicles, images of militarism have spilled over into private motor-vehicle use. The jeep, "the original American SUV," has taken on a modernized form in the Jeep Cherokee, which is the "bearer of Manifest Destiny, doing God's work finding and dominating new lands in the American West" while at the same time appropriating a Native American name that "only reflects a more general pattern of such appropriation of what had been destroyed by European colonization" (Patterson and Dalby 2006:5). The ultimate SUV is the Hummer, an adaptation of the military transport, the Humvee, brought to public attention by its use in the 1991 Gulf War.

Automobiles constitute the second most expensive commodity (after homes) that Americans purchase. In 1990, Americans spent 31.3 percent of their income on motor vehicles (Freund and Martin 1993:16). Indeed, as Simpson (1994:3) so aptly observes, automobiles have "increasingly become extensions of home: radio, stereo, CD players, telephone and a whole range of other home comforts are not matched by local public transport," all of which ingeniously seduce people away from public transportation. In recent decades, automobile firms have been searching for new markets in the third world and, with the collapse of the Soviet bloc, in Eastern Europe. During the cold-war era of the 1950s and early 1960s, General Motors (GM) urged patriotic U.S. citizens to "see the USA in your Chevrolet." Such advertisements on the part of the automobile industry served to seduce North Americans away from what was once a relatively well-developed mass transportation system, that included passenger trains, numerous intercity bus lines, and extensive urban and interurban trolley or tramlines. Indeed, a consortium called National City Lines, consisting of General Motors, Standard Oil of New Jersey, and the Firestone Tire and Rubber Company, spent $9 million by 1950 to obtain control of street railway companies in 16 states and converted them to less efficient GM buses. The companies were sold to operators who signed contracts specifying that they would buy GM equipment.

National City Lines in the 1940s began buying up and scrapping parts of Pacific Electric, the world's largest interurban electric rail system, which by 1945 served 110 million passengers in 56 smog-free Southern California cities. Eleven hundred miles of Pacific Electric's track were torn up, and the system went out of service in 1961, as Southern California commuters came to rely primarily on freeways (Flink 1973:220). Unfortunately, Henry Huntington, the owner of Pacific Electric, used his interurban trolley company more as a scheme for promoting his real estate endeavors than providing a public service and often alienated citizens in various ways, including his failure to provide lines that connected suburbs to each other as opposed to strictly city centers (Bottles 1992). A similar process in which a consortium of road interests colluded to destroy efficient trolley or tram systems occurred throughout the United States and Australia (Goddard 1994; Davison 2004). According to Hunter (2003:50), General Motors and its allies managed to destroy more than 100 trolley systems in 45 North American cities, with Ford and Chrysler having engaged in "mop-up operations." Whereas large cities such as New York, Boston, Philadelphia, and Chicago developed and still operate public transportation, Detroit—the capital of the motor vehicle industry—never did so, for obvious reasons.

In the 1950s, with the assistance of the Eisenhower administration, the development of an interstate highway system resulted in enormous profits for corporations and benefits to supportive politicians, while hindering the development of public transportation, and thereby forcing the general public to purchase and use cars (Leavitt 1970). Indeed, Lewis Mumford (1963) argues that the federally funded highway programs of the 1950s contributed to the creation of a "one-dimensional transportation system." According to Crawford,

> the Interstates gave truckers a subsidized route network that allowed them to compete successfully with railroads despite the labor and energy inefficiency of trucking. It also gave real estate developers the high-speed arteries leading to downtown that made large-scale suburban sprawl possible. (Crawford 2000:88)

A powerful lobby consisting of the automobile industry, the American Automobile Association, petroleum companies, trucking companies, and tire companies continues to pose a barrier to the development of an effective public transportation system in the United States. Whereas heavy trucks contribute more than 95 percent of the highway deterioration in this country, trucking companies pay only 29 percent of the highway bill (Freund and Martin 1993).

Various U.S. cities, such as Houston, Detroit, and Phoenix, as well as cities in other parts of the world, such as Perth and Canberra in Australia and Bangkok in Thailand, have developed into what Newman and Kenworthy (1999:31–33) term "automobile cities." In describing the economic situation in U.S. society during the 1970s, Sweezy (1973:7) contends that the "private interests which cluster around, and are directly or indirectly dependent upon, the automobile for their prosperity are quantitatively far more numerous and wealthy than those similarly related to any other commodity or complex of commodities in the U.S. economy."

Although the United States has long assumed the lead in the promotion of motor vehicles as a means of transporting both people and consumer products, "automobilization" has become a global phenomenon (Sweezy 1973:7). Down Under, war bonds posters urged Australians to save for a post–World War II car (Davison 2004:3) and the Holden station wagon became in the late 1950s a "mobile embodiment of a middling-class suburb family life" (Davison 2004:21). Indeed, the American architect Walter Burley Griffin designed Canberra, the national capital, with its elaborate road system consisting of concentric circles and turnarounds, with the automobile in mind rather than trains or trams. Although Canberra has grown to a sprawling city of some 310,000, with a bus system vastly superior to that of most U.S. cities of roughly the same size, politicians, urban planners, and a substantial number of residents postpone the inevitable day of reckoning in terms of traffic congestion by arguing that a light-rail system would be prohibitively expensive. Simpson (1994:1) reports that the number of licensed automobiles in Britain increased from 13,399,000 in 1974 to 19,737,000 in 1991, an increase of 47 percent.

Along with industrial pollution, motor vehicles have transformed cities around the world, particularly ones in underdeveloped nations, into environmental disaster areas accompanied by a wide array of health problems. Over a decade ago, Zuckerman (1991) itemized the following components of the "world car crisis": 1) 500 million vehicles on the road; 2) mounting traffic congestion; 3) the impact of pollution on health and climatic change; 4) a heavy dependence on fossil fuels; 5) 250,000 traffic deaths per year; and 5) producing 50 million new vehicles each year. Needless to say, these problems have intensified as humanity has entered the 21st century.

The revolving-door syndrome between the U.S. motor vehicle industry and the state is illustrated by the fact that both Charles Wilson, a former General Motors president, and Robert McNamara, a former Ford president, both served as secretaries of defense, and that Thomas Mann, a high-ranking State Department official, became president of the Automobile Manufacturers Association. A massive highway lobby consisting of vehicle manufacturers and dealers, petroleum companies, the United Auto Workers, the American Automobile Association, and highway construction companies heavily influenced party politicians in the federal, state, and local governments to pass legislation that promotes the culture of automobility. Although various American cities, such as Portland; San Diego; St. Louis; Baltimore; Washington, D.C.; San Francisco; Los Angeles; and Dallas have embarked upon improvements in mass transportation systems, these function as supplements to automobiles.

In Australia, the motor vehicle lobby and the Liberal Party eventually convinced the Labor Party to join them in the promotion of road construction rather than prop up a deteriorating public transportation system (Davison 2004:125). According to Davison (2004:261), "by the 1990s more than 80 percent of daily journeys in Melbourne were made by car, and more than 50 percent of households had two or more cars." Indeed, every city in Australia, except Melbourne, lost its trams and trolley buses between 1950 and 1970 (Ponting 1992:337).

Nazi Germany constitutes another example of the close ties between the automobile industry and the state. Hitler unveiled his strategy to rejuvenate the declining German auto industry at the International Automobile and Motor Cycle Exhibition in Berlin a few days after coming to power in 1933 by announcing plans for the development of the Volkswagen and the autobahn. The Volkswagen plant produced military jeeps and Daimler-Benz and BMW produced aircraft engines, tanks, and armored trucks (Wolf 1996). Opel, owned by General Motors, and Ford also manufactured products for the Nazi war apparatus (leading to U.S.

government payments to these companies for damages as a result of U.S. bombing of Germany during the war).

While corporations often assert that they favor minimal government involvement, in reality the collusion between the motor vehicle industry and governments around the world constitutes an example of *state capitalism par excellence*. As Dicken (2003:353) observes,

> the state has played an extremely important role in [the automobile industry's] evolution. In particular, trade barriers have exerted an extremely important influence in both developing and developed economies. At the same time, national governments have struggled to outbid one another . . . to secure the large manufacturing industries. . . . The giant TNCs of the industry have developed consummate skills in playing governments off against one another.

Western European governments in particular have been extensively involved in their domestic motor vehicle industries. Indeed, until recently, the French, British, and Italian states owned automobile manufacturing operations.

In 1990 there were reportedly approximately 550 million motor vehicles in the world, a number that continues to rise with population increase and consumer demand spurred on by corporate advertising (Graedel and Allen 1998:115). In Eastern European countries, for example, which used to rely heavily upon trolley cars as a form of public transportation, the wave of consumerism that followed in the wake of the collapse of the Soviet Union resulted in a massive increase in the number of automobiles as well as in resulting traffic congestion. Former Eastern bloc countries have subsequently embarked upon large-scale programs of highway construction and have abandoned railway lines as more and more people turn to cars for transportation. Table 3.1 provides statistics on the number of motor vehicles manufactured in various world regions and selected countries in 2003 and 2004.

Automobile production has been concentrated in Europe, Japan, and North America, with production and utilization on the rise in developing nations. According to Dicken (2003:359),

> in the Americas, both Canada and Mexico are tightly enmeshed with the US automobile industry . . . while Brazil remains the major automobile

Table 3.1. Motor Vehicles Manufactured in 2003 and 2004 in World Regions and Selected Countries

	2003	*2004*	*% Change*
Europe	20,000,286	20,829,774	4
North and South America	18,280,312	18,826,944	3
USA	12,114,971	11,989,387	−1
Brazil	1,827,791	2,210,062	21
Asia-Oceania	21,986,694	24,086,520	10
Australia	413,261	411,406	0
China	4,443,686	5,070,527	14
India	1,161,523	1,511,157	30
Japan	10,286,218	10,511,518	2
Africa	395,933	422,017	7

Source: Adapted from data presented by the International Organization of Motor Vehicle Manufacturers, www.oica.net.

> production centre in Latin America. The most striking new development of recent years has been the sudden emergence of South Korea as an important producer. As recently as the early 1980s, Korea was producing only 20,000 automobiles; In 2000 Korean output was 2.4 *million* (6 percent of the world total).

Thailand has evolved into the "car capital" of Southeast Asia with many major foreign automobile companies having manufacturing facilities there. The Chinese automobile industry consists of state companies as well as a number of joint operations between these companies and foreign companies, including Volkswagen, Toyota, Nissan, Honda, Hyundai, and General Motors (Dicken 2003:396–397).

In terms of motor vehicle utilization, annual travel by private passenger cars (passenger kilometers per capita) in 1990 stood at 19,004 in Houston; 16,686 in Los Angeles; 9,417 in Sydney; 4,482 in Paris; 3,175 in Tokyo; 6,299 in Kuala Lumpur; 4,634 in Bangkok; 2,464 in Seoul; and 1,546 in Jakarta (Newman and Kenworthy 1999:84). The most dramatic instance in the growth of motor vehicles in the developing world is China (Spellerberg 2002:7). Diamond reports:

> The number of motor vehicles (mostly trucks and buses) increased 15-fold between 1980 and 2001, cars 130-fold. In 1994, after the number of motor vehicles had increased 9 times, China decided to make car production one of its four so-called pillar industries, with the goal of increasing production (now especially of cars) by another factor of 4 by

> year 2010. That would make China the world's third largest vehicle manufacturing country, after the U.S. and Japan. (Diamond 2005:362)

Motor vehicles along with coal-powered power plants are contributing to air pollutants such as nitrogen oxides and carbon dioxide in China. As even less developed countries than China gain more purchasing power in the global economy, the number of cars and resulting pollution in these countries are bound to grow as well.

Anthropologist Daniel Miller (1995) has written a fascinating account of the centrality of automobiles in one third-world community, namely the town of Chaguanas in central Trinidad, the fastest growing urban center within Trinidad and Tobago. Although most residents of Chaguanas achieved affordability of a car, even if only a reupholstered older one, in the wake of the oil-boom of the late 1970s it has come to dominate the Trinidadian self-image:

> People are constantly recognized through their cars. . . . Street dialogue constantly asserts that men are attractive to women as much through the body of their cars as their own bodies and there are abundant metaphors based on car parts. (Miller 1995:286–287)

Furthermore, many residents cease walking once they have acquired a car, which has developed into a significant marker of modernity.

The Impact of Motor Vehicles on the Environment

Along with industrial pollution, motor vehicles have transformed many cities around the world, particularly ones in the third world such as Mexico City, into environmental disaster areas (Robinson 1971). Of the estimated 4.4 million tons of human-generated pollutant emitted into the air of Mexico City in 1989, 76 percent were produced by motor vehicles (Freund and Martin 1993:67). Continued degradation of air quality caused the Union of Concerned Scientists in 1991 to shift its primary concern from nuclear energy to the internal combustion engine and the Natural Resources Defense Council to declare the following year that the automobile was "the worst environmental threat in many U.S. cities" (Kay 1997:80).

Cities vary greatly in terms of carbon dioxide (CO_2) emission and other motor vehicle pollutants. Whereas the transportation-produced CO_2 in the New York metropolitan area totaled 3,378 kilograms per capita in 1990, it was 5,193 kilograms in the Houston area (Newman and Kenworthy 1999:120). In contrast, Toronto has 46 percent less CO_2 per capita than the average U.S. city, largely due to an extensive public transportation system.

Motor vehicles have contributed to the destruction of ozone in the stratosphere as a result of a catalytic process in which chlorofluorocarbons and other chlorine-containing gases produce chlorine. Another major by-product of gasoline exhaust is benzoapyrene, a carcinogenic chemical that is suspended in urban air. Motor vehicles also emit carbon monoxide, sulfur oxides, nitrous oxides, benzene, and formaldehyde, which in turn contribute to acid rain and human respiratory complications and in some cases cancer.

Despite improvements in car fuel economy and emissions controls standards, a doubling of miles driven during the 1980s and the 1990s by and large negated the impact of these innovations. Furthermore, while the catalytic converter "effectively breaks down the various nitrous oxides [NO_x] that contribute to smog and local air pollution . . . it creates nitrous oxide [N_2O], benign in smog creation but 300 times more potent than carbon dioxide as a greenhouse gas" (Porter 1999:81).

The Clinton administration's creation of a Partnership for a New Generation of Vehicles provided funding to national laboratories and auto-parts companies with the objective of creating a midsized automobile that would get 80 miles to the gallon, but the growing popularity of gas-guzzling, expensive sports utility vehicles (SUVs)—which the U.S. government classifies as "light trucks," and so are subject to less stringent emissions standards—significantly added to air pollution during this period (Bradsher 2002:70). Ironically, SUVs have particularly appealed to baby boomers, many of whom view themselves as sensitive to environmental issues, as well as movie stars, directors, singers, and other entertainment idols. Nevertheless, SUVs reportedly produce up to five and a half times as much exhaust fumes per mile as do standard automobiles.

While the overall automobile pollution problem is greatest in the United States and other industrialized countries, the situation in less-developed countries is problematic at the individual vehicle level. In resource-poor settings, limited funds exist to maintain emission control equipment on vehicles and to enforce any regulations that may exist (which are often nonexistent). One just has to walk through the streets of Quito, Ecuador, or Lagos, Nigeria, to experience this firsthand.

The Impact of Motor Vehicles on Health

When automobiles first began to appear, various public health reformers viewed them as a panacea to the manure and urine deposited by horses in cities. In contrast, motor vehicles have evolved into a major source of accidents around the world and an enemy to the environment. In 1990 420,000 people were killed and some nine million were injured around the world as a result of motor vehicle accidents, and between 1960 and 1994 approximately five million died as a result of motor vehicle accidents. Road traffic accidents are reportedly the leading cause of death worldwide among males between ages 15 and 44 (Crawford 2000:70). In contrast, between 1894 and 1994, 9,678 people died in railroad disasters.

Motor vehicle accidents are the leading cause of death in the 15-to-24-year-old age category in the United States (Wright 1992:101). Crawford (2000:70) observes:

> The USA is one of the safest countries in the world in terms of deaths per distance driven, but in 1998, despite safer cars and highways, US motor vehicle crashes caused almost one death per 100 million vehicle-kilometers traveled, for a total of 41,471 lives lost.

In addition to alleging that automobile manufacturers had resisted legislation and public pressure to build safer cars, O'Connell and Myers (1965) assert that they attempted to shift responsibility for the increasing number of accidents to driving behavior and road conditions. Motor vehicles also pose hazards for pedestrians and cyclists. The National Safety Council reported some 6,600 pedestrian deaths and 800 cyclist deaths in 1989 in the United States (Freund and Martin 1993:102). In their survey of cities in various parts of the world, Newman and Kenworthy (1999:118) report that traffic deaths in 1990 in U.S. cities, "despite their highly developed road systems, strictly regulated traffic, and a population generally well educated in traffic safety issues," were the highest at 14.6

per 100,000, compared to 12.0 per 100,000 in Australian cities, 6.5 in Toronto, 8.8 in European cities, 6.6 in "wealthy" Asian cities, and 13.7 in "developing" Asian cities. Toronto's relatively low rate is due to the fact that this city has a good public transportation system. Furthermore, "Amsterdam, at 5.7, and Copenhagen, at 7.5 deaths per 100,000, have among the lowest rates in Europe and have among the highest rates of bicycle usage" (Newman and Kenworthy 1999:119).

In addition to the greater gas emissions rate associated with SUVs mentioned in the previous section, they also are a major contributor to accidents and deaths not only the United States, but also increasingly in other parts of the world, including Australia (despite higher gasoline prices). Although they are often perceived as safe due to their large size, particularly the early models of SUVs, such as the Bronco II, they were prone to rollovers that killed and injured occupants at an alarming rate. Bradsher (2002:163) reports that SUV rollovers killed some 12,000 people in the United States alone during the 1990s. Despite design improvements that have made SUVs safer for occupants, their large size continues to pose a hazard to other car drivers and pedestrians. Whereas standard automobiles with their low bumpers often flip pedestrians onto a relatively soft hood, SUVs hit them higher up, thereby inflicting worse injuries.

Speed constitutes a major contributing factor to motor vehicle deaths and accidents. The implementation of a short-lived 55 miles per hour speed limit in the United States reduced highway fatalities 20 percent (Wolf 1996:172). Germany is famous or infamous, depending upon one's perspective, for the lack of a speed limit on its autobahns, a policy that was first established during the Nazi era. Whereas the German Democratic Republic (former East Germany) had a speed limit on its autobahns, the unification of 1990 resulted in the eradication of this restriction and a doubling of the number of highway fatalities (Wolf 1996:172).

The American Lung Association estimates that in 1985 motor vehicle pollution contributed to some 120,000 deaths in the United States (Freund and Martin 1993:29). Sixty percent of the residents of Calcutta, India, were found to have pollution-related respiratory diseases (Freund and Martin 1993). Additionally, some brake linings contain asbestos, a well-known carcinogen.

Motor vehicle emissions contribute to elevation of ozone levels, of which Greater Atlanta is a prime example. The city has evolved into the leading U.S. metropolitan area in vehicle miles traveled per person per day at 34.1, as opposed to other leaders, such as Dallas (30.1); Washington, D.C. (22.6); and Los Angeles (21.5). The result is massive air pollution, including ozone, which contributes to various respiratory complications, including asthma. Research Atlanta, an institute affiliated with Georgia State University, has reported that asthma-related visits to the pediatric emergency clinic at Grady Memorial Hospital increase by a third during high ozone days (Doyle 2000:3). The Centers for Disease Control and Prevention estimates that the number of asthmatics in the United States increased from 6.8 million in 1980 to 17.3 million in 1998, in part due to ozone pollution (Doyle 1998:4). An estimated 100 million Americans live in places that do not meet the EPA's eight-hour air-quality standard for ozone (Doyle 1998:5).

The situation is not any better internationally. In Athens, for instance, the death rate increases as much as fivefold on the most polluted days (Nadis and MacKenzie 1993:23), and Mexico City reportedly exceeds EPA ozone standards virtually every day of the year.

Pollution is not the only health problem associated with cars. Motor vehicle driving, particularly under congested conditions, induces stress and heightened blood pressure, contributes to medical complications such as lumbar disk herniation, or "motorist's spine," and contributes to sedentarization. Truck drivers in particular suffer a high rate of back injuries.

Automobilization also impacts psychological health. Auto transportation discourages patterns of social interaction vital to mental well-being in that most motorists, especially in advanced capitalist societies, drive alone. As Wolf (1996:192) so aptly observes, "the car society reproduces an elementary phenomenon of the capitalist mode of production: the depersonalization and reification of human relationships." With the decline of public transportation, especially in the United States, mothers in particular function as chauffeurs for their children as they transport them hither and yon in sprawling suburbs and developments. In fact, in less than ten years after 1983, women's automobile travel reportedly quadrupled in the United States (Kay 1997:22). Ironically, at the same time, low-income people living in inner cities often find themselves with inadequate transportation to jobs, medical clinics, and hospitals, all of which are increasingly located in suburban areas. As Kay so aptly observes,

> the car culture has thus become an engine of inequity, raising high the barriers of race and class. Transportation that is difficult at best, nonexistent at worst, darkens their lives in myriad ways and adds to the financial and social inequality they suffer. (Kay 1997:38)

Elderly people often continue to drive because the automobile is necessary to maintaining social connections with friends and family scattered about urban areas. Finally, various studies have indicated that automobile driving, particularly in conditions where traffic congestion is moderate to light, may contribute to "road rage" because drivers feel frustrated by the inability to reach their destinations in the shortest time possible (Smith 2002:34–41).

Challenges to the Technology Hegemony of Motor Vehicles

Despite the existence of massive corporate support for the ongoing use of motor vehicles, in the form of advertisements and other promotional campaigns, there have been some counterhegemonic efforts, particularly within the green movement in Western Europe, to resist the automobilization of society by emphasizing the need for people to rely on other forms of transportation. Environmental groups, car safety activists, bicyclists, and other social activists in the United States and other parts of the world have extracted some concessions from the corporate class and its political allies on issues such as emissions control standards, motor vehicle design, highway construction, and public expenditures for mass transit systems.

Public awareness of some negative aspects of motor vehicle transportation reached new heights with the publication of Ralph Nader's book *Unsafe at Any Speed* (1965). Environmentalists and other social activists began to challenge the pollution, health hazards, traffic, sprawl, and fragmentation of social life resulting from motor vehicles and highways during the 1970s (Golten et al. 1977). Such efforts contributed significantly to the passage of both federal and state regulatory laws in the United

States. Such legislation offered a technological fix that mandated catalytic converters and periodic car inspections. Rajan (1996), however, asserts that mandatory pollution-control devices and emissions testing do not significantly reduce pollution.

The Energy Policy and Conservation Act of 1975 forced the U.S. automobile industry to improve fuel economy in passenger cars, making them more like those manufactured in Europe and Japan. Unfortunately, despite various reforms, the sanctity of the automobile as an integral component of U.S. political economy and culture has generally gone unchallenged. Nevertheless, an increasing number of scholars over the past decade or so have made suggestions for reducing reliance upon automobiles. Wright (1992), for example, proposes the following steps: 1) switching from private motor vehicles to trains and buses; 2) increasing the distance that transport vehicles can travel per energy unit; 3) manufacturing engines that are less polluting; 4) implementing road designs, traffic regulations, and vehicle operations that contribute to more efficient vehicle utilization; and 5) relying upon less polluting sources of fuel.

Furthermore, pockets of resistance to the motor vehicle hegemony are manifested in the slow but steady development of a "global auto city protest movement" (Newman and Kenworthy 1999:60–62). Indeed, Kay (1997:286) asserts "that deposing the car from its dominion over the earth is a radical, even revolutionary, move" and argues that those who participate in this still burgeoning "countercultural rescue movement" must act as "promobility advocates: pro-walking, pro-cycling, pro-transit" (Kay 1997:286). Kay (1997:356–357) advocates a strategy of antiautomobile activism at the local, regional, state, and national levels that challenges "moribund highway-based plans" and the "vehicle-first policies promoted by long-entrenched forces."

Grassroots groups opposed to highway construction projects that threaten stable and historic neighborhoods and rural landscapes have formed in states such as Oregon, Kansas, California, Indiana, and New Hampshire. Grassroots groups in both Toronto and Vancouver prevented freeways from being built in the inner city (Newman and Kenworthy 1999), and over 900 antifreeway groups have emerged throughout Britain (Newman and Kenworthy 1999). The Link-Up Conference and other similar events have served as forums for antifreeway groups in Australia.

Critical Mass, an organization of procycling activists, has engaged in probicycle and antiautomobile mass actions in cities such as San Francisco; Austin; Washington, D.C.; and Edmonton. The green movement in Western Europe has mobilized opposition to the automobilization of society by emphasizing the need for people to rely on cycling and other forms of transportation. Unfortunately, notwithstanding this progress, U.S. greens have not systematically challenged the environmental damage created by the world's leading car culture.

Like Critical Mass in North America, environmentalists in Germany attempt to promote cycling as a form of transportation by sponsoring demonstrations consisting of bikers riding through otherwise busy city streets. Ironically, while cycling constitutes an "environmental" mode of transportation, as well as a healthy means to provide the body with aerobic exercise, it will remain a highly dangerous activity as long as the streets and highways are filled with fast-moving motor vehicles. However, grassroots groups in Copenhagen, Amsterdam, and other Dutch cities have done much to create bikeways, marked paths for cyclists on roads, and a "culture of respect" for cyclists (Newman and Kenworthy 1999:206). Simon Batterbury (2002:2–3) reports that Copenhagen and the community of Frederiksberg situated within the city limits has 307 kilometers of bike paths and that in 2000 "34% of home to place-of-work trips were made by bicycle." In the U.S. some 20 pedestrian advocate groups have formed a coalition called America Walks, and citizens consisting of walkers and bicyclists have pressured cities to create greenways and bike paths in communities around the country (Kay 1997).

Illustrating the dialectic of automobile use, Simon Maxwell (2001) conducted focus-group discussions in order to ascertain how residents of Cambridge, England, juxtapose their utilization of automobiles with their concerns about their impact on social life and the environment. Although he found that many participants held other car users and the government as being responsible for the negative consequences of reliance upon automobiles, he also found that:

> Many people had also made great efforts to limit or reduce their car use. For these participants, the social and environmental benefits of finding alternatives to the car intersect with other varied concerns, ranging from personal health to general quality of life. (Maxwell 2001:209)

Newman and Kenworthy (1999:144–189) propose five policies for overcoming automobile dependency: 1) traffic calming in which speed plateaus, neck-downs, and other strategies are employed to slow down traffic in order to make streets safer, particularly for pedestrians, cyclists, shoppers, and residents; 2) the construction of quality transit systems as well as bike and walking paths; 3) the development of "urban villages" or multinodal centers with mixed, dense land use; 4) growth management to counter urban sprawl; and 5) and increasing taxes on motor vehicle transportation in various ways. Elsewhere, J. H. Crawford (2000) offers a radical solution to the multifaceted problems associated with motor vehicles in cities. While recognizing that transportation is a key component of modern cities, he maintains that the automobile is the "most space-intensive form of urban transport ever devised and has forced cities to expand into rural areas" (Crawford 2000:24). He additionally contends that it "has isolated the young, the elderly, and anyone who does not drive, particularly in suburban areas lacking any other form of transport" (Crawford 2000:73). Dismissing traffic management as an unsuitable solution, Crawford (2000) maintains that rail transport offers a cheaper, cleaner, faster, and more comfortable alternative to cars. The denser settlement pattern of car-free cities would help restore a sense of community missing in suburban areas and allow for nearby parks and other green spaces. He does admit, however, that cars can improve mobility in rural areas and small towns.

The significance of relying on trains rather than cars for transportation is by no means a utopian idea. According to Newman and Kenworthy (1999:155), "hundreds of cities, both large and small, in Europe, North America, Australia, and other nations, have joined the light rail revolution in recent years." In the United States, light rail systems have been developed in Baltimore, St. Louis, Dallas, Portland, Salt Lake City, and San Diego. In contrast to Crawford (2000), Newman and Kenworthy believe that buses are an important component and have three roles to play in the development of efficient public transportation systems: "(1) as an inferior solution before a rail spine is built, to fulfill the same line-haul function; (2) as a local distributor for flexible linkage systems to the line-haul route; and (3) as an effective local service in areas of lower demand where there is little possibility or need for rail service." While such efforts are commendable and should continue to be supported, in most instances the ongoing emphasis on automobile utilization continues to quickly counteract the former. Despite the creation of the Metropolitan Atlanta Rapid Transportation Authority (MARTA), for example, the Atlanta area has continued to evolve into a motor vehicle nightmare where the average commute has reached 35 miles per day, about 50 percent greater than that in the Los Angeles area, and which had 69 smog alert days in 1999 (Kunstler 2003:51). Conversely, MARTA has become a "second-class transportation system for second-class citizens" (Kunstler 2003:68), while commuter highways continue to be widened.

In contrast to Atlanta, various cities, including Singapore, Hong Kong, Zurich, Copenhagen, Freiburg (Germany), Vancouver, Toronto, and Boston have created innovative strategies for reducing motor vehicle utilization and encouraging residents to rely on various forms of public transportation. Copenhagen has adopted various traffic calming strategies, including the creation of extensive pedestrian zones in the city center and extensive 30-kilometer-per-hour zones; alternate forms of transportation, including bike paths; extensive reduction of parking areas; extremely high motor vehicle registration and parking fees; and urban villages around train lines and mixed-land use in centers (Newman and Kenworthy 1999:204–208). Copenhagen is one of the world's most bike-friendly cities.

> One-third of the city goes to work by bike. Like many European cities, Copenhagen had a lot of bicycle use early this century, but unlike other cities, it has not abandoned bicycling as it has modernized and become wealthy. (Newman and Kenworthy 1999:206)

Copenhagen has designated bike right-of-ways and has fostered an ethos of respect for cyclists.

Conclusion

The centrality of motor vehicles is an integral part of the capitalist world system. Fueled by profit seeking, political complicity, and promotion of a consumptive culture, car ownership has grown worldwide and has become a symbol of both freedom and status. While the culture of automobility is most advanced in developed countries, it also is quickly spreading to developing countries. These countries, however, generally lack the necessary resources to pay for the infrastructure that accompanies motor vehicles as well as strict environmental protection laws.

Unfortunately the convenience that the automobile may confer on people at various times is counteracted by congestion, social isolation, high costs, and loss of time. Based upon a detailed historical study of automobility in Melbourne, Davison (2004:xii) poses the following dilemma:

> Mass motorisation was a kind of Faustian bargain. It promised its followers much, but the promises were often negated by the unanticipated consequences of their fulfillment. By attempting to universalize individual mobility the car created congestion. By building freeways to bring communities closer together it often endangered the cohesion of the communities itself. By feeding the desire for speed it caused death and injury. Now, it seems, like Dr. Faustus, we are so deeply in thrall that we cannot escape the bonds of the car, even if we wished to.

Yet, for the sake of the planet, ultimately for the sake of both the ecological body and the human body, it is imperative that we turn back, despite the fact that this will be no easy task. In the long run, the contradictions associated with automobility, including those associated with the environment and health, can only be adequately addressed through the creation of global democratic ecosocialism, a system premised upon meeting human social needs and creating a sustainable environment (Baer, Singer, and Susser 1997). Such a change obviously requires time and the exertion of our agency, both at the individual level and collective levels. In the short run, the challenges to motor vehicle hegemony by academics, grassroots groups, and progressive politicians constitute examples of what Andre Gorz (1973) terms "non-reformist reforms" which challenge existing power relations and pave the way for more revolutionary social changes. The starting point for de-automobilization of society is recognition of the automobile as a killer commodity: a cruel, mindless killer of health and environmental quality.

References

Baer, Hans A., Merrill Singer, and Ida Susser
1997 *Medical Anthropology and the World System: A Critical Perspective.* Westport, CT: Bergin & Garvey.

Barnet, Richard, and John Cavanaugh
1994 Global Dreams: Imperial Corporations and the New World Order. New York: Simon & Schuster.
Batterbury, Simon
2002 Cycling in Copenhagen. Electronic document, www.simonbatterbury.net.
Bottles, Scott L.
1992 Mass Politics and the Adoption of the Automobile in Los Angeles. *In* The Car and the City: The Automobile, the Built Environment, and Daily Urban Life. Martin Wachs and Margaret Crawford, eds. Pp. 199–203. Ann Arbor: University of Michigan Press.
Bradsher, K.
2002 High and Mighty: The World's Most Dangerous Vehicles and How They Got That Way. New York: PublicAffairs Books.
Crawford, J. H.
2000 Carfree Cities. Utrecht: International Books.
Davison, Graeme
2004 Car Wars: How the Car Won Our Hearts and Conquered Our Cities. Sydney: Allen & Unwin.
Diamond, Jared
2005 Collapse: How Societies Choose to Fail or Succeed. New York: Penguin.
Dicken, Peter
2003 Global Shift: Reshaping the Global Economic Map in the 21st Century, 4th ed. New York: Guilford Press.
Domhoff, G. William
1990 The Power Elite and the State: How Policy Is Made in America. New York: de Gruyter.
Doyle, Jack
2000 Taken for a Ride: Detroit's Big Three and the Politics of Pollution. New York: Four Walls Eight Windows.
Flink, James J.
1973 The Car Culture. Cambridge, MA: MIT Press.
1988 The Automobile Age. Cambridge, MA: MIT Press.
Freund, Peter E. S., and George Martin
1993 The Ecology of the Automobile. Montreal: Black Rose.
Gilroy, Paul
2001 Driving While Black. *In* Car Culture. Daniel Miller, ed. Pp. 81–104. Oxford: Berg.
Goddard, Stephen B.
1994 Getting There: The Epic Struggle Between Road and Rail in the American Century. Chicago: University of Chicago Press.

Golten, Robert J., Oliver A. Houck, and Richard Munson, eds.
1977 The End of the Road: A Citizen's Guide to Transportation Problem Solving. Washington, DC: National Wildlife Federation.
Gorz, Andre
1973 Socialism and Revolution. Garden City, NY: Anchor.
Graedel, Thomas E., and Braden R. Allen
1998 Industrial Ecology and the Automobile. Upper Saddle River, NJ: Prentice-Hall.
Hunter, Robert
2003 Thermageddon: Countdown to 2030 . New York: Arcade Publishing.
Kay, Jane Holtz
1997 Asphalt Nation: How the Automobile Took Over America and How We Can Take It Back. New York: Crown.
Kunstler, James Howard
2003 The City in Mind: Notes on the Urban Condition. New York: Free Press.
Leavitt, Helen
1970 Superhighway—Superhoax. New York: Doubleday.
Lee, Martyn
1993 Consumer Culture Reborn: The Cultural Politics of Consumption. London: Routledge.
Lynd, Robert S., and Helen Merrell Lynd
1929 Middletown: A Study in American Culture. London: Constable.
1937 Middletown in Transition: A Study in Cultural Conflict. New York: Harcourt, Brace.
Maxwell, Simon
2001 Negotiations of Car Use in Everyday Life. *In* Car Cultures, Daniel Miller, ed. Pp. 203–222. Oxford: Berg.
Miller, Daniel
1995 Consumption Studies as the Transformation of Anthropology. *In* Acknowledging Consumption: A Review of New Studies. Daniel Miller, ed. Pp. 264–295. London: Routledge.
Mills, C. Wright
1956 The Power Elite. New York: Oxford University Press.
Moorhouse, H. F.
1983 American Automobiles and Workers' Dreams. Sociological Review 31:403–426.
Mumford, Lewis
1963 The Highway and the City. New York: Harcourt, Brace.
Nader, Ralph
1965 Unsafe at Any Speed: The Designed-In Dangers of the American Automobile. New York: Grossman.

Nadis, Steve, and James J. MacKenzie
1993 Car Trouble. Boston: Beacon Press.
Newman, Peter, and Jeffrey Kenworthy
1999 Sustainability and Cities: Overcoming Automobile Dependence. Washington, DC: Island Press.
O'Connell, Jeffrey, and Arthur Myers
1965 Safety Last: An Indictment of the Auto Industry. New York: Random House.
Patterson, Matthew, and Simon Dalby
2006 Empire's Ecological Tyreprints. Environmental Politics 15(1):1–22.
Ponting, Clive
1992 A Green History of the World: The Environment and the Collapse of Great Civilizations. New York: St. Martin's.
Porter, Richard C.
1999 Economics at the Wheel: The Costs of Cars and Drivers. San Diego: Academic Press.
Rajan, Sudhir
1996 The Enigma of Automobility: Democratic Politics and Pollution Control. Pittsburgh: University of Pittsburgh.
Robinson, John
1971 Highways and Our Environment. New York: McGraw-Hill.
Simpson, Barry J.
1994 Urban Public Transport Today. London: E & FN Spon.
Smith, E. O.
2002 When Culture and Biology Collide: Why We Are Stressed, Depressed, and Self-Obsessed. New Brunswick, NJ: Rutgers University Press.
Spellerberg, Ian F.
2002 Ecological Effects of Roads. Enfield, NH: Science Publishers.
Sweezy, Paul
1973 Cars and Cities. Monthly Review 24(11):1–18.
Taebel, Delbert A., and James V. Cornehls
1977 The Political Economy of Urban Transportation. Port Washington, NY: Kennikat Press.
Wolf, Winfried
1996 Car Mania: A Critical History of Transport, trans. Gus Fagan. London: Pluto Press.
Wright, Charles L.
1992 Fast Wheels—Slow Traffic: Urban Transport Choices. Philadelphia: Temple University Press.
Zuckerman, W.
1991 End of the Road: From World Car Crisis to Sustainable Transportation. Vermont: Chelsea Green Publishing.

CHAPTER FOUR

LAY ME DOWN TO SLEEP

SIDS, Suffocation, and the Selling of Risk Reduction

Martine Hackett

In October 2005, the American Academy of Pediatrics (AAP) released a set of recommendations that were intended to reduce the risk of sudden infant death syndrome (SIDS), the major cause of death of infants aged one month to one year in the United States. Many of these recommendations reinforced the first set of SIDS risk-reduction messages that were developed in 1992: Babies should be put to sleep on their backs; they should not be overdressed; and women should not smoke during pregnancy. There was also one recommendation in the list of ten that was new and stood out compared to the others, which centered on behavioral activities. This recommendation advised parents and caregivers of infants to "[a]void commercial devices marketed to reduce the risk of SIDS: Although various devices have been developed to maintain sleep position or to reduce the risk of re-breathing, none have been tested sufficiently to show efficacy or safety" (Task Force on Sudden Infant Death Syndrome 2005). These products, often marketed to new parents as SIDS prevention devices, were declared as potentially harmful by the AAP. But what led to the creation of these products, and how could they create harm when they were intended to prevent it?

Throughout history, the identification of the sudden death of infants was influenced by how Western culture constructed it as a risk and what was determined to be its cause. As hypotheses about its etiology came and went, so did different methods to prevent these deaths from occurring.

Unfortunately, sudden infant death risk-reduction interventions and products have also created harm and even death to the infants they were designed to protect. Also, as research into the cause of SIDS developed in the early 1990s, previously harmless bedding products were discovered to be deadly. Responsibility for removing these products and regulating their risk in the United States falls to the Consumer Product Safety Commission, a government entity with limited enforcement powers against industries that continue to produce and promote these dangerous products. What is a concerned mother or father to do when the products they buy are assumed to be safe and they are not? What role does the state, in the form of the Consumer Product Safety Commission, have in regulating this sense of safety when it comes to potentially deadly products? These issues are brought together under the harrowing search for the cause and cure of the sudden death of infants.

Though the cause of SIDS still remains unknown, one constant epidemiological factor is that these deaths occur during periods of sleep. However, SIDS can only be diagnosed after the death has occurred, and there are few warning signs that it will occur. The diagnosis is arrived by a process of elimination, not of positive identification, and the official definition illustrates this uncertainty: "the sudden death of an infant under one year of age which remains unexplained after a thorough case investigation, including performance of a complete autopsy, examination of the death scene, and review of the clinical history" (Willinger et al. 1991). SIDS is sometimes referred to as a "garbage can diagnosis," since any cause of death that is not identifiable can be considered a SIDS death.

Due to the uncertain nature of the cause of SIDS, there has been a history of attempts to prevent it from occurring that has varied from harmless to life threatening. As research developed to investigate the source of SIDS and the aspects that contribute to it, dangerous products have been identified along two sides of the production cycle: products that already existed in the home—specifically infant bedding—were found to be deadly, and products that were created to reduce the risk of SIDS, from apnea monitors to X-rays, were discovered to be potentially harmful. In this chapter I argue that due to the unknown character of SIDS and the surrounding concern with it as a dangerous public health problem as it relates to the cultural and symbolic notions of risk, two separate but related trends emerged. The first is that products marketed to promote the comfort and well-being of infants, particularly pillows and comforters, have been found to contribute to hundreds of infant deaths, yet they continue to be sold and presented by manufacturers to parents and other consumers as desirable items, sending a mixed and potentially deadly message. The second is that new consumer products that were created to protect infants from SIDS and offer peace of mind to anxious parents were not safe.

Ironically, this increased attention to reducing the risk of SIDS is taking place at a time when the number of reported SIDS deaths has been dropping. Between 1983 and 1992, the average number of SIDS deaths ranged from 5,000 to 6,000. Over the past few years, especially since the late 1990s, the number of SIDS deaths has declined significantly. The National Center for Health Statistics reported that in 2002 in the United States, 2,295 infants under one year of age died from SIDS (Mathews et al. 2004). This significant reduction in SIDS deaths has been attributed to the success of the public health campaign to reduce the risks of SIDS, known as Back to Sleep. The campaign was effectively implemented in Australia, New Zealand, England, and other countries with high SIDS rates before it was established in the United States in 1994, and it primarily recommends that infants sleep on their backs, not on their stomachs, which was the prevailing infant sleep position at the time. Although the overall SIDS rates have declined in all populations throughout the United States, disparities in SIDS rates and prevalence of risk factors remain in certain groups. SIDS rates are highest among African Americans and American Indians and are lowest among Asians and Hispanics (National Institute of Child Health and Human Development 2001). Clearly, any infant death is a tragedy, and regardless of the relative numbers of infants who die each year, there is still no definitive cause or cure, and SIDS remains as a significant public health issue in the United States.

The identification and negotiation of the risk factors for SIDS also can be seen through the lens of contemporary risk theory. Since the early 1980s, there have been three major theoretical frameworks on risk that have been identified as the cultural/symbolic, risk-society, and governmentality approaches (Lupton 1999). Though these perspectives have major differences, they all see risk as a concept that is a central aspect in human existence in Western society, that risk can be managed through intervention, and that risk is not random, but connected to individual responsibility and choice (Lupton 1999). The cultural/symbolic approach refers to the work of cultural anthropologist Mary Douglas (Douglas 1985; Douglas and Wildavsky 1982), and these theories look at how concepts of risk are used to establish boundaries between groups and institutions. Each culture determines which individuals or events are risky and are to be avoided, and risk is also seen as a way to explain why adverse events occur. Within this framework, SIDS is seen as something that happens to those who engage in the known risk factors, and that can be forestalled through the use of risk reduction techniques.

The sociological theory of "risk society" focuses on the larger, structural factors that influence modern society's concerns about risk. The work of Beck (1992) and Giddens (1991) exemplifies this perspective, which critiques the way in which social structures in late modernity (i.e., capitalism, the government, science) produce many of the risks we are concerned with. In this view, risk is not a result of a twist of fate but something that can be identified and controlled by human action. Here the sudden death of an infant is not seen as an outcome of the dangers associated with having babies that may or may not live until their first birthday, but with risks identified by modern scientific research and investigation.

The rationalization of risk and how it is distributed in modern society is also seen in the governmentality perspective, described in the work of Michel Foucault (1984) and others. From this perspective we see the designation of risk as occurring through a series of calculations of "normal" behavior and health outcomes of a society that is monitored and disciplined by institutions created by modern liberal government. Within this system, expert knowledges are constructed to determine who is deviating from the norm and is considered at risk, and these same expert knowledges can be used by individuals to control risks for themselves. Governmental actions and the associated discourse to regulate dangerous products associated with SIDS are a way to manage a population and control its risk. It is this concept of risk that is most useful in examining how the changing notions of SIDS, efforts to reduce its risk, and the regulation of deadly products intersect. From this perspective, the risk of SIDS serves as a symbol of maintaining vigilance over infants through the regulation of their physical environment and the development of products to protect them. It is also a venue for the surveillance of how successful individual parents or caregivers are at keeping the risks of SIDS at bay, with those who fail to protect their child ultimately seen as responsible for not protecting the infants in their care.

Historical Claims about Sudden Infant Death

Most new mothers today cannot avoid hearing the terms *sudden infant death syndrome*, *SIDS*, or *crib death*. SIDS is now a well-known and well-established member of the constellation of parental fears, though this was not always the case. Particularly in the last 50 years, the definition, diagnosis, and acceptance of these silent deaths of seemingly healthy infants have changed from being seen as an act of neglect to an accident to a crime to a medical mystery. In the past, medical professionals were unable to find any evidence of fatal disease or injury and attributed these deaths to undetermined causes, pneumonia, or accidental suffocation. The suddenness of these infant deaths coupled with the uncertainty of its origin caused parents to be occasionally stigmatized by the criminal justice system and members of the community (Bergman 1986). Because the causes of these deaths were unknown, there was the suspicion that it must be due to neglect or abuse by the parents, especially if everything else had been ruled out. A well-known expert in the field warned that intentional suffocation could not be excluded at autopsy with certainty, further blurring the line between abuse and disease (Valdes-Dapena 1967). Criminal investigations were not uncommon in these cases, particularly when poverty and race were factored in. Accusations against parents, whether explicit or unsaid, fueled the desire to find the external cause of these deaths, one that the community could understand and that could help to make sense of this mystery. Parents were also left feeling guilty for what they could have done to prevent these deaths from occurring.

There have been three major hypotheses about the cause of sudden death of infants: overlaying, the thymus hypothesis, and the apnea hypothesis. Along the way, consumer products were developed that paralleled the prevailing theories to help parents feel like there was something that they could do to reduce the risk of this terrible fate from occurring.

Overlaying

History is littered with tales of infants not surviving to their first birthday, of small headstones in cemeteries, of babies not given names until parents were sure that they would make it into childhood. In the literature on SIDS, the Bible is often referenced as evidence of the long history of sudden infant deaths. In the story of King Solomon in the Old Testament (1 Kgs 3:19) two women, most likely prostitutes, were each sleeping in bed with their infants. One woman's child "died in the night because she overlaid it" and the grieving mother replaced her dead infant with the other woman's live one. Each claimed to be the living child's mother, and King Solomon's threat to cut the baby in two settled the dispute. This parable is often used as an example of Solomon's wisdom in resolving the argument, with little attention paid to the reason behind the baby's death. For centuries afterward, the cause of sudden infant deaths was blamed on the unfortunate (but not always illegal) act of overlaying, or rolling over on a sleeping baby who shared the bed, and smothering it. This problem prompted the creation of a preventative device in Florence in the 17th century to protect infants. An *arcutio* was an arched cover made of wood and iron that was placed over babies during sleep to protect them from their mothers, but still allowed them to be nursed during the night (Limerick 1992).

By the end of the 19th century, infants who died during sleep were scientifically associated with the ills of urban poverty. The first systematic epidemiological study of sudden death in infants in the industrial city of Dundee, Scotland, was conducted by the local police-surgeon in 1892 (Guntheroth 1995). The study found that babies tended to die at night, during the winter and before the age of three months, and that the children from poor families were more likely to die. The study contended that overlaying was the principal cause due to the ignorance, carelessness, and drunkenness of the mothers, who lived in overcrowded conditions. The police-surgeon also suggested that the illegitimacy and life insurance on the infants should be taken into consideration (Bergman 1986). This study concluded with the recommendation that mothers be prosecuted for negligence. Overall, the diagnosis of overlaying as the cause of the sudden deaths of infants at this time was seen as an unavoidable part of life, especially for the poor.

Thymus Hypothesis

Mining the history of the medical explanations for the sudden death of infants inevitably reflects the prevailing medical approaches during the time in which they were discovered (Starr 1986). The early 19th century saw the rise of pathological anatomy as a means to make sense of disease and to impose a framework in which to understand it. In 1842, an article was published in the *American Journal of Medical Science* on the abnormally large thymus gland in infants as a possible cause of sudden infant deaths (Guntheroth 1995). This hypothesis, labeled status thymicolymphaticus, became the official cause of death until the early part of the 20th century. The cause of death was said to be due to an enlarged thymus—a gland in the neck—which obstructed airways for breathing. In the 1930s and 1940s the preventative measure for concerned parents made use of the most up-to-date technology of the time, which was to irradiate and shrink the thymus in children via X-ray. It took almost 100 years to prove to doctors that "normal-size" glands were actually based on autopsy specimens of infants who had died of malnutrition and who therefore had shrunken thymus glands. It did not take that long to discover that this cure caused thyroid cancer as some of those children got older (Golding, Limerick, and Macfarlane 1985).

The eventual discounting of the thymus hypothesis and the dismissal of deaths due to overlaying as a province of the poor left room for a new negotiation of the diagnosis of the sudden death of infants by the mid-1940s. The belief that was held for centuries, as previously described, was that infants who were found dead in their beds suffered from accidental suffocation, even though bed sharing was no longer a common practice in the United States. Indeed, by the middle of the 20th century, more babies, particularly those of the middle and upper classes, had rooms of their own. This social shift from bed sharing to baby's own bed led to a new distinction in the accidental suffocation diagnosis. No longer were they said to have been overlaid by their mothers who they shared a bed with, but infants instead were said to have suffocated on the sheets and blankets in their cribs (Guntheroth 1995). Even the name that these deaths were given at this time—crib death—reflects the shift in the location of where infants were put to sleep. Though the crib-death diagnosis also left the impression that the parents were neglectful, physicians generally considered these deaths to be accidents and did not follow up with an autopsy to determine the cause of death. However, the criminal justice system got involved with many cases, and the police would interrogate the parents as to the specifics of the baby's death, occasionally with arrests being made for infanticide (Bergman 1986). During this period, a crib death in the family was not only an individual tragedy, but one that carried with it the taint of neglect and crime.

This change in the location of where infants sleep, from sharing an adult bed to sleeping in their own bed in a separate room, is relatively recent in terms of its evolution and one that is particular to Western culture. Some have argued this shift has contributed to higher SIDS rates in countries where parent-infant cosleeping is not the norm. In particular, McKenna, a medical anthropologist who has extensively studied infant sleep under laboratory conditions (1986; McKenna 1996) argues that the regulation of breathing and arousal patterns during sleep between mothers and newborns who share a bed is protective against SIDS for vulnerable infants. However, this hypothesis and its encouragement of infant bed sharing has met with resistance as a major hypothesis of the cause of SIDS, due in part to the norms and values associated with independent sleeping for infants in Western cultures (Anders and Taylor 1994).

The Apnea "Breakthrough"

By January 1974, legislation was passed to fund SIDS research on a national level, and the Sudden Infant Death Syndrome Act of 1974 was passed by the U.S. Congress. The law assigned responsibility to the National Institute of Child Health and Human Development (NICHD) to conduct SIDS research and the Maternal and Child Health Bureau was delegated the information and counseling component of the legislation. There would be a $6-million, three-year program that would develop public information and professional educational material related to sudden infant death syndrome and $12 million for direct federal support for research into the cause of these deaths (New York Times 1974). This phase of SIDS research would occur as a result of this federal funding and would represent its establishment as a public health issue, not (solely) a personal tragedy.

With the availability of federal funding for research into the physiological causes of SIDS, new hypotheses were promoted by scientists with research agendas. One hypothesis broke through in the early 1970s in a promising direction, particularly because it offered the possibility of identifying vulnerable infants and the possibility of preventing their deaths. The hypothesis was that SIDS was related to a pause in breathing during sleep, known as apnea. The study, titled "Prolonged Apnea and the Sudden Infant Death Syndrome: Clinical and Laboratory Observations," was published in 1972 in *Pediatrics* by Alfred Steinschneider. The article described five patients with abnormally prolonged periods of apnea, two of whom were siblings who eventually died of SIDS, and the paper provided support for the hypothesis that prolonged apnea and SIDS are linked and was possibly hereditary. The apnea study was considered a significant scientific step, a breakthrough in SIDS research because of Steinschneider's hypothesis that a developmental abnormality, not a mysterious disease, was the cause of SIDS (Hufbauer 1986). It also left open the possibility for further clinical and physiological investigation.

The apnea hypothesis stated that infants who experienced prolonged apnea spells were at risk for SIDS, and that their deaths could be prevented if they were wired to apnea monitors. During the mid-to-late 1970s, the NICHD supported the apnea hypothesis with generous research funding for efforts to locate the pathological abnormalities in SIDS victims, to find the psychological indicators for identifying high-risk infants, and to develop home monitors to warn parents of dangerous apnea episodes (Hufbauer 1986). Apnea monitors were prescribed for at-risk infants and used every time they slept, and an alarm would sound whenever they stopped breathing, signaling a "near miss" which was thought to precede death by SIDS.

By 1977, Dr. Steinschneider received a federal grant for $2.4 million to monitor over 4,000 infants born in the University Hospital in Maryland. His study looked to develop a profile of the typical SIDS victim, by monitoring them in the hospital and at home for their feeding habits, breathing and heart rates, and crying patterns. The apnea hypothesis also was seen as a technological breakthrough to prevent SIDS from occurring. Ten percent of the study participants were sent home with an apnea monitor for parents to observe and record their infants' breathing during sleep. The alarm would sound, warning parents if the monitor determines that the infant has not taken a breath for a period of time, and parents were taught mouth-to-mouth resuscitation to revive their infants if needed. The reality of what this meant for a parent is highlighted in a statement by a nurse at another hospital that was conducting a similar study: "A parent can be no more that 10 seconds away from the baby 24 hours a day when it is on the monitor. They can't shower, go to the mailbox, put out the garbage or care for other children unless someone else is around" (Charles 1981). All of this effort was determined to be necessary. According to Steinschneider, "if we're really crazy lucky, at the end of five or ten years we may know if we're headed in the right direction" (Colen 1977). This uncertainty did not stifle the market's exploitation of the apnea hypothesis. During this period, the electronic-baby-monitoring industry that manufactured and sold apnea baby monitors for $2,500 each to hospitals and to parents was launched. By 1983, the infant monitor market reached $40 million in sales and was considered to be a rapidly growing industry that was "good for stockholders" (New York Times 1983).

Though apnea research was well supported by the federal government and was seen as a positive direction for the future of SIDS prevention, there were many issues revealed that shook the foundations of the scientific SIDS industry. In their book, *The Death of Innocents: A True Story of Murder, Medicine and High Stake Science*, published in 1997, husband and wife authors Richard Firstman and Jamie Talan uncover the unconventional methods that Steinschneider used to come to his conclusions and chronicled the tragic misuse of the SIDS diagnosis. In his 1972 study, Steinschneider based his findings on his documentation of five patients with repeated apnea incidents, two of which were siblings who eventually died of SIDS. These were the children of Waneta Hoyt, who also had three other children who died suddenly without explanation. At the time, all of these deaths were seen as suspicious, but Steinschneider's findings legitimated them, and they were retrospectively said to have probably died of SIDS. It was not until 1995, almost 25 years later, Firstman and Talan explain, that Hoyt was convicted of murdering all of her children, including the siblings who were the basis of Steinschneider's landmark study. The authors also reveal that Steinschneider ignored warnings from nurses that Hoyt may have been responsible for the deaths of her infants and from other researchers who questioned his data. Though millions of dollars went to the study of the apnea hypothesis, subsequent studies failed to support these findings. The federal government also concluded there was no proof that apnea monitors could prevent SIDS (Keens and Ward 1993). The desire for a biomedical explanation for SIDS superseded the science, and left researchers and parents open to receive the next big thing.

Since the discovery of the popular apnea hypothesis, millions of dollars were spent on research and thousands of babies were fitted to apnea monitors, but there was no change in the rate of SIDS deaths in the United States. According to the physician who was responsible for coming up with the term *sudden infant death syndrome*, Bruce Beckwith, "SIDS researchers are in shock from the loss of their favorite pet hypothesis. The situation is verging on the chaotic. We've had lots of ideas but few hard facts" (Blakesbee 1989). The quest for next the SIDS solution continued.

By the late 1980s, a turning point in the approach to SIDS risk reduction arrived. Studies from the Netherlands, Australia, England, and other countries implicated the stomach sleeping position as being associated with a greater risk of SIDS (DeJonge et al. 1989; McGlashan 1989; Fleming et al. 1990, Guntheroth 1995). As a result of these studies, communication campaigns that promoted back sleeping and SIDS risk reduction were quickly carried out in the United Kingdom, Holland, New Zealand, and five other countries. These campaigns utilized national media coverage as well as doctors and health service providers and were successful in significantly reducing the number of SIDS deaths (Mitchell et al. 1991, Engelberts et al. 1991; Wigfield et al. 1992, Guntheroth 1995).

After all of the biomedical research into the causes of sudden infant deaths, the millions of dollars of funding, and the abject failure of the apnea monitors, could something as simple and untechnical as infant sleep position—a behavior change which cost nothing—solve the mystery of SIDS? American SIDS researchers were initially skeptical of the validity and applicability of a health promotion for back sleeping to reduce the risk of SIDS in the United States. At the time, scientific studies of sleep positions in the United States didn't show any adverse effect on breathing in the prone position or any advantage to sleeping in the supine (back) position (Orr et al. 1985; Peirano et al. 1986). Critics pointed out that it was difficult to make a direct correlation between a change in sleep position and a decrease in SIDS rates in the countries that promoted back sleeping. They also questioned the applicability of studies conducted in these smaller, less ethnically and economically diverse countries that had some form of national health insurance, unlike in the United States.

In addition, the decision to go with recommending back sleep confronted conventional child-care wisdom in the United States, where the most common sleep position for infants was prone (on their stomachs). For decades, pediatricians had advised parents to avoid putting their children to sleep on their backs for fear that their children might choke on their vomit. It was also the experience of many parents that babies slept better on their stomachs. Indeed, Dr. Benjamin Spock in his best-selling book, *Baby and Child Care*, strongly advocated this sleep position as the safest for infants (Spock 1985).

Despite these concerns, the advisory group of the AAP felt that they could not ignore the dramatic reduction in SIDS deaths in the countries that promoted back sleeping. In 1992 the AAP issued a statement recommending that infants, when being put down for sleep, be positioned on their back. By 1994, the national Back to Sleep campaign was launched, which alerted parents, pediatricians, and caregivers across the country that babies should be put on their backs to sleep.

Today, SIDS is recognized as a physiological entity that is explained by the "triple risk model," where a vulnerable infant (perhaps born with underlying defects in the parts of the brain that control breathing, heartbeat, and arousal) is placed in an environment with exogenous stressors (soft bedding, prone sleep position, secondhand smoke) during a critical development period (about age two to four months) where rapid changes in sleep and wake patterns, breathing, and heart rate occur (Filiano and Kinney 1994). Though the cause of SIDS was still not determined, this development in SIDS research proved to be the most promising by far, and soon other research into an infant's sleep environment continued.

SIDS, Suffocation, and Lethal Products

Modern consumer culture prepares parents before the birth of a child by presenting lists of the most essential, best, and safest items every infant needs upon entering the world. Baby showers are rites of passage for new mothers where they are "showered" with gifts, often from registered lists from chain stores that specialize in products for a baby's every need. In exchange, consumers accept an unspoken and increasingly uneasy trust between the product manufacturers and the government that the products that they are bringing into their home are safe and that there is a larger system in place to ensure this security.

However, in 1991, two medical researchers, James Kemp and Bradley Thach, published findings in the *New England Journal of Medicine* from their research about SIDS, sleep position, and the infant's sleep environment that concluded that at least 37 infant deaths that had been attributed to SIDS in autopsy reports were actually most likely due to suffocation by the cushions they slept on (Kemp and Thach 1991). These infant cushions were soft and resembled beanbags—cotton covering loosely filled with plastic foam beads—and when infants were placed on them in the prone position, their cushions conformed to their heads, and their faces were buried in the cushions, causing them to rebreathe lethal amounts of carbon monoxide and suffocate. Though these findings were significant in pointing out the harm that these cushions could cause, they also reflected the constantly conflicting nature of SIDS diagnosis. Dr. Kemp is quoted as saying, "Our findings challenge the basic assumptions used to distinguish SIDS from accidental suffocation and emphasize the need for new safety regulations for [all] infant bedding" (Raloff 1991:407). The risk of SIDS, which had gone through decades of building and dismissing theories, had a new wrinkle. Though the cause of SIDS was still unknown, here was a lethal product, a piece of bedding, which caused death to infants. These deaths looked like SIDS but were really due to suffocation. Now parents' fear of infant death shifted from an unknown entity to a product designed to provide comfort. The term *crib death* now took on another ominous meaning.

The possibility that these cushions could be a cause of death raises the issue of how much security parent's can feel about the products that their infants come in contact with. The names of the cushions were soothing: Mother's Helper, Comfort Tote, Cozy Baby, and Cushie Comfort, and they were initially created by a NICU (Neonatal Intensive Care Unit) nurse to provide support for premature infants (Squires 1990). Though these products were commercially available, they were not necessarily safe, and could be used in ways that made them deadly.

Though the scientific study by Kemp and Thach in 1991 provided evidence that the cushions were responsible for infant deaths, there were earlier anecdotal reports of their fatal risks. In 1990, the Consumer Products Safety Commission (CPSC) began investigating the cushions when Charles Odom, an assistant medical examiner in Dallas, reported that three babies died while sleeping face down on the pillows (Squires 1990). The CPSC warned medical examiners and coroners nationwide, but the difficulty was that autopsies cannot distinguish between infants who die of suffocation and those who die of SIDS. However, by late 1990, the CPSC issued a press release that stated, "Because of recent infant deaths, the U.S. Consumer Product Safety Commission today issued an urgent warning not to place infants, especially those under six months of age, to sleep on small pillows or cushions filled with plastic foam (polystyrene) beads because of a suffocation risk" (CPSC 1990). In the CPSC press release it was observed that "it is unusual for so many deaths associated with a relatively new product to occur over such a short period." The manufacturers of the cushions were asked to voluntarily remove the products from stores, but what about the 950,000 cushions that had already been purchased by the time the statement was released? Warnings were issued to consumers that the products should not be used any longer, which raises issues about who was made aware of this message, for how long, and what would keep these types of products from being produced in the future. The questions reflect the limited abilities the CSPC has over the regulation of potentially deadly products.

The Consumer Product Safety Commission was established in 1972 as part of the Consumer Product Safety Act to "assist consumers in evaluating the comparative safety of consumer products; to develop uniform safety standards for consumer products and to minimize conflicting state and local regulations; and to promote research and investigation into the causes and prevention of product related death, illnesses, and injuries" (CPSC 2006). The CPSC is an independent regulatory agency that has the authority to issue and enforce mandatory standards, ban products if no standard could protect the public, order recalls of unsafe products, and institute labeling requirements in order to protect consumers from risk of injury. The way that the agency makes the public aware of these dangerous products is by informing and educating consumers through the media, by contacting state and local governments, by working with private organizations, and by responding to consumer inquiries (CPSC 2006). Though some products for infants and children have mandatory federal standards—car seats, cribs, pacifiers, and sleepwear, most products that infants come in contact with are unregulated. For all of these other products, a recall of the product issued by CPSC is the only means of regulation, which occurs after there have been reports of injuries and even deaths.

The concept of recalling or alerting the public to dangerous products for children would appear to follow a certain logic. There are items that, at first glance, seem to be dangerous for children. Products like battery-powered scooters, doorway baby jumpers, walkers, paintball markers, and even sweatshirts with drawstrings. Indeed, all of these products have been cited as having the potential to cause harm by the CSPC. But a look at the nonprofit organization International SAFE KIDS website from just June 2005 to March 2006 shows a listing of over ten products that are meant to *protect* young children that have been recalled by the CSPC due to safety concerns. These include two different brands of child safety seats which may cause harm in a crash due to flaws in their design, a bicycle helmet that poses a risk of head injury, sunglasses that contain high levels of lead, two brands of multivitamins that do not have a childproof cap and "could cause serious injury or death," tub seats made by a manufacturer called Safety First that "can break and tip over, causing the child to fall in water," inflatable arm bands for the pool that can "tear, deflate and pose a drowning hazard," and even organic baby food that was recalled because glass was found inside the jars (SafeKids USA 2006). The monitoring of the safety of these items relies on voluntary standards created and enforced by manufacturers and trade groups. This has led to a tacit acceptance of an agreement between the creators of the products and the consumers that states something like, "if you don't see a problem, then it does not exist. . . . Until there is a recall."

The recall process has been criticized on several levels as a method of controlling the safety of products for infants and children, particularly because of the lengths that the infant product industry goes to conceal their safety records (Felcher 2001). First, the process is a reactive one. Each year, there are over 10,000 complaints about hazardous products that are investigated by a limited staff, and juvenile products other than toys send an estimated 65,400 young children to emergency rooms each year; some 87 die (Spake 2001). According to testimony presented in 2006 to Congress by Donald Mays, senior director of the Product Safety and Consumer Sciences of Consumer Union (the creators of *Consumer Reports* magazine), in the 2005 fiscal year, the CPSC administered 397 recalls of unsafe products that were already in stores (Mays 2006). When the CSPC initiates the recall of an item, it generally persuades the manufacturer to notify retailers that the product can no longer be sold (Felcher 2001). The agency relies on a company's willingness to report safety problems. There is also concern that the CPSC is underfunded and understaffed, and indeed the staffing level of the CPSC has been steadily dwindling. The budget for fiscal 2007 culminates a two-year reduction of full-time positions from 471 to 420—a total loss of 51 employees, down from over 800 originally (Mays 2006).

A second issue involves how recalls are announced. Usually recalls are done in the form of a press release, issued jointly by the CSPC and the product's manufacturer. These press releases are often negotiated with the manufacturers of the products, the manufacturers' lawyers, product engineers, and public-relations professionals as to the description of why the product has been recalled and what people who own it should do (Felcher 2000). The result of this collaboration is that the releases are written in language that can seem rather unexciting, which minimizes the newsworthiness and ability to get covered as a news story. Also, when a press release does happen (the CPSC also has a website and sends out e-mails to those who sign up for them), it is usually not enough for all parents who purchased the items to get the information. When issues of ethnicity and class are factored into who receives messages from the CPSC and who does not, there are sure to be some differences in who hears about a recall before buying the item. Indeed, people who get the products secondhand may not know because there is no connection between the recall and the product when it is resold or passed down and even parents who bought the recalled product new can miss the message (Spake 2001). A 1999 CPSC survey of thrift stores showed that at least one dangerous children's product was on sale in 69 percent of them (CPSC 1999).

The CPSC also collaborates on original research into the potential danger of products being sold to consumers. This was the case with a study that was based on the research that found that infants suffocated to death on soft cushions and that these deaths were often diagnosed as SIDS. A 1998 study conducted by the CPSC found that about 30 percent of the 206 infants in the study who died of SIDS were found with their noses and mouths covered by soft bedding (Scheers, Dayton, and Kemp 1998). The study indicated that this bedding could be responsible for as many as 900 infant deaths a year, deaths that were attributed to SIDS but were in fact due to suffocation on the bedding. Most of those infants had been placed on their stomachs to sleep and were found lying on top of soft bedding such as pillows, comforters, and sheepskins. It was the first epidemiologic evidence that directly linked the rebreathing of carbon dioxide trapped in bedding to infants found dead in the prone sleep position. These findings were another reason to recommend that infants be put to sleep on their backs, since these specific bedding items were associated with an increased risk for death for infants who slept in the prone position (Scheers, Dayton, and Kemp 1998). This study led the CPSC to release a warning in 1994 against having any soft bedding in an infant's crib at all. This recommendation was soon supported by SIDS organizations and the government and was added as an important means of risk reduction for sudden infant death syndrome.

The warnings advised that the only thing in the infant's crib, besides the infant, should be a fitted sheet around the mattress. Only a light blanket, if one was to be used at all, was suggested, and it should be tightly tucked in all around the mattress. Considering the danger of these products and the recommendations not to use them for their intended purpose as bedding, the clearest reaction would be to recall the items that were already in stores and to prevent them from being sold and marketed as products for infants. Though the warning issued to the public that the use of pillows, blankets, and comforters was dangerous for infants and increased the risk of death, shoppers looking for cribs and bedding would have observed a completely different message. In the stores and in catalogs, displays of the latest patterns of bedding sets show matching pillows, comforters, and bumpers luxuriously filling the cribs. Many parents, unaware of the risk, would not know that these products that promised to comfort their babies could be the cause of their death. The ominous nature of this soft bedding again provided a stark contradiction for parents between soothing intent and potentially deadly consequences. Indeed, the Juvenile Products Manufacturers Association, the trade group responsible for the infant bedding market, initially did not react to the CPSC's warnings about the risk of infant death related to their products. Since the CPSC has no regulatory power over the creators of the products, they were powerless to stop the items from being sold or even displayed in a way that encouraged the risky practices. Also, bedding products are a multimillion-dollar industry, making it almost impossible to negotiate a voluntary regulation or removal.

Without the cooperation of the product's manufacturers, the CSPC had limited options as to what actions it could take. In 2000, the CPSC took a different tack and approached the retail chains that sold the bedding products and got 75 percent of the soft-bedding market to join a "safety initiative" that was not a recall of the potentially dangerous products, but a change in how bedding was displayed in cribs from the overstuffed look to one that matched the more austere style recommended by public health officials (Brown 2000). By 2002, the Juvenile Products Manufacturers Association joined the CPSC and advocacy organizations and launched an information campaign called Sweet Dreams . . . Safe Sleep for Babies, that provided safety tips to parents and caregivers to create a "safe sleep environment" for babies. The tip about bedding products is listed after admonishments to not share an adult bed with an infant (buy a crib instead), to always put babies to sleep on their backs to reduce the risk of SIDS, and then in order "to reduce the risk of suffocation, remove all soft bedding, such as pillows, thick quilts, and comforters before placing your baby to sleep" (CPSC 2002). This compromise allows the soft bedding manufacturers to still sell their products and appear concerned for the safety of infants by warning parents about the potential harm in using their products. Buyers are left with the burden of securing the safety of infant bedding that once purchased, cannot actually be used without putting babies at risk for SIDS. This arrangement goes beyond traditional warnings of "buyers beware" to buying products that are in effect useless.

The recommendation to reduce the risk of SIDS by limiting infant bedding reflects a particular set of middle-class norms and values and poses a dilemma to those in different circumstances. Providing a warm and safe environment for an infant, especially during sleep, is a common desire in most societies around the world. How this is done varies, and in the United States, this type of protection is assumed to come from central heating systems in private homes or apartments. However, those with limited incomes who may have trouble maintaining their home at a warm temperature due to the cost may wind up covering their infants with several blankets instead. In this scenario, does the risk of SIDS outweigh the risk of the baby sleeping in the cold? Are concerns about SIDS perhaps a luxury of relatively affluent people in developed societies whereas poor people in developed and developing societies have to worry more about whether their infants have access to warmth, food, clean water, sanitary living conditions, shelter, and other more basic concerns? Certainly a hierarchy of needs exists in most situations that have to do with providing for an infant. Nevertheless, recommendations to reduce the risk of SIDS make no mention of this, and can add anxiety to an already stressful situation among parents who fall outside of the campaign's intended audience.

The Sweet Dreams campaign also caused protest from parenting advocates and others who promote sharing a bed with infants to facilitate breastfeeding and bonding. These groups were skeptical of the relationship between the CSPC and the Juvenile Products Manufacturers Association, an association that benefits from parents buying more cribs and the accessories to go with them. There was also mistrust based on a previous announcement by the CSPC in 1999 that categorically stated that cosleeping was dangerous and the adult bed was unsafe for infants, a study that was later criticized for the data used and the conclusions that were drawn (Bernstein 2002).

With a history of reacting to the safety of products that caused infant deaths only *after* they occurred, in March 2000 the CPSC became proactive. It was then that the agency went after manufacturers that made products that claimed to prevent SIDS. These products were advertised mainly on the Internet and included the BabeSafe mattress cover that claimed that it was "proven to be 100% effective in preventing SIDS" and even that "your baby can sleep on his/her tummy" (thediaperlady.com 2006). Other products included "breathable" mesh-topped mattresses and mattress covers—one even came with an air pump—that promoted their safety and ability to remove the risk to infants who used them. Signifying a change in direction with how the safety of infant products were monitored, the CPSC said that despite the claims, it was not aware of any evidence that babies can safely be placed to sleep on their stomachs on these products, or that using the products would reduce the risk of SIDS. Though there have been no deaths associated with these products, the CPSC succeeded in stopping the firms that manufactured and distributed these products, as well as request that stores stop selling them (CPSC 2000). The difference between the actions to regulate the safety of these products as compared to soft bedding comes down to issues of power. The manufacturers of the products targeted by the CPSC's action were small companies that were not aligned with a trade organization with the reach and impact of the Juvenile Products Manufacturers Association and were unable to lobby for a compromise. Also, the claims made by the products that babies were safe from harm when placed on their stomachs directly contradicted the prevailing public health advice about infant sleep position and reducing the risk of SIDS. These claims led the Food and Drug Administration to also investigate these products (CPSC 2000).

Since SIDS is still an entity with an unknown cause or causes and it still holds anxiety and uncertainty for parents and caregivers of infants, there continue to be products that are developed and sold that claim to prevent SIDS, like infant sleep positioners, which are meant to keep infants on their backs in a crib when asleep, and one-piece wearable blankets that zip around an infant so that additional bedding is not needed. Also, even though it was discounted as a possible cause of SIDS, there are now reconfigured apnea monitors on the market, which are designed to sound an alarm if they detect a stop in an infant's breathing. However, these monitors have been known to cause more anxiety than comfort to new parents as they tend to go off frequently. The AAP 2005 recommendation not to purchase these products has yet to have an effect, and they are still available for sale at your local baby superstore.

Conclusion

Parents want to protect their infants from risk of SIDS, but products that they buy to do this can kill or injure the infants and protections that exist can't stop this from happening, especially as new risks are being discovered. The burden of responsibility for removing potentially deadly products should not rest on the parents of infants, but should be shared by the manufacturers and retailers. There is no regulation that calls for testing products aimed at children, and the danger is often not known until there has been an injury or a death. Retailers sell these products without guarantees to consumers that they are safe, and there is no accountability on their part if the products are found to be hazardous. The CPSC is limited in its ability to be effective in its charge to protect consumers from dangerous products, and is often left playing a deadly game of catch up to warn the public about them.

The changing nature of what is the cause and cure for sudden infant death syndrome throws a curve into an already precarious system. As new scientific findings indicate potential risks to infants, parents are left questioning what is safe and whom they can trust. Issues of ideology, ethnicity, and class also influence how this biomedical advice is interpreted among different groups, a consideration not usually accounted for in these recommendations. Risks already lurk just about everywhere for a new parent. Having to worry about the safety of the products that are meant to protect, comfort, and soothe babies is enough to lose much more than sleep over.

References

Anders, Thomas F., and Teresa Taylor
1994 Babies and Their Sleep Environment. Children's Environments 11(2):66–84.
Beck, Ulrich
1992 Risk Society: Towards a New Modernity. London: Sage.
Bergman, Abraham
1986 The "Discovery" of Sudden Infant Death Syndrome: Lessons in the Practice of Political Medicine. New York: Praeger.
Bernstein, Margaret
2002 Where Is Baby Safe? Family Bed Advocates Say Campaign Is Slanted Toward Crib Makers. Cleveland Plain Dealer, September 16: C1.
Blakesbee, Sandra
1989 Crib Death: Suspicion Turns to the Brain. New York Times, February 14: C1.
Brown, Ann
2000 Speech presented at SIDS Alliance Conference. Salt Lake City, April 8.
Charles, Eleanor
1981 Drop Indicated in Crib-Death Rate. New York Times, July 26: section 11:7.
Cohen, B.
1977 Md. School Gets $2 Million to Seek Cause of Crib Death. Washington Post, October 14: C1.
CPSC (Consumer Product Safety Commission)
1990 CPSC Issues Urgent Warning about a Suffocation Risk. Press release # 90-042. Washington, DC: Consumer Product Safety Commission.
1999 CPSC Finds Hazardous Products Being Sold in Thrift Stores. Press release # 00-018. Washington, DC: Consumer Product Safety Commission.
2000 CPSC Warns Against Baby Mattresses, Pads That Make Unfounded Claims about Reducing SIDS. Press release # 00-079. Washington, DC: Consumer Product Safety Commission.
2002 Sweet Dreams . . . Safe Sleep for Babies. CPSC, Industry and Safety Groups Mark Baby Safety Month with Safe Sleep. Press release # 02-245. Washington, DC: Consumer Product Safety Commission.

2006 Who Are We—What We Do for You. Electronic document, www.cpsc.gov/about/who.html, accessed March 18.

De Jonge, G., A. Engelberts, A. Koomen-Liefting, and P. Kostense
1989 Cot Death and Prone Sleeping Position in the Netherlands. British Medical Journal 298:722.

Douglas, Mary
1985 Risk Acceptability According to the Social Sciences. New York: Russell Sage Foundation.

Douglas, Mary, and A. Wildavsky
1982 Risk and Culture: An Essay on the Selection of Technical and Environmental Dangers. Berkeley: University of California Press.

Engelberts, A., G. de Jonge, and P. Kostense
1991 An Analysis of Trends in the Incidence of Sudden Infant Death in the Netherlands 1969–89. Journal of Pediatric Child Health 27:329–333.

Felcher, E. Marla
2000 Children's Products and Risk. Atlantic Monthly:36–42.
2001 It's No Accident: How Corporations Sell Dangerous Baby Products. Monroe, ME: Common Courage Press.

Filiano, J., and H. Kinney
1994 A Perspective on Neuropathologic Findings in Victims of the Sudden Infant Death Syndrome: The Triple-Risk Model. Biological Neonate 65(3–4):194–197.

Firstman, R., and J. Talan
1997 The Death of Innocents: A True Story of Murder, Medicine and High-Stakes Science. New York: Bantam.

Fleming P., R. Gilber, Y. Azaz, P. Berry, P. Rudd, A. Stewart, and H. Hall
1990 Interaction between Bedding and Sleeping Position in the SIDS: A Population-Based Case-Control Study. British Medical Journal 301:85–89.

Foucault, Michel
1984 The Politics of Health in the Eighteenth Century. *In* The Foucault Reader. P. Rainbow, ed. New York: Pantheon Books.

Giddens, Anthony
1991 Modernity and Self-Identity: Self and Society in the Late Modern Age. Cambridge: Polity Press.

Golding, J., Sylvia Limerick, and Aidan Macfarlane
1985 Sudden Infant Death: Patterns, Puzzles and Problems. Seattle: University of Washington Press.

Guntheroth, Warren G.
1995 Crib Death: The Sudden Infant Death Syndrome, 3rd ed. Armonk, NY: Futura.

Hufbauer, Karl
1986 Federal Funding and Sudden Infant Death Research, 1945–1980. Theme issue, "Funding and Knowledge Growth." Social Studies of Science 16(1):61–78.

Keens, T., and S. Ward
1993 Apnea Spells, Sudden Death, and the Role of the Apnea Monitor. Pediatric Clinician North America 40:897–911.

Kemp J., and Bradley Thach
1991 Sudden Death in Infants Sleeping on Polystyrene-Filled Cushions. New England Journal of Medicine 324(26):1858–1864.

Limerick, Sylvia
1992 Sudden Infant Death in Historical Perspective. Journal of Clinical Pathology 3(6):3–6.

Lupton, Deborah
1999 Risk. London: Routledge.

Mathews, T., F. Menacker, and M. MacDorman
2004 Infant Mortality Statistics from the 2002 Period Linked Birth/Infant Death Data Set. National Vital Statistics Reports 53(10). Hyattsville, MD: National Center for Health Statistics.

Mays, Donald L.
2006 Defective Products: Will Criminal Penalties Ensure Corporate Accountability? Testimony presented before the Senate Judiciary Committee. Washington, DC, March 10.

McGlashan, N.
1989 Sudden Infant Deaths in Tasmania, 1980–1986, a Seven Year Prospective Study. Social Science Medicine 29:1015–1026.

McKenna, J.
1986 An Anthropological Perspective on the Sudden Infant Death Syndrome (SIDS): The Role of Parental Breathing Cues and Speech Breathing Adaptations. Medical Anthropology (special issue) 10(1):9–53.
1996 Sudden Infant Death Syndrome in Cross-Cultural Perspective: Is Infant-Parent Cosleeping Protective? Annual Review of Anthropology 25:201–216.

Mitchell E. A., R. Scragg, A. W. Stewart, D. M. O. Bencroft, and B. J. Taylor
1991 Results from the First Year of the New Zealand Cot Death Study. New Zealand Medical Journal 104:71–76.

National Institute of Child Health and Human Development
2001 From Cells to Selves. Targeting Sudden Infant Death Syndrome (SIDS): A Strategic Plan. Bethesda, MD: National Institute of Child Health and Human Development.

New York Times
1974 House on Jan. 21 Approves 4 Health Bills Authorizing Total of $533.2 Million. New York Times, January 22: A11.
1983 Healthdyne Gains with Crib Monitor. New York Times, March 5: section 1:31.

Orr, W. C., M. L. Stahl, J. Duke, M. A. McCaffree, P. Toubas, C. Mattice, and H. F. Drous
1985 Effect of Sleep State and Position on the Incidence of Obstructive and Central Apnea in Infants. Pediatrics 75:832–835.

Peirano, P., S. Guidasci, and N. Monod
1986 Effect of Sleep Position on Transcutaneous Oxygen Tension in SIDS Siblings. Early Human Development 13:303–312.

Raloff, Janet
1991 Do Some SIDS Victims Actually Suffocate? Science News 139(26):405–408.

SafeKids USA
2006 Product Recalls. Electronic document, www.usa.safekids.org, accessed June 10, 2006.

Scheers, N., C. Dayton, and J. Kemp
1998 Sudden Infant Death with External Airways Covered. Archives of Pediatric and Adolescent Medicine 152:540–547.

Spake, Amanda
2001 Kids' Safety Is on the Line as Recalled Products Stay in Use. U.S. News & World Report, August 13: 48–50.

Spock, Benjamin
1985 Baby and Child Care. New York: Pocket Books.

Squires, Sally
1990 Warning on Baby Pillows; Manufacturers Withdraw Cushions After Deaths. Washington Post, April 24: Z7.

Starr, Paul
1986 The Social Transformation of American Medicine. New York: Basic Books.

Steinschneider, Alfred
1972 Prolonged Apnea and the Sudden Infant Death Syndrome: Clinical and Laboratory Observations. Pediatrics 50(4):646–654.

Task Force on Sudden Infant Death Syndrome
2005 The Changing Concept of Sudden Infant Death Syndrome: Diagnostic Coding Shifts, Controversies Regarding the Sleeping Environment, and New Variables to Consider in Reducing Risk. Pediatrics 116(5):1245–1255.

thediaperlady.com
2006 BabeSafe Mattress Covers. Electronic document, www.thediaperlady.com/BabeSafe.htm, accessed April 12.

Valdes-Dapena, Marie
1967 Sudden and Unexpected Death in Infancy: A Review of the World Literature 1954–1966. Pediatrics 39:123–138.
Wigfield, R., P. Fleming, P. Berry, P. Rudd, and J. Golding
1992 Can the Fall in Avon's Sudden Infant Death Rate Be Explained by Changes in Sleeping Position? British Medical Journal 304:282–283.
Willinger M., L. S. James, and C. Catz
1991 Defining the Sudden Infant Death Syndrome (SIDS): Deliberations of an Expert Panel Convened by the National Institute of Child Health and Human Development. Pediatric Pathology 11:677–684.

CHAPTER FIVE

MELANOMA WHITEWASH

Millions at Risk of Injury or Death Because of Sunscreen Deceptions

Brian McKenna

That "beauty mark" may appear innocuous, but if it's dark with irregular borders and about the size of a pencil eraser, it might be malignant melanoma. If not caught early, there's a good chance that it will metastasize and kill you. It was caught early enough for John McCain, Troy Aikman, and Sam Donaldson. But sadly it was not for Maureen Reagan, Bob Marley, and rising folk-musician star Eva Cassidy, gone at 33.

In 1930 melanoma was rare, with a lifetime risk of just one in 1,500 people. Since then, it has grown exponentially, with a lifetime risk in the United States of 1 in 250 in 1980, 1 in 120 in 1987, 1 in 75 by 2000 (Etzel and Balk 2003), and 1 in 32 today (Swetter 2007). The black cells of melanoma struck an estimated 59,940 in the United States in 2007 and killed a projected 8,110 (American Cancer Society 2007). Worldwide it yearly strikes an estimated 132,000 people with an estimated 48,000 deaths (Lucas 2006). It is one of the fastest growing cancers in the world.

Although the exact causes of melanoma are complex, the consensus of biomedical research and opinion is that it is strongly related to exposure to ultraviolet radiation, type A (UVA), the long solar waves (320 to 400 nanometers along the sun's spectrum) that travel beneath the skin's surface to damage melanocytes, the pigment-making cells. In contrast, UVB (290 to 320 nanometers along the sun's spectrum) causes red sunburn and is a major contributor to the more easily curable basal and squamous cell skin cancers. No problem, just lather on the white creamy sunscreen before taking to the beach and you are protected, right?

It turns out that U.S. sun-care manufacturers—who had $1.9 billion in sales in 2005 (Marketresearch.com 2005)—do not tell people the full truth about their sunscreen products in their advertising, labeling, websites, or commercials. Sunscreen makers willfully take advantage of the ambiguity of the term *skin cancer* in their marketing, avoiding any open reference to the term *melanoma* while strongly appealing to melanoma fears, since 79 percent of all skin cancer deaths are due to melanoma (Etzel and Balk 2003). Over the past half century, as the frequency of melanoma exploded, so has sunscreen production, with apparently little or no preventive effect. It is a powerful correlation that alarms epidemiologists and other researchers, suggesting causal linkages, but to many biomedical practitioners, it's just an irony. Schools, sports teams, supermarkets, and the media vigorously promote the idea—through their actions, emphases, and omissions—that sunscreen is the first and most important choice in fighting skin cancer and melanoma. Incredibly, pediatricians rarely counsel sun protection in office visits even though they provide health care to a population, children, that receives up to 80 percent of its total sun exposure before the age of 18 (Etzel and Balk 2003). According to one study, doctors broach the issue in only 1 percent of clinical visits and when they do, sunscreen is the most recommended cancer precaution (Easton et al. 1997). In fact, the most effective prevention sunscreen is not found in an expensive four-ounce, $8.99 bottle. It is simple avoidance of the sun between 10 a.m. and 4 p.m., proper clothing and eyewear, wide-brimmed hats (four inches or more), and shady structures.

This chapter explains why it is appropriate to call sunscreen a killer commodity. Employing critical ethnography (Kincheloe and McLaran 1994), this study reports on the social forces that promote sunscreen use even in the face of massive evidence against it as a melanoma preventive.

Theoretical Considerations

Responsibility for this crisis lies primarily with the pharmaceutical corporations that profit directly from these deceptions. But they are not the villains pure and simple. Drug companies could not sustain their campaigns without the support of allies in government, in the medical establishment, and in the media, as we shall see. Public health and medical social science researchers are also partly responsible since they are in privileged positions to investigate the issue and to work as scholars and public pedagogues to counter this and other pressing health issues with the urgency that these topics require. Citizens also bear a small measure of responsibility for not being critically attentive to the facts.

Questions of responsibility cannot be separated, however, from the overarching fact that we live in a very powerful neoliberal capitalist culture that saturates everyday life with commodities, to a degree unsurpassed in human history. These commodities have reified (or "naturalized") and fetishized (or "magical") associations (Marx 1887). Reification points to a form of social amnesia about a commodity, a blinded stance in which citizens, as consumers, do not reflect on a product's social history, the actual production processes behind its creation, the concealed labor within it, the possible toxicity of it, and the ways it expresses cultural power. What does this mean for the concept of sunscreen? When people think of sunscreen, few think about the ozone layer, about which sunscreen is the most important, or about skin pigmentation, clothes, shady structures, or hats. All are hidden "remainders" in the concept of sunscreen. In this chapter I analyze these remainders and demonstrate that the dominant culture's use of the term *sunscreen* actually comes to mean the very opposite of what it is usually taken to mean. That is, the white creams screen from consciousness the darker meanings—and pigments—associated with being in the sun. In other words, sunscreen creams, to a significant degree, literally and figuratively whitewash melanoma.

This chapter provides an up-to-date account of how an avowed melanoma precaution—sunscreen lotion—is, more often than not, an iatrogenic danger to the world's light-skinned peoples who use it. The chapter details multiple levels of contestation—educational, regulatory, legal—against neoliberal capitalist hegemony. It argues for the precautionary principle (or "taking action without certain proof of harm") as a necessary front in forging safer alternatives for melanoma prevention.

A Journey into the Kingdom of the Sick

"You've got two melanomas," Dr. White, my oncologist, told me. "You have a 70 percent chance of surviving the next five years." That was back in 1992. I was diagnosed just six months after arriving at Michigan State University (MSU) to pursue a PhD in medical anthropology. I was the one in 32 U.S. individuals who gets melanoma in his or her lifetime. There were two independent skin cancers, one on my right calf and the other in the center of my back, common areas for the disease.

If I was going to get cancer, there wasn't a better scholarly field to study than anthropology, which "studies what's behind what's behind," as my friend Dr. Harry Raulet used to say. One theoretical point emergent from medical anthropology is that biomedicine tends to conceal the social origins of sickness and, as a result, operates to suppress protest and, generally, to support the ideological and cultural hegemony of dominant classes. The sunscreen scandal is a poster child for this claim. A melanoma diagnosis jolts the victim. "How did I get this?" I gasped. Aside from an initial feeling of dread, there was a strong desire to understand the etiology of the disease and how I could stop it from spreading. I was soon disheartened to learn that another MSU graduate student, Ron Hart, had died of melanoma a few years earlier, soon after returning from fieldwork in Yemen. I recognized that I would have to use all my available intellectual, financial, social, and anthropological resources to beat melanoma, if I could. And so I began the ultimate participant observation journey, one where the stakes were highest. Many anthropologists have written about their "journeys into the kingdom of the sick," and I now join them (DiGiacomo 1987).

Sunscreen, I was told by dermatologists, oncologists, and surgeons who treated me, was essential to my survival, especially given that my chances of getting a new primary skin melanoma were at least twice as high as the general population, they said. Of course sunscreen would have absolutely no effect on what my oncologist referred to as "the hundreds of millions of melanoma cells that might be within you now" should they metastasize to my lungs or brain, common sites of reoccurrence from the original skin lesion.

I became a "walking fieldnote" (Sanjek 1990), crossing borders into multiple spheres of knowledge, pursuing alternative disciplines and experiences while adopting a critical stance on everything before me. Following below is some of what I wish I had been told in 1992.

False Sense of Security

The essential truth about sunscreen was first brought to light by epidemiologists Frank and Cedric Garland in 1990 after their soon-to-be-published work was profiled in a *New York Times* article (Angier 1990). The two brothers investigated the use of sunscreen on military populations and concluded that "sunscreens give you a false sense of security," because they did not sufficiently block out UVA rays (Angier 1990; Garland et al. 1992; Segrave 2005). The American Academy of Dermatologists quickly denounced the Garlands' research, arguing that it would inhibit sunscreen use and result in more cancers. Alarmed at the attacks and afraid it would affect future research funding, the Garlands decided to avoid journalists and keep out of the public eye (Segrave 2005). Thus did the biomedical establishment successfully ostracize them and their conclusions were mostly forgotten for three years (Segrave 2005:113).

In 1993 science writer Michael Castleman changed everything, propelling the issue into the culture permanently. In the now-classic 1993 *Mother Jones* article, "Beach Bummer," Castleman investigated the historical evidence, including the Garlands' work, and found that sunscreens offer a false sense of security and prolong people's time in the sun by preventing the only natural melanoma warning system human skin has—sunburn (Castleman 1993).

A growing number of researchers have advanced the Garlands' discovery and assert that sunscreen does not protect you from melanoma. That was the conclusion of research by epidemiologist Marianne Berwick of the prestigious Memorial Sloan-Kettering Cancer Center in 1998. "It's not safe to rely on sunscreen" to protect you from malignant melanoma, she told the media (Berwick 1998). The American Academy of Dermatology denounced Berwick's conclusions (Segrave 2005). In the December 16, 2003, issue of *Annals of Internal Medicine*, Dr. L. K. Dennis of the University of Iowa added that "no association was seen between melanoma and sunscreen use," after she and her colleagues conducted a comprehensive MEDLINE search of articles published from 1966 to 2003 that reported information on sunscreen use and melanoma in humans (Dennis et al. 2003). The *Journal of the National Cancer Institute* is also critical. In a July 2003 article, Damaris Christensen quoted Olaf

Gefeller, PhD, of the University of Erlangen-Nuremberg in Germany who said that given the failure of studies to date to demonstrate a protective effect of sunscreen against melanoma, the rigorous tests of evidence-based medicine suggest that "as a pharmaceutical product marketed for melanoma protection (instead of the prevention of sunburns), sunscreens would have failed the tests of efficacy during the approval procedure" (Christensen 2003).

"Messages about prevention may need to shift the emphasis still further toward covering up and staying out of the sun if the trend of [increasing melanoma] incidence is to be reversed," said Dr. Julia Verne, director of the South West Cancer Intelligence Service in Bristol, England, in 2003 (Fry 2003:114). But, as I'll show, that shift is not taking place to any significant degree. That is because, by default, the chief educators about skin cancer prevention are the drug companies who profit enormously from what Castleman calls "a cynical sleight of hand" (Castleman 1993). Four major manufacturers dominate the sunscreen market: Schering-Plough, makers of Coppertone; Playtex (Banana Boat); Neutrogena (a subsidiary of Johnson & Johnson since 1994); and Tanning Research, Inc., producers of Hawaiian Tropic (Shaath 2005:935–936). Market analysis of the industry is privatized; it costs $1,995 for a detailed analysis from Marketresearch.com. But a review of the data that they make public reveals that Schering-Plough dominated the market in 2005 with about a 33 percent market share.

What Is Sunscreen?

Sunscreen is not just a white creamy emollient. But if one listens only to the drug companies, one might think so. According to *Webster's* Dictionary, sunscreen is "a screen to protect against sun." In hominid natural history, the two most important sunscreens were the stratospheric ozone layer and the human skin. Anthropologists point out that hominid ancestors most likely had darkly pigmented skin to protect them from the sun (Jablonski 2004). Lighter-skinned humans evolved in northern latitudes of the earth, their skin permitting them to capture and synthesize vitamin D, which was necessary for bone growth and the prevention of rickets, or so it has been hypothesized (Jablonski 2004). Various cultures have explored botanicals, clothes, ointments, and shady structures to protect themselves from the sun's harsh rays. The ancient Egyptians used aquatic lotus oil and rice-bran extracts as sunscreens (Shaath 2005). Women of ancient Greece used lead paints, which no doubt had their own iatrogenic effects.

Anthropologist Marvin Harris investigated the history of the parasol and found that royalty considered it a privilege to be able to avoid the heat and glare of the direct rays of the sun, which is why parasols were readily adapted by the kings of West Africa, by Chinese emperors, and by the popes of Rome. Harris notes that everywhere ordinary people were forbidden to protect themselves with such devices, "pallid skin became a marker of upper-class status" (Segrave 2005:8). At the beginning of the 20th century, in the United States, lighter-skinned people avoided the sun. Parasols and long-sleeved clothes were in abundance at the beach. Tanned skin was considered lower class. But by the 1920s, a cultural transformation in favor of sun tanning took place. This was the result of a number of factors, including the new view by the biomedical community that the sun was a healer (curing everything from tuberculosis to rickets), increased leisure time by the bourgeois classes (where outdoor sports like tennis and golf rose in importance), and the entrance of a growing class of proletarians into dark factories (Segrave 2005). Sun therapy was also popular in naturopathic circles during this period.

Sunscreens in the United States came of age in the 1940s. The first sunscreens were for tanning and sunburn prevention and had little or nothing to do with skin cancer prevention. In the post–World War II era increased attention was placed on the dangers of the sun. Segrave (2005) shows how this was reflected in the number of public articles written about skin cancer. The number of articles reflecting these worries increased slowly but then grew dramatically from about 1980 onward (Segrave 2005). Tanning became less fashionable and a plethora of sun creams and sunscreens came on the market with a variety of exaggerated claims (Segrave 2005).

How to Read a Sunscreen Bottle: Sun Protective Factor (SPF) Is Not Related to Melanoma

Millions of consumers zero in on the high sun protective factor (SPF) rating of a sunscreen and feel comforted that it will ensure protection against skin cancer of any type. But the fact is that the SPF factor only pertains to UVB protection for sunburn; the greater the SPF, the more protection. For example, a person who would normally experience sunburn in ten minutes can be protected from sunburn for about 150 minutes with an SPF-15 sunscreen (10 × 15). But protection is not total. According to skin research studies, sunscreens with a SPF of 15 or more will theoretically filter more than 92 percent of the UVB responsible for erythema. Sunscreens with a SPF of 30 filter out about 97 percent of the UVB (Etzel and Balk 2003:380).

Again, these SPF numbers have absolutely nothing to do with melanoma. An SPF value for melanoma would have to be: SPF 0.

Given the wide variety of claims and the vague use of advertising language, it is not surprising that most people are confused about the proper use and effectiveness of sunscreens or confused even about "tanning" as well (Segrave 2005). This was evident, for example, in a recent trip to a local supermarket where the blond, three-year old Little Miss Coppertone greeted me on a huge cardboard display. The pigtailed child is still having her bathing suit tugged down by a mischievous little dog after 50 years in the business. But where there was once a tan line above the buttocks on this famous advertising trademark, I noticed, there is now just one tone, and it was not copper, but a consistent shade of ivory. The visual message contradicted the written label: the child had a sunless pale look since she wore "sunblock," a cream that blocks out all the sun's rays. Below her were rows of Schering-Plough's Coppertone sunblock lotion with labels that read "SPF 15, UVA/UVB Protection, Waterproof." It is a carefully crafted ambiguous message. The subliminal point is: you can be practically naked having fun in the sun all day long, get a Coppertone tan but still also be pale and be protected from skin cancer. It is an impossible outcome, but it's everything you want, so buy it.

Continuing on my ethnographic journey, I turned into the snack food aisle, where I spotted another sunscreen display. This one had rows of Johnson & Johnson's "Neutrogena Healthy Defense Sunblock Oil-Free UVA/UVB SPF 45" for $7.39 each. Later, near the checkout, I found yet another sunscreen center that included Hawaiian Tropic Ozone Sport Sunblock SPF 60+ packaged with a travel size bottle of ten ounces for $11.99. It said that "This 'Triple Play Action' formula is non-migrating, so it won't run into your eyes, sweatproof, and waterproof. Developed specially for a sports enthusiast's active lifestyle, so it's non-greasy and won't affect a sports grip. Protects against the sun's burning UVB/UVA rays." The trouble is that there is no SPF system for UVA. But it's not surprising that consumers often think so, given the juxtaposition of UVA with other acronyms as in Neutrogena's promise of UVA/UVB SPF 45 protection.

In fact, manufacturer claims that its products are "sunblocks," are "waterproof," and "offer broad spectrum UVA/UVB protection" are untrue for any sunscreen and patently misleading and deceptive when it comes to melanoma. Industry scientists behind the scenes often admit as much. Joseph Stanfield, the president of Sunscreen Research Laboratories, says there is no agreement on the level of UVA protection needed, no test that actually predicts water resistance in actual use, and no standard for photostability (Jeffries 2006).

2006 Sunscreen Lawsuit Shakes Industry

On March 29, 2006, the nation's most successful class action law firm, Lerach, Coughlin, Stoia, Geller, Rudman & Robbins LLP, filed a class-action lawsuit that brought many of these issues into the legal domain. "Sunscreen is the Snake Oil of the 21st Century and these companies that market it are Fortune 500 Snake Oil salesmen," asserted Samuel Rudman, a partner with the New York firm. "False claims such as 'sunblock,' 'waterproof,' and 'all-day protection' should be removed from these products immediately," he said (Goldstein 2006). The 104-page suit was filed in the Superior Court of the State of California, County of Los Angeles, on behalf of several plaintiffs who ask for $74,999 in compensation. There are seven defendants, who together produce five brands of sunscreen, including Schering-Plough (Coppertone), Sun Pharmaceuticals and Playtex Products (Banana Boat), Tanning Research Laboratories (Hawaiian Tropic), Neutrogena Corp. and Johnson & Johnson (Neutrogena), and Chattem Inc. (Bullfrog). The Skin Cancer Foundation (SKF) has taken this lawsuit to heart. In 2006, when consumers went to its website, they were greeted with a banner headline that read: "Lawsuit may discourage sunscreen use." The site continued, "This lawsuit is especially disturbing because it may cause people to stop wearing sunscreen." Importantly, the SKF is led by a corporate council comprised of seven groups that include the lead defendant in the lawsuit, Schering-Plough HealthCare Products, Inc.

FDA Defeated in Behind-the-Scenes Corporate Battle over "Commercial Speech"

The Federal Trade Commission (FTC) and the Food and Drug Administration (FDA) addressed the overreaching claims of the sunscreen industry in the late 1990s. In 1997 the FTC reached an agreement with Schering-Plough, Coppertone's manufacturer and the corporation with the industry's largest market share, to cease its deceptions about the efficacy of its products, but Schering-Plough never complied with the agreement (Segrave 2005; Goldstein 2006).

Later, in 1999, the FDA drafted new, more stringent language to specifically restrict the use of misleading claims. The FDA was about to crack down on labels with "unsupported, absolute, and/or misleading and confusing terms such as 'sunblock,' 'waterproof,' 'all-day protection' and 'visible and/or infrared light protection'" (Brune 2005), but over the next few years there was an intensive lobbying effort by sunscreen manufacturers and their trade group, the Cosmetics, Toiletries and Fragrance Association, and the FDA was persuaded not to implement the rules. Lobbyists argued that "commercial speech" protection for sunscreen manufacturers was more important than truthful consumer protection for the public.

Leading the lobbying charge was John Roberts, a White House lawyer who had convinced President Ronald Reagan in 1985 to tell the public that science had not yet proven that casual contact or simple touch was safe enough to ensure protection from AIDS, thus setting back HIV prevention and education efforts for a significant period (Simone 2006). According to FDA records, Roberts met with FDA officials, including FDA chief counsel Daniel Troy, a strong Bush supporter, on January 4, 2000, and on October 29, 2001 (OMB Watch 2005). A few months after the last meeting, the FDA suspended the stricter rules for labeling sunscreen products. Between 1998 and 2004 Schering-Plough spent $28 million in lobbying efforts (Lobbywatch 2006). Roberts's future successes are illuminating. In September 2005 he was appointed chief justice of the U.S. Supreme Court.

In a telling irony which underscores the continuing assault on First Amendment rights in the United States, on May 30, 2006, Roberts ruled with the 5–4 Supreme Court majority that approximately 20 million governmental employees no longer have full free speech rights. The implications are chilling. In effect this ruling means that the sunscreen industry is free to continue deceiving the public under "commercial speech" protections while, at the same time, an employee within the FDA, CDC, NIH, or any other governmental agency who witnesses corruption between his superiors and corporations like Schering-Plough is not free to blow the whistle without the risk of being fired or prosecuted. Thus, "commercial speech" has made gains over "free speech" as the United States slips closer to authoritarianism (Giroux 2004). According to social theorist Henry Giroux, "within neoliberalism's market-driven discourse, corporate power marks the space of a new kind of public pedagogy, one in which the production, dissemination, and circulation of ideas emerges from the educational force of the larger culture" (Giroux 2004:106).

It is unlikely that the FDA will reverse itself. In a Federal Register notice published on May 16, 2002, the FDA states that "recent case law has emphasized the need for not imposing unnecessary restrictions on speech." However, in a surprising move, on May 29, 2007, Connecticut attorney general Richard Blumenthal filed a formal petition with the FDA urging that it implement its 1999 rules. "The FDA is AWOL—enabling false labeling and encouraging overexposure to the sun," Blumenthal said in a press release. "It has shelved rules that could save lives. Reliance on voluntary compliance has led to pervasive deception," he said. "The FDA's delay is unfathomable and unconscionable. Claims to block 'all harmful rays,' and 'waterproof' are mostly truth proof. The FDA has put new sunscreen standards in bureaucratic limbo, making them dead letter, useless and unenforceable" (Blumenthal 2007).

European Union Intervenes to Confront Sunscreen Deceptions

In May 2006 the European Union (EU) acted to do for European citizens what the FDA has not done for U.S. citizens, launching a dramatic initiative to improve its sunscreen labeling system. Commissioner Markos Kyprianou, who is responsible for health and consumer protection, said,

"Consumers must be made fully aware that no sunscreen product can provide 100% protection against hazardous UV-radiation. There are serious health risks, such as skin cancer, linked to insufficient protection from the sun. EU citizens need to be fully informed about what sunscreens will and will not do for them" (Medical News Today 2006:1).

The EU argues that claims like "sunblockers" and "total protection" are untrue. The commission is especially alarmed at claims for which no standardized research evidence exists: broad spectrum; broad extra UVA, UVB, 100 percent anti UVA/UVB/IR; keeps short UVA radiation away; UVA of 30A, strengthened protection UVA (Medical News Today 2006). The recommendations were scheduled to take effect in 2007 and include imported sunscreens. Only 12 percent of the European sunscreen market is comprised of non-European companies. Indications are that this initiative will have a great impact (Medical News Today 2006). It remains to be seen whether or not U.S. sunscreen manufacturers will begin telling more of the truth on their European products in order to continue having access to those markets, and if so, whether that will have any relationship to what they tell the American people.

From Tanning Creams to Vending Machines

Not much has changed since the emergence of sunscreen products in the United States in the 1920s which promised you a "healthy tan," an oxymoronic term since tans indicate skin damage. Sunscreens do not expedite the tanning process. Tanning happens on its own timeline from prolonged sun exposure. The earlier sunscreens helped stop the sunburn (UVB rays), but had little or nothing to do with the tanning UVA rays, which would have accumulated at the same rate in any case (Segrave 2005).

Sunscreen manufacturers today know about the dangers of their commodities but do not talk about the limits of their products in their labeling or marketing. But critical information about some products is available from the industry even though much of their research is proprietary. For example, sunscreen chemists admit that the photostability of Avobenzone is a problem, but they claim it is one they can rectify with quenchers and emollients (Shaath 2005). In addition to Avobenzone, other ingredients within sun creams are temporarily effective in blocking some UVA light. These include physical screens like titanium oxide and zinc oxide, often worn by lifeguards on their noses (why not the rest of their bodies?). Currently one product, mexoryl, is also reported to have some efficacy against UVA rays (Bryant 2004). It has been available in Europe since 1993 but not in the United States until July 2006 when the FDA permitted L'Oreal to market it in a formula called Anthelios SX. La Roche-Posay also markets a form of it. Canadian dermatologist Robert Bissonnette recommends mexoryl but admits, "there are not many studies comparing sunscreens with and without mexoryl to determine how much benefit you actually get" (Bryant 2004). Sunscreen manufacturers will no doubt continue to search for a magic bullet cream while ignoring the social context of use and marginalizing other less expensive, but more effective protections as are discussed below.

A growing literature questions the safety of many of the specific UVA protective ingredients, especially the increasing use of nanoparticles in the formulae (Korting 2005; Montague 2004; Chiang 2005). The Environmental Protection Agency (EPA) claims to be monitoring them and says that regulations will emerge if detrimental effects are found (Chiang 2005). But the pharmaceutical companies do not concern themselves with the dangers of nanotechnology; they celebrate it. They hope to make sunscreen as accessible as candy bars. Playtex (Banana Boat) has placed vending machines at golf courses, swimming pools, resorts, water parks, marinas, and other outdoor recreation facilities where they "offer and deliver a convenient sun protection solution for the consumer" (USA Technologies 2003). Even sunscreen advocates like Dr. Martin A. Weinstock (2001), a professor of dermatology at Brown University, argue that for sunscreen to work it must be applied very heavily and reapplied every few hours. That can amount to a full 12-ounce bottle per person per day at the beach, a very expensive proposition.

There is little ethnographic research on the social context of sunscreen use, especially at the beach. But available studies are not encouraging. For example, Dr. Joseph Grob, a dermatologist, conducted research on Mediterranean beaches and found that few people even knew what SPF meant and that this contributed to the misapplication of sunscreens. "People don't know what they are doing," he said. "They think that they can get both get a tan and be protected from long-term complications—which is impossible" (Nash 2005). In a 2002 survey, 39 percent of teenagers claimed that they were using a broad-spectrum sunscreen when they got their worst sunburns (Shane 2003). Importantly, many citizens have no knowledge of melanoma. In a 1996 random-digit dialed survey of 1,001 persons, reported by the Centers for Disease Control and Prevention, a high proportion of respondents (42 percent) had no knowledge about melanoma (CDC 1996). Only 16 percent of those ages 18 to 24 were aware that melanoma is a type of skin cancer (CDC 1996). They probably concluded, as I once did, that the distinction between the three types of skin cancer is not that important since sunscreen companies do not make such a distinction in their marketing—and the government does not require them to do so. The idea that skin cancer is easily curable reinforces this false conclusion.

Capital's Treadmill of Production, Consumption, Disease, and Pollution

Back in 1992, I sat on a hospital gurney waiting to have my leg "resectioned" (i.e., a deep wedge of flesh removed around my lesion to capture any melanoma cells that may still be there), and my surgeon, aware of my critical interest in medicine, handed me a professional biomedical journal article which listed ozone depletion as a probable contributing factor to melanoma. He winked at me, as if to say, "when you're up to it, go investigate this."

I appreciated Dr. Jones's effort to legitimize my quest to understand the larger social context of my disease. At the same time I was aware that he made a lucrative career from disease care and spent little or no time in preventive education activities outside of the clinic. I felt like a diseased product on an assembly line, and I wondered about the thousands of casualties who did their time in the hospital mill, oblivious to the larger treadmill of capital (Schnaiberg 1980:205–250).

The chance of death riveted my attention to the etiologies and solutions to the threat. The ozone connection focused my attention on one aspect of it. As I lay there, I wondered, "Am I a victim of pollution? Is my skin cancer related to the larger culture?" In fact, the threat to the ozone layer had been known for years. In 1974 the first clear and credible early warning came out regarding the ozone layer and increased skin cancer (Harremoës 2001). The cause was a "miracle compound" of capitalist culture, chlorofluorocarbons (CFCs), first identified in 1927. One CFC, freon, became common in household refrigerators and air conditioners. The ozone layer is nature's sunscreen, blocking about 94 percent of all ultraviolet radiation from the sun (Blatt 2005). A simple molecule with three atoms of oxygen, ozone inhabits the earth's stratosphere, a layer 10 to 22 miles above Earth. Colder air helps to separate chlorine atoms from the CFC. Each chlorine atom can destroy about 100,000 ozone molecules.

In the 13 years after 1974, a contentious battle took place over ozone depletion led by chemical companies who fought against restrictions against products like aerosol sprays (NRDC 2005). The Natural Resources Defense Council brought a lawsuit against the EPA to force tighter restrictions on CFCs. Aerosol sprays containing CFCs were banned in 1978. Then suddenly in the mid-1980s, scientists found shocking proof of the theory, a dramatic ozone hole above the Antarctic. The result was the historically momentous Montreal Protocol of 1987. It was the first-ever global environmental agreement, signed by 57 nations. It halted the production of CFCs in industrial countries by 1996. Today more than 180 nations have signed on.

One reason for unanimity was almost universal recognition of the potential threat. In 1991 the EPA estimated that even if everyone phased out CFCs right on schedule, ozone loss would cause 12 million skin cancers in the United States and 200,000 deaths over the next 50 years (Montague 1991). EPA's worldwide estimates put skin cancer almost in league with AIDS, projecting a billion skin cancers from ozone loss, including 17 million deaths by 2031 (Montague 1991). In 2000, the Montreal Protocol's scientific assessment team stated that without the global agreement, ozone depletion would be at least 50 percent in the mid latitudes and as a result, ultraviolet radiation would double in the mid latitudes in the Northern Hemisphere and quadruple in the middle latitudes in the Southern Hemisphere. The result? By the year 2060, it is estimated that there will be an additional 19 million cases of nonmelanoma skin cancer and 1.5 million more cases of melanoma. In addition, there will be several other less quantifiable effects such as lower immunity against disease, a drop in crop productivity, and ecosystem damage (Baker 2000).

Other regions of the earth are currently affected. Ozone loss over the Arctic averaged between 25 and 30 percent between 1971 and 1997. Ozone loss is most severe at the poles because the chemical reaction that destroys ozone is catalyzed by very cold temperatures, particularly below −110 degrees Fahrenheit. The stratospheric layer over Antarctica averages −144 degrees Fahrenheit, while the Arctic averages −108 Fahrenheit. Ozone loss in the mid latitudes averages 6 to 7 percent (Blatt 2005:181).

In 2006 the Antarctic hole had stabilized and, according to some scientists (Blatt 2005), the trend is that it will begin to shrink in a few years and may recover fully by 2050. But there are several mitigating factors, like global warming, that may prevent this from happening. Global warming increases ozone destruction because the warmer gases in the lower atmosphere lead to cooling in the upper atmosphere, resulting in colder temperatures and a higher rate of ozone destruction (Blatt 2005:184). A thinned layer is now much larger than Antarctica and extends to southern South America and New Zealand to 40 degrees latitude. New Zealand and Australia experience the highest melanoma rates in the world. New Zealand signed the Kyoto Protocol in 2003, and Australia in 2008, to reduce the emission of greenhouse gases which delay the recovery of the ozone layer.

Other epidemiological evidence is unsettling. In a creative study, the Garland brothers decided to study the relationship between ozone exposure and melanoma mortality rates around the world (Garland, Garland, and Gorham 2003). They obtained UVA and UVB radiation and age-adjusted melanoma mortality rates for all 45 countries reporting cancer data to the World Health Organization. Stratospheric ozone data were obtained from NASA satellites. They found that UVA radiation was associated with melanoma mortality rates after controlling for UVB and average pigmentation. It is important to point out that more than 80 percent of UV rays get through light clouds on a summer day and up to 40 percent of UV rays penetrate water down to a half-meter depth (European Union 2006).

"Ozone acts like the stuff you smear on yourself at the beach," said Blatt, a geologist (2005:178). And yet nature's "sun cream" is incredibly fragile. If it were all brought to sea level it would only be as thick as two pennies (Blatt 2005:178).

Ferocious Market Expansion

Sunscreen corporations are very aggressively expanding their wares across multiple domains seeking to overcome a short summertime window of consumption and integrate it as a "need" in everyday life (Shaath 2005). There are now sunblock tube sticks on key chains that people "on the go" can carry. They are "especially for people who want to protect kids at any time" (Toth 2006:17). There are continuous aerosol spray applications so parents don't have to be troubled with rubbing cream on kids but can "run around and chase them with a spray. It's all about convenience" (Toth 2006:17) for the customer so he'll be more likely to buy it. At stake are billions of dollars in profits, not only from sunscreens, but lip balms, shampoos, cosmetics, and a vast array of new products as manufacturers "cross over the traditional boundaries that once restricted ultraviolet filters to summertime sunbathing applications and infiltrate the daily wear skin care market" (Shaath 2005). As part of this strategy, sun-care companies are now appealing to "a major green movement sweeping the country," making strong efforts to associate sun-cream products with good health. They are adding a vast array of "natural ingredients" to their formulae, including green tea, pomegranate, and "extracts of galanga, green coffee, licorice, oat, annatto . . . that improve the solubility of UV filters, preserve the formulations, and improve the feel and elegance of natural cosmetics" (Shaath 2005). The sunscreen industry is but a smaller subset of the sun-care and lip-care industry, which recorded $2.2 billion in sales in 2004 (Marketresearch.com 2005). This includes the growing sunless-tanning products industry, for those who desire a "healthy glow" look without the dangers of the sun. "This is a responsive industry, continually growing to responsibly meet the needs of the consumer" (Shaath 2005). Of course they prefer not to respond to the FDA and consumer protection groups. Geographically, the sunscreen market has grown significantly in Eastern Europe and China, where cosmetics registered a 12 percent growth in 2004. According to Cosmeticsdesign.com (2005), an industry group, "the fashion for whiter skin in China has also prompted significant growth in the sunscreen market."

Biomedical researchers are often too eager to help expand this iatrogenic market. For example, Dr. Alan Geller, a research professor at Boston University's School of Medicine, reviewed sunscreen advertisements in 24 magazines spanning 579 issues from September 1997 to 2002 and found that there is a dearth of sunscreen ads in parent and family magazines (less than one ad per issue) and less that one every six months in outdoor-recreation magazines, reaching mostly men.

"There's a huge opportunity for an untapped market [in sunscreen consumption]," Geller says (Forbes.com 2006). Schering-Plough was once even successful in getting "green window dressing" to support its urgent cry for sunscreen. A public relations firm called Hill and Knowlton lined up a number of environmental groups behind a coalition called Partners in Sun Protection Awareness (Partners). The PR firm convinced the Natural Resources Defense Council and the Sierra Club to add their names to its letterhead. Partners did not offer any proposals for preventing further thinning of the ozone layer, and their key goal was to sell more sunscreen. It was later discovered that Partners was a front group for Schering-Plough. Environmental groups said they were ignorant of the connection. Hill and Knowlton have also worked on behalf of corporate clients who hired them to belittle the environmental risks of global warming (Stauber 1995).

Sunscreen corporations fund many scientists and technicians who work around the clock to improve formulae, test new ingredients, make sun cream more stable, and vigorously expand their commodity into already existing product lines and world cultures. This work is represented in a 2005 industry book called *Sunscreens: Regulation and Commercial Development*, which boasts 48 chapters and 941 pages. It is written by "prominent scientists and practitioners from appropriately varied disciplines including academia, industry, the medical community, marketing, the press, scientific organizations and regulatory agencies" (Shaath 2005). It is very clear from reading this text that the industry is not concerned with public health therapies, like clothing, ozone recovery, protective structures (like tents), or with changing sun-related behavioral habits. None of these more effective sun protections creates as good a return on investment as bottled chemical creams. The stated goal is to "research the underlying causes of skin cancer from a cellular and molecular biology perspective, uncarth markers for early detection, and ultimately assist marketers in producing superior, more natural sunscreen [*sic*] products" (Shaath 2005:15). Of the 48 chapters, there is only one on sun-protective clothing. The reader comes away from the book thinking that there is no controversy over sunscreen other than the fear of government regulation. "Creativity in innovation," it asserts, "has been hindered only by regulatory agencies and patent restrictions worldwide" (Shaath 2005:iii).

Skin Cancer Education in the Clinic: Cookbook Medicine?

As noted earlier, pediatricians focus on sunscreen, not clothing, on those occasions when they counsel children about sun safety (Easton et al. 1997). A survey, reported in the journal *Pediatrics* in 2004, confirmed this. It revealed that pediatricians considered the following prescriptions to be "most important": using a sunscreen with an SPF of 15 or greater (64.4 percent) and avoiding the sun during the peak hours of 10 a.m. to 4 p.m. (22.7 percent). Other effective preventive factors were practically ignored. Only 5.4 percent of pediatricians believed that wearing long-sleeved shirts and other protective clothing was most important, and only 5.4 percent said seeking shady structures was the most important. When asked about the chief barriers constraining them to counsel patients on sun protection, 57.8 percent of pediatricians responded that there is a "lack of sufficient time in health maintenance visits to address sun care/skin cancer prevention" (Balk et al. 2004).

Dermatological ignorance is rampant. According to a 2006 study in the Archives of Dermatology (Moore et al. 2006), 43.4 percent of 934 students graduating from seven U.S. medical schools had never examined a patient for skin cancer. Only 28.2 percent rated themselves as somewhat or very skilled in skin cancer examination, a rate that dropped to 19.7 percent among 553 students who had not completed a dermatology elective (Moore et al. 2006). Segments of the public health community have reinforced this practice. In 2003 the U.S. Preventive Services Task Force updated its research and reached the disappointing conclusion that the evidence is insufficient to recommend for or against routine counseling by primary care clinicians to prevent skin cancer (Helfand and Krages 2003). Dr. Ruth Etzel, an environmental pediatrician, strongly disagrees. The coauthor of the groundbreaking *Pediatric Environmental Health* "green book" (Etzel and Balk 2003:378) argues that "pediatricians have an important role in [sun safety] education beginning in infancy, and later when developmental stages result in new patterns of sun exposure."

Sun-Wise Precautionary Principle

"Better safe than sorry" is the mantra of the precautionary principle, the movement dedicated to preventing harm to humans and the environment by encouraging action even when absolute scientific proof is lacking. Australia is far ahead of the United States in creating a precautionary sunscreen infrastructure, out of necessity. Two out of every three Australians develop some form of skin cancer and one in 25 develops melanoma. While Australia only makes up about 0.3 percent of the world's population, 6 percent of all lethal forms of skin cancer are diagnosed there.

Australia has a "No Hat, No Play" rule. Every child must wear a hat to play outside. Recess times are often scheduled outside the 11 a.m. to 3 p.m. time frame (although many schools have strongly resisted such recommendations). Children have begun wearing neck-to-knee swimsuits on beaches and at pools. Lifeguards are directed to set an example by wearing sunglasses, wide-brimmed hats, long-sleeved shirts, zinc oxide, and sunscreen as well as sitting in the shade (Lombard et al. 1991). Many pools and playgrounds are now covered by expansive tents or newly planted trees (Gies et al. 1998). The government also recruits popular athletes as fashion models for sun-smart behaviors. In one campaign, Olympic swimming gold medalist Dawn Fraser illustrates the above lifeguard fashions (Borland et al. 1991). These campaigns are associated with an increase in the use of protective clothing and shade in adults and children.

In response to its own crisis, the New Zealand Ministry of Health released an important document in 2003 called "What Works in Cancer Prevention?" Among their recommendations are campaigns to increase the provision of shade and to influence the timing of outdoor events.

Private Fashion Advances, But Not Much Else

There is an emerging market of sun-smart design clothing and furniture (e.g., long awnings and boat tops) that is important though it is not a serious challenge to sun-cream dominance. This includes Lands' End and some other popular retailers that are now promoting sun-protective clothing in their stores. The quality of the fabric is not uniformly protective from manufacturer to manufacturer; however, the cultural phenomenon of associating clothing with sunscreen is a significant improvement. One manufacturer that has been involved in the business for over a decade is Sun Precautions, which markets over a hundred quality products for active wear, including shade caps with neck drapes, pants, ultrasun hats with four-inch brims, beach tunics, kids' full-zip swimsuits, pullover surf shirts, and balaclavas (knit caps that cover the entire head and neck with an opening for the eyes). All are made with dense, lightweight, well-ventilated weaves that the manufacturer says offer the equivalent of 30+ SPF all-day UVA and UVB sun protection. One eye-catching ad shows a sun-drenched ultramarathoner wearing Sun Precautions' Solumbra clothing from head to toe in the grueling Badwater Ultramarathon, a 135-mile race that traverses Death Valley in midsummer where temperatures can soar to 130 degrees. "Solumbra versus Sunscreen," they caption, "which would you choose?"

Can You Wear a Sun Hat at Work? How about a Sun Drape?

Perennial presidential candidate John McCain is rarely photographed wearing a hat even though he has had serious bouts with melanoma. One can speculate on reasons why. Fashion is a form of communication and most likely politicians and celebrities want to communicate that they are fit and healthy. They do not want to be a walking advertisement that communicates cancer victim or worrywart. A wide-brimmed hat may not be perceived as being cool. The hat breaks a cultural denial mechanism. However, if McCain and other well-known melanoma victims wore hats and modeled sun-smart behavior, they would perform a valuable public service.

Wearing hats on the weekend, during one's free time is one thing, but what about wearing a hat at work? Not just during the journey to work, but at work? In the 1920s through 1940s, during the period when UV radiation was seen as a healthy panacea for everything from TB to the common cold, several companies intentionally saturated their indoor workers with UV radiation in the belief it would improve productivity and thwart absenteeism (Segrave 2005). That diminished after concerns about UV started to become widely known. However, today fluorescent lighting is common in office settings and it emits UVA, UVB, and sometimes UVC emissions. Intensities of some emissions were of similar magnitude to those in sunlight (Sayre 2004). According to several studies (Walter 1992; Sayre 2004), fluorescent light exposure remains a potential risk factor for melanoma (Walter 1992:749) and "chronic exposure to indoor lighting may deliver unexpected cumulative UV exposure to the skin and eyes" (Sayre 2004). This means that it would be legitimate—even necessary—to wear a sun hat and full-face drape inside an office setting. It also requires worker efforts to petition against the use of fluorescent lighting and find better alternatives. But what effect might that have on one's career trajectory, even if one was permitted to do so? Employers need to develop a formal sun protection program in order to promote a safe work environment. In 1992 the Occupational Safety and Health Administration (OSHA) wrote an interpretation of their Personal Protective Equipment Standards (1910.132(A)) stating that employers have a duty to protect workers who are overexposed to solar radiation on the job because this could result in serious physical harm or death. But most corporations and employers have no such policy. Unfortunately, there is only limited research in this area.

Conclusion: Challenging Sunscreen Hegemony and the Culture of Denial

Sunscreen lotions are, contrary to common sense, one of the means by which melanoma is induced. The white creams are largely fetishes that cover up the real causes of melanoma, even as they act, ironically, as vehicles that help produce it. Responsibility for the sunscreen falsehoods and the resulting rise in melanoma lies primarily with the pharmaceutical corporations that profit directly from these deceptions. They must be held accountable. So must the federal government which has protected them since the FDA's 1999 recommendations were shelved. The crisis is extremely urgent. As Connecticut attorney general Blumenthal put it in May 2007, "these false claims dangerously deceive consumers into believing they are protected when they may be exposing themselves—and their children—to harmful sunrays that can lead to deadly skin cancer and other harmful conditions" (Blumenthal 2007).

Melanoma must also be understood as a disease that occurs within a wider holistic context. The exponential leap in melanoma incidence over the past 50 years conjoined with the evidence herein presented indicates that serious political, economic, environmental, and cultural causes are at root. Melanoma is a by-product of the "terror of neoliberalism" (Giroux 2004), which transfers responsibility back to the individual as the state diminishes its role in areas such as health care, public education, and social services. In summary, the culture of neoliberal capitalism helps to induce melanoma by:

- Sunscreen products that are deceptive, mislabeled, and iatrogenic.
- Ozone depletion caused by chlorine atoms from CFCs.
- Global warming from fossil fuel cultures and the refusal of the United States to sign on to the Kyoto Protocol.
- A youth-oriented "healthy-glow" conception of beauty that reproduces consumers' feeling of imperfection, propels the cosmetics industry, promotes tanning, and undervalues health.
- Lack of public resources, like tent-covered tennis courts to shield against UVA
- Poor governmental regulation of occupational settings, schools, and tanning salons.
- Compulsory outdoor activities at work and play during the most dangerous parts of the day without any policy or protective clothing.
- Commercial speech's dominance over free speech.
- Commodity fetishization (i.e., the magic cream) over critical inquiry and its corollary, technocratic rationality over democratic education.
- Cultural denial of history, social processes, and modes of cultural resistance.
- The dominance of biomedicine in state-supported medical education.
- Poor funding of public health and primary care.
- The melanoma whitewash of sunscreen capital abetted by government support.

SURGEON GENERAL'S WARNING: Sunscreen does not sufficiently protect you from melanoma, the most deadly skin cancer, responsible for about 80 percent of all skin-cancer deaths. Sunscreen may actually cause melanoma by giving you a false sense of security in the sun. People are at risk of injury or death by using these creams, which pharmaceutical companies misrepresent in their quest for profits. The most immediate way to protect yourself from ultraviolet rays is simple sun avoidance between 10 a.m. and 4 p.m., sun-protective clothing, UV-protective sunglasses, and a wide-brimmed hat. On a public health level, important protections include education about ozone depletion, the greenhouse effect, and the ways corporate culture endangers human health; also required are new recreational and workplace norms, sun-smart signage, and shady structures. Public education on the precautionary principle is necessary to encourage action even in the absence of scientific certainty of harm, as with the Montreal Protocol of 1987, in which over 50 nations (more than 180 signatories) agreed to ban chlorofluorocarbons, which destroy nature's sunscreen: the ozone layer.

What is required is a cultural transformation in how we think and act about "sunscreens" and the sun. As part of this undertaking, a vast educational campaign is required. I suggest that efforts be made to establish a surgeon general's warning on sunscreen bottles.

References

ABC News
2006 Sunscreen Makers Sued, but Doctors Defend Products. ABC News, March 30.
American Cancer Society
2007 Cancer Facts and Figures 2007. Atlanta: American Cancer Society.
Angier, Nathalie
1990 Theory Hints at Sunscreens Raise Melanoma Risks. New York Times, August 9: B10.
Baker, Linda
2000 Think the Ozone Layer Is Yesterday's Issue? Think Again. Earth Action Network. Farmington Hills, MI: Gale.
Balk, Sophie, Karen O'Connor, and Mona Saraiya
2004 Counseling Parents and Children on Sun Protection: A National Survey of Pediatricians. Pediatrics, October.
Berwick, Marianne
1998 Sunscreens and Skin Cancer: The Epidemiologic Evidence. Meeting of the American Association for the Advancement of Science in Philadelphia. February.
Blatt, Harvey
2005 America's Environmental Report Card, Are We Making the Grade? Cambridge, MA: MIT Press.

Blumenthal, Richard
2007 Attorney General Demands FDA Action to Stop False and Misleading Claims by Sunscreen Makers. Press release, Connecticut Attorney General's Office. May 29.
Borland, R. M., B. Hocking, G. A. Godkin, et al.
1991 The Impact of a Skin Cancer Control Education Package for Outdoor Workers. Medical Journal of Australia 154:686–688.
Bowman, Chris
2006 Aerojet to Pay $25 Million to Settle Pollution Lawsuit. Knight Ridder Business News, May 17: 1.
Brune, Tom
2005 Roberts Omits Stint with Cosmetics Group. Newsday, August 3.
Bryant, Rebecca
2004 Popular Sunscreen Seeks U.S. Approval. Dermatology Times, September 1.
Castleman, Michael
1993 Beach Bummer. Mother Jones 18:32–37.
CDC (Centers for Disease Control and Prevention)
1996 Morbidity and Mortality Weekly 45(17):346–349.
Chiang, Chuck
2005 EPA Outlines Plans for Researching Nanomaterials. Knight Ridder Tribune Business News, December 14: 1.
Christensen, Damaris
2003 Data Still Cloudy on Association between Sunscreen Use and Melanoma Risk. Journal of the National Cancer Institute 95(13):932–933.
Conlan, Kathleen
2003 The Sun, Another Construction Site Hazard. Proof #5. Electronic document, www.coppertone.com/summers_suncare.aspx.
Cosmeticsdesign.com
2005 China Cosmetics: The Gold Rush Is On. Decision News Media. Cosmeticsdesign.com.
Davis, Devra
2007 The Secret History of the War on Cancer. New York: Basic Books.
Dennis, Leslie, Laura Beane Freeman, and Marta VanBeek
2003 Sunscreen Use and the Risk for Melanoma: A Quantitative Review. Annals of Internal Medicine 139(12):966–978.
DiGiacomo, Susan M.
1987 Biomedicine as a Cultural System: An Anthropologist in the Kingdom of the Sick. *In* Encounters with Biomedicine: Case Studies in Medical Anthropology. Hans A. Baer, ed. Pp. 315–346. New York: Gordon and Breach Science Publishers.

Easton, A., J. Price, K. Boehm, and S. Telljohann
1997 Sun Protection Counseling by Pediatricians. Archives of Pediatric Adolescent Medicine 51:1133–1138.
Egilman, David, and Susanna Rankin Bohme
2005 Corporate Corruption of Science. International Journal of Occupational and Environmental Health 11:331–337.
Etzel, Ruth, and Sophie Balk, eds.
2003 Pediatric Environmental Health, 2nd ed. Elk Grove Village, IL: American Academy of Pediatrics, Pp. 371–391.
European Union
2006 Sunscreen Products: What Matters? May 4.
Ferrini, Rebecca L., Monica Perlman, and Linda Hill
1998 Physician Recommendation of Protection from UV Light Exposure. American Journal of Preventive Medicine 14(1):83–86.
Forbes.com
2006 Not Enough Men Getting the Message on Sunscreen. Forbes.com, May 29.
Fry, Allison, J. Verne
2003 Preventing Skin Cancer. British Medical Journal 326:114–115.
Garland, C. F., F. C. Garland, and E. D. Gorham
1992 Could Sunscreens Increase Melanoma Risk? American Journal of Public Health 82(4):614, 615.
2003 Epidemiologic Evidence for Different Roles of Ultraviolet A and B Radiation in Melanoma Mortality Rates. Annals of Epidemiology 13(6):395–404.
Gies, P. H., C. R. Roy, S. Toomey, and A. McLennan
1998 Protection against Solar Ultraviolet Radiation. Mutation Research 422:15–22.
Giroux, Henry
2004 The Terror of Neoliberalism. Boulder: Paradigm.
Goldstein, Joseph, v. Schering-Plough et al.
2006 Amended Master Complaint Filed with the Superior Court of the State of California for the County of Los Angeles.
Harremoës, P., David Gee, Malcolm MacGarvin, Andy Stirling, Jane Keys, Brian Wynne, and Sofia Guedes Vaz
2001 Late Lessons from Early Warnings: The Precautionary Principle 1896–2000. Environmental Issue Report no. 22. Copenhagen: European Environment Agency.
Haywood, R., P. Wardman, and C. Linge
2003 Sunscreens Inadequately Protect against Ultraviolet-A-Induced Free Radicals in Skin: Implications for Skin Aging and Melanoma? Journal of Investigative Dermatology 121(4):862–868.

Helfand, M., and K. Krages
2003 Counseling to Prevent Skin Cancer: A Summary of the Evidence for the U.S. Preventive Services Task Force. Rockville, MD: Department of Health and Human Services, Agency for Healthcare Research and Quality.
IARC (International Agency for Research on Cancer)
1992 Solar and Ultraviolet Radiation: IARC Monographs on the Evaluation of Carcinogenic Risks to Humans. Lyon: IARC Press.
Jablonski, Nina G.
2004 The Evolution of Human Skin and Skin Color. Annual Review of Anthropology 33:585–623.
Jeffries, Nancy
2006 SPF Test Debate Sizzles. Global Cosmetic Industry 174(2):40–42, 44.
Kincheloe, Joe, and Peter McLaran
1994 Rethinking Critical Theory and Qualitative Research. *In* Handbook of Qualitative Research. Norman Denzin and Yvonna Lincoln, eds. Beverly Hills, CA: Sage.
Knapp, Thomas
1999 Texas Workers Compensation Board, appeal no. 990654.
Korting, Maier T.
2005 Sunscreen—Which and What For? Skin Pharmacology and Physiology 18(6):253–262.
Lee, Eric T., David O'Riordan, Susan M. Swetter, Marie-France Demierre, Katie Brooks, and Alan C. Geller
2006 Sun Care Advertising in Popular U.S. Magazines. American Journal of Health Promotion 20(5):349–352.
Lobbywatch: The Center for Public Integrity
2006 Schering-Plough. Electronic document, www.publicintegrity.org/lobby/profile.aspx?act=clients&year=2003&cl=L002674.
Lombard D., T. E. Neubaner, D. Canfield, and R. A. Winett
1991 Behavioral Community Intervention to Reduce the Risk of Skin Cancer. Journal of Applied Behavior Analysis 24:677–686.
Lucas, R.
2006 Global Burden of Disease of Solar Ultraviolet Radiation, Environmental Burden of Disease Series, July 25, 2006; No. 13. News release, World Health Organization.
Manson, J. E., K. M. Rexrode, F. C. Garland, and M. A. Weinstock
2000 The Case for a Comprehensive National Campaign to Prevent Melanoma and Associated Mortality. Epidemiology 11:728–734.
Marketresearch.com
2005 Market Trends: Sun Care and Lip Care Products. Marketresearch .com, September 1. Pub. ID: LA1097889.

Marx, Karl
1887 Capital. London: Lowrey.
Medical News Today
2006 Sunscreens: European Commission Moves to Improve Labeling. Dermatology News, May 8.
Ministry of Health
2003 What Works in Cancer Prevention? Wellington: Ministry of Health.
Montague, Peter
1991 Dismantling Our Life-Support Systems. Rachel's Hazardous Waste News #246, August 14. http://www.ejnet.org/rachel/rhwn246.htm.
2004 Welcome to NanoWorld: Nanotechnology and the Precautionary Principle Imperative. Multinational Monitor 25(9):16–19.
Moore, Megan M., Alan Geller, Zi Zhang, Benjamin Hayes, Kendra Bergstrom, Julia E. Graves, Andrea Kim, Juan-Carlos Martinez, Ladan Shahabi, Donald R. Miller, and Barbara A. Gilchrest
2006 Skin Cancer Examination Teaching in U.S. Medical Education. Archives of Dermatology 142(4):439–444.
Nash, Karen
2005 Sunscreen Warnings Must Be Clearer to Be Effective, M.D. Says. Dermatology Times 26(8):86–87
New York Times
2005 Nominee Discloses Questionnaire Error. August 4: A14.
New Zealand Herald
2005 Sunscreen Suppliers Defend Products. New Zealand Herald, December 17.
NRDC (Natural Resources Defense Council)
2005 Healing the Ozone Layer. Electronic document, http://www.nrdc.org/globalwarming/ozone.asp.
OMB Watch
2005 High Court Nominee Admits Lobbying OMB, FDA. August 8.
Sanjek, Roger, ed.
1990 Fieldnotes, the Makings of Anthropology. Ithaca: Cornell University Press.
Sayre, Robert M., John C. Dowdy, and Maureen Poh-Fitzpatrick
2004 Dermatological Risk of Indoor Ultraviolet Exposure from Contemporary Lighting Sources. Photochemistry and Photobiology 80(1):47–51.
Schnaiberg, Allan
1980 The Environment: From Surplus to Scarcity. New York: Oxford University Press.
Segrave, Kerry
2005 Suntanning in 20th-Century America. Jefferson, NC: McFarland.

Shaath, Nadim, ed.
2005 Sunscreens, Regulations and Commercial Development, 3rd ed. Boca Raton, FL: Taylor & Francis.
Shane, Scott
2003 Sunscreen May Not Help Prevent Melanoma. Baltimore Sun, July 14.
Simone, Renata, and William Cran
2006 The Age of AIDS. Presidential briefing memo. PBS, aired May 30.
Stauber, J. and S. Rampton
1995 Toxic Sludge Is Good for You: Lies, Damn Lies and the Public Relations Industry. Monroe, ME: Common Courage Press.
SunPrecautions
2006 Advertising booklet. Everett, WA.
Swetter, Susan
2007 Malignant Melanoma. Emedicine Clinical Knowledge Base from Web MD.
Toth, Wendy
2006 Sun Safety Net. Supermarket News 54(7):17.
U.S. Environmental Protection Agency
2001 The Burning Facts. Air and Radiation EPA430-F-01-015. : U.S. Environmental Protection Agency.
USA Technologies
2003 USA Technologies' Intelligent Vending(TM) Solution Chosen to Enable Vending of Banana Boat Suncare Products. PRNewswire, September 11.
USPSTF (United States Preventive Services Task Force)
1996 Guide to Clinical Preventive Services, 2nd ed. Report of the U.S. Preventive Services Task Force. Baltimore: Williams and Wilkins.
Walter, Stephen, Loraine Marrett, Harry Shannon, Lynn From, and Clyde Hertzman
1992 The Association of Cutaneous Malignant Melanoma and Fluorescent Light Exposure. American Journal of Epidemiology 135(7):749–762.
Weinstock, Martin
2001 Sunscreen Use Can Reduce Melanoma Risk. Photodermatology, Photoimmunology, Photomedicine 17:234–236.

CHAPTER SIX

BUILDING WITH POISON
Toxicity and CCA-Treated Lumber

Terence Love

Chromated Copper Arsenate (CCA) treatment is the most widely used wood preservative (Nico et al. 2005). Like all wood preservatives, it is toxic. Arsenic is its main constituent and is particularly harmful to humans as a poison and a carcinogen (ATSDR 2005). Nonetheless, CCA-treated lumber is used in picnic tables, decks, fences, patios, outdoor furniture, and building construction, uses that put humans in regular close proximity to this product. CCA-treated lumber is known to cause health risks for children and adults in their home, work, and leisure environments (EPA 2006b; HBN 2001a; Sharp et al. 2001).

There is a well-documented history of the increasing use of CCA-treated lumber in the public realm and its recent fall from grace because of citizen pressure. Comprehensive sources of references are available from Bancca (2005), Beder (2003), the Environmental Research Foundation (2006), particularly two articles by Steingraber (2004a; 2004b), the U.S. Consumer Products Safety Commission (CPSC 2006), the Environmental Protection Agency (EPA 2006a), the Healthy Building Network (HBN 2001b), Lansbury Hall and Beder (2005), and the Bad Developers website (Bad Developers 2005).

Taken together, the picture that emerges from the very large number of documents available about CCA-treated lumber and its problems is its similarity to many other killer commodities. Ultimately, the marketing of CCA-treated lumber was, like many other killer commodities, driven by greed. Managers in lumber preservation and retailing exhibited business callousness as they ignored health risks to the public and workers in favor of maximizing profits. Safer alternatives to CCA-preservative treatment are available, but are more costly and thus are less attractive to manufacturers, constructors, and retailers (Cookson 2005; Freeman et al. 2003).

It is clear, in the United States at least, that CCA-treatment businesses and retailers were aware of the adverse health effects of CCA-treated lumber since the 1970s (McArdle 2002; Prager 2003). This information was likely to be widespread through the industry. The industry mainly comprises a small number of multinationals such as Osmose and Koppers-Arch that are in close communication (Rebstock 2006), with industry members tightly linked through highly active national wood preservation associations such as the American Wood Preservers Association (AWPA 2006); the Western European Institute for Wood Preservation (WEI-IEO 2006); the Canadian Institute of Treated Wood (2006), which is closely related to the Canadian Forest Network (n.d.); and the Timber Preservers Association of Australia (TPAA 2006).

Regulators long resisted public concern about CCA-treated lumber until public pressure reached the media and citizen-driven lawsuits began to impact manufacturers directly (Beder 2003; McArdle 2002; Steingraber 2004a). In the three countries that dominate CCA-treated timber use, the United States, Australia, and New Zealand, the response was half-hearted. Recent take up of the public concerns by the media, with public airing of the adverse effects and risks, together with increasing success of litigation has pressured regulators and CCA-treated lumber manufacturers and retailers into making tentative steps to improve their image. Initially, this comprised an arrangement to make consumer health and safety information available from retailers and more recently resulted in a voluntary halt in production of CCA-treated lumber for domestic use and public use in situations in which the public might unknowingly be contaminated. This voluntary cessation of production has occurred in the United States (since 2004) and Australia (since early 2006). The agreement allows for the sale of existing retail stocks and so toxic CCA-treated lumber potentially remains available in many depots.

This chapter uses the lens of *path dependence* to reveal a deeper understanding of the way CCA-treated lumber became so widely established in built environments and so weakly regulated. Path dependence provides a tool for understanding how historical factors shape the design and uptake of new products. The use of path dependence analysis reveals how the use of CCA-treated lumber as a replacement material influenced its application in the *design* and uptake of other products such that its use increased significantly.

This chapter has five parts:

- Section one provides an overview of the chapter.
- Section two describes CCA-treated lumber and its dual role both as a product and as a component of other products, outlines its health and safety problems, and the history of industry-driven misinformation and weak regulation that lead to the ongoing use of CCA-treated lumber in situations that compromise public health.
- Section three uses path dependence to discover insights into the uptake of CCA-treated lumber in preference to less toxic solutions, particularly in the ways that designers, constructors, and users subconsciously came to use toxic CCA-treated timber as if it were nontoxic.
- Section four reviews the liability issues.
- Section five describes how and why a different health and safety approach is needed for this class of killer commodity that has a dual role as a product and as a component of other products. This section also points to the range of agencies with potential roles in health and safety management of CCA-treated lumber and similar types of products.

To recap, this chapter goes beyond a historical analysis of the failure of the health and safety regulation regime of CCA-treated lumber. It reviews misinformation techniques used by manufacturers and retailers of CCA-treated lumber to maximize their sales and minimize regulatory action. These outcomes were at the expense of public health, particularly of children, the environment, and workers' occupational safety. This chapter describes how path-dependent factors influenced design and construction processes in ways that extended the application of CCA-treated timber beyond simple product substitution. Several examples show mechanisms that unhelpfully commodified CCA-treated lumber in other areas of the built environment. The chapter concludes by pointing to the need for a different way of understanding and regulating killer commodities such as CCA-treated lumber.

Overview of CCA-Treated Lumber

The technique of CCA treatment of lumber was developed in 1933 by an Indian scientist, Dr. Sonti Kamesam, to preserve structural lumber supports in mines (Cooper 1999; Steingraber 2004a). His breakthrough was to combine the arsenic and copper compounds used as preservatives in the pressure treatment of wood with chromium to bind the arsenic and copper to the wood cells and reduce leaching (Cooper 1999; Rahman et al. 2004). All three of these constituents are toxic to humans. The element of main concern to human health is the arsenic, which is toxic in very small quantities and carcinogenic at low doses.

The emergence of CCA-treated lumber as a killer commodity resulted from repurposing this lifesaving breakthrough in mining engineering as a product for use by designers and constructors in the public realm. CCA-treated lumber was initially sold as an inexpensive substitute for hardwoods that were intrinsically resistant to borers and mold. After the 1970s, however, domestic and public use of CCA-treated lumber expanded dramatically when its profit advantages were recognized by wood-preserver businesses, architects and designers, building constructors, and manufacturers producing outdoor timber items such as play sets, picnic tables and benches, and garden furniture.

CCA-treated lumber looks very similar to other lumber; green or yellow tinted or occasionally dyed brown. When weathered, CCA-treated lumber often appears *identical* in appearance to other softwood. CCA-treated lumber can be effortlessly cut, drilled, nailed, bolted, and jointed with conventional woodworking tools in a similar manner to any other softwood. Typically, CCA-treated lumber is cut to section before being pressure-treated with the CCA-preservative chemicals and is available in round logs and common building construction sections. CCA-treated lumber can be found in almost any structure that is made of wood that requires protecting from fungal, bacterial, or borer attack or the elements. It is widely used in the framing and cladding of houses, in children's play equipment, sheds, gazebos, pergolas, fences, and power poles. Unseen, and often unlabeled, its payload of toxic and carcinogenic arsenic, chromium, and cooper compounds is waiting to leach into the environment, to be removed from its surface by touch, or ingested in some other way. If CCA-treated lumber is used, for example, in building a deck on the back of a home, even if the original owner is aware that it is constructed of CCA-treated lumber, subsequent buyers are not likely to know and would treat the desk as if regular, safe lumber were used.

History of Use

By the 1960s, CCA-treated lumber was in use internationally in a variety of domestic indoor and outdoor settings, such as picnic tables, decks, playgrounds, structural lumber in buildings, and as wood cladding. In the mid-1970s, Germany banned the use of CCA-treated lumber. During the 1980s, demand for CCA-treated lumber soared. Around 14.5 million cubic meters of CCA-treated lumber were manufactured in the United States each year (Clausen 2003; Freeman et al. 2003; Nico et al. 2005). Projected to 2015, the disposal rates are expected to be about the same (Cooper 1999). Currently in the United States, there are estimated to be 300,000 tons of arsenic in circulation in CCA-treated lumber (Nico et al. 2005) comprising around 90 percent of the United States' annual use of arsenic (CPSC 2006).

As CCA-treated timber has accumulated in the public environment, there have emerged increasing health and safety concerns. These have centered on health effects on workers in manufacturing, the risks of burning CCA-treated lumber (e.g., in disposing of waste), and the risks to children playing on or around CCA-treated playgrounds and other outdoor structures. During this time, the CCA-treated wood industry and government health and safety organizations avoided controlling the use of CCA-treated lumber and instead attempted to transfer the responsibility for safe use of CCA-treated lumber to the public and small-scale businesses by making available consumer health and safety information sheets at retailers. In the 1990s, through the efforts of individuals and consumer groups, there emerged increased evidence about the severity of arsenic contamination and an awareness that the safety information program had failed (Sharp et al. 2001). These factors together with the difficulties in distinguishing between CCA-treated wood and normal wood deeply compromised health and safety management of CCA-treated wood. Following behind-the-scenes negotiations, producers of CCA-treated lumber in countries such as the United States and Australia voluntarily halted production for use in domestic situations. CCA-treated lumber is still produced for industrial, marine, and rural purposes and is still used in urban public environments.

Health Concerns

The arsenic, copper, and chromium that are the basis of the CCA-treatment process are significantly hazardous to health through a variety of ingesting and absorption mechanisms and activities. The CCA poisons that are pressure-injected into the lumber in the CCA-treatment process remain toxic for the lifetime of the wood and do not readily decay in the environment. Arsenic is the main focus of concern. The CCA poisons can contaminate adults and children, land, water, and air through a wide variety of routes. They can be absorbed from CCA-treated lumber by direct contact with the skin; from touching lumber and mouthing (i.e., touching lumber and then putting hands in one's mouth, touching lumber and handling food or other items that are put in the mouth such as cigarettes, and chewing the lumber—important in the case of children); direct contact between food and the CCA-treated lumber, for example by using CCA-treated lumber as tables, chopping boards, or food containers; through eating or breathing CCA-treated lumber dust from manufacturing or construction processes, involving, for example, sawing or sanding CCA-treated lumber; from splinters of CCA-treated lumber; from drinking water that has passed over CCA-treated lumber, such as runoff; from the fumes and smoke from burning CCA-treated lumber; from the ashes of burned CCA-treated lumber; and by breathing, touching, or absorbing by other means such as eating food grown in soil that has been contaminated by CCA-treated lumber leachate or ash residues.

In children's play equipment, the easy access to arsenic is particularly significant because children are sensitive to poisons developmentally. Children touch the CCA-treated lumber equipment and absorb the poisons directly through their skin, or ingest the poisons from licking their hands, handling food, or through playing in soil or in the barrier compounds that are under play equipment to reduce accidents from falls. The soil near CCA-treated wooden play equipment becomes contaminated via rainwater runoff that has leached arsenic, chromium, and copper from the CCA-treated lumber. In some cases, the ground covering in play areas comprises mulch made from chippings of waste CCA-treated lumber. Concern about these issues has been central to the increasing regulation of CCA-treated lumber (ATSDR 2005; Beder 2003; CPSC 2003; Lewis and Heeringa 2004; Natali et al. 2003; Nico et al. 2005; Sharp et al. 2001).

The carcinogenic effects of arsenic from CCA-treated lumber are only evident after a period of time (CPSC 2003). Arsenic is associated with multiple physical consequences and hence, immediate neurological and physiological toxic consequences, particularly to children, can be masked or attributed to other events (Lansbury Hall and Beder n.d.-b) such as childhood diseases or behavioral problems.

Commercial Greed, Misinforming Consumers, and Unethical Behavior

The history of the promotion of CCA-treated timber and its regulation is a story of greed in the wood industry.

Five factors characterize CCA-treated lumber as a killer commodity. The way these factors have been managed were influenced by greed and are indicative of poor business ethics and lack of due care required of all parties in the manufacturing and regulation chain.

The CCA-preservative treatment was known at the outset to be poisonous and carcinogenic. It contains arsenic, chromium, and copper and wood treated with it can poison adults and children via direct contact, via leaching, from cutting it, or from fumes or ash from burning it. The potential adverse health consequences are serious. They involve acute and chronic poisoning, neurological damage, and cancer. The effects can be fatal in the long- and short-term. For example, children playing on CCA-treated lumber play sets may in two weeks of play absorb sufficient arsenic to exceed their lifetime cancer risk levels (Sharp and Walker 2001).

Second, CCA-treated lumber is indistinguishable in most cases from untreated, safe lumber, especially when weathered. For normal lumber, all of the above activities are regarded as unproblematic in health terms. Those manufacturing and retailing CCA-treated timber were clearly aware that toxic CCA-treated lumber was almost indistinguishable in appearance from untreated lumber. In fact, this was used as a selling point in terms of its application in outdoor settings. The lack of a distinguishing appearance from normal wood reduced consumers' purchasing resistance by reducing their potential awareness of its toxicity.

Third, it was self-evident to manufacturers, regulators, and constructors that health and safety advice was not resulting in widespread awareness of the toxicity of CCA-treated lumber (Sharp et al. 2001). It could be readily observed that essential safety practices were not widely used by those interacting with CCA-treated timber or its poisonous residues.

Four, CCA-treatment plant managers and CCA-treated lumber retailers used misinformation and marketing sleights of hand to reduce consumers' and workers' awareness of health risks and essential safety practices that might reduce sales. This compromised the risks to consumers and workers. Manufacturers resisted regulation and the distribution of information about adverse health effects and necessary safety procedures. There was an initial refusal by manufacturers and retailers to label CCA-treated lumber. As a compromise, manufacturers were pressured by government agencies into making available consumer safety information brochures at retailers (Bancca 2004; Lansbury Hall and Beder n.d.-a; Sharp et al. 2001). In reality, however, these safety brochures were rarely made available and attention was not drawn to them by manufacturers or retailers (Lansbury Hall and Beder 2005; Sharp et al. 2001). Worse, these consumer data sheets were carefully worded to minimize concern, portraying CCA-treated timber as safe, as identical to using ordinary lumber, and encouraging its use in situations cautioned against by authorities such as the EPA and contradicting the information provided in Materials Safety Data Sheets provided by the Occupational Health and Safety Adminstration (Sharp et al. 2001). A parallel means of disinformation was the renaming of CCA-treated lumber as "salt-treated" or "pressure-treated" wood or using new names such as "LifeWood" to make it appear to be a different product from that containing arsenic and to direct attention away from its poisonous nature. More disingenuously for consumers, retail lumber sales personnel, perhaps through poor training, often misinformed the public of the risks of CCA-treated lumber, sometimes claiming that there was no risk, that the CCA-treated timber didn't contain arsenic, or that it was a different product (Lansbury Hall and Beder n.d.-a). These practices were widespread; for example, one of the larger CCA-treatment companies, Osmose, was accused of intentionally misleading customers that CCA-treated lumber is similar to ordinary wood; of avoiding to inform customers that the wood contains arsenic; of being aware that workers had been injured, and more workers were likely to become injured, but not informing the U.S. Environmental Protection Agency (EPA); of withholding information from consumers that CCA-treated wood is toxic when burned; and of intentionally delaying the start of the customer safety information program (Natali et al. 2003).

Five, the use of CCA-treated lumber has become ubiquitous as a key design element in public space, outdoor settings, and building construction. Wood in most outdoor settings from around 1970 is likely to be CCA-treated. This marks a difference in exposure to risk compared to other pathways for arsenic contamination of humans. For example, only about 10 percent of water supplies in the United States reach the safety limits set for arsenic, yet most American children play on arsenic-treated lumber from which they potentially get much larger doses than they would through drinking the water (Sharp and Walker 2001).

The CCA-wood-treatment industry's response to these issues has been less than ethical. They operated to maximize sales of a product by whatever means regardless of the fact that it exposed direct users and bystanders to health risks whilst keeping from them the knowledge that they were at risk or that they were being poisoned.

This unethical approach to business seems to be characteristic of the CCA-treated-lumber industry. Members of the industry were, in 2005, also charged with cartel price fixing and misleading government investigation agencies by conducting a deliberate strategy of withholding documents, removing them from company premises, and storing them in a secret location (Rebstock 2006).

Regulation Issues

The regulation issues relating to CCA-treated lumber are typical of a product that requires carefully managed health and safety procedures. Yet CCA-treated lumber has become a *commodity* of the built environment: an environment relatively difficult to control in health and safety terms. The process by which CCA-treated lumber becomes part of families' lives and is used in public situations as decks, fences, play equipment, and power poles comprises mainly small subcontractors (joiners and small workshops), small businesses, and individuals using CCA-treated lumber at home. Partly as a result of the misinformation strategies of CCA-treatment businesses, CCA-treated lumber has been widely used in ways that routinely expose people and children to toxic and carcinogenic doses of arsenic (McArdle 2002; CPSC 2006).

When CCA-based lumber preservative treatment was originally submitted for permits for manufacture and sale, it was well known that CCA treatment comprised high loads of toxic compounds and understood that care would be needed to avoid long- and short-term health problems adversely impacting those producing it, manufacturing items with it, using it directly, or being indirectly affected. The differences in use between CCA-treated lumber and any other softwood are the additional health and safety precautions needed to protect the health of those involved in the construction, those using the CCA-treated products, and those incidentally and perhaps unknowingly potentially exposed to toxins from CCA-treated lumber either in the construction processes or later. The EPA, for example, requires workers to be provided with Material Safety Data Sheets and advises consumers of a range of precautions (EPA 2005). Official safety advice is that "CCA-treated lumber is safe to use, so long as *all* [emphasis added] safety precautions are followed" (Cookson 2005).

There is another story. CCA-treated lumber belongs to the class of killer commodities that has two aspects: as a product in its own right and as a component of other products. This dual purpose of CCA-treated lumber results in its having multiple roles as a killer commodity across multiple product life cycles. The analyses presented later suggest that regulators and commercial enterprises have ignored the complexity and taken an oversimplistic view of CCA-treated lumber in human environments.

This simplistic view ignores the path-dependent influences increasing the uptake of CCA-treated timber that are due to traditional historical use of wood and wood-related technologies. In effect, this view has compromised health and safety. By taking an oversimplistic view of the factors shaping CCA-treated timber use, those producing CCA-treated lumber, constructing products from it, and regulating it have gained commercial advantage and reduced their health and safety costs by avoiding addressing difficult issues relating to regulation of the design of products, contamination management, safe-use practices, and whole of life disposal issues across multiple different product life cycles.

Until the "voluntary" reduction in CCA treatment by manufacturers, it was clear to many individuals and consumer groups that the regulatory approaches that have been used had failed to act in the public's interest. Significant regulatory problems remain in relation to the disposal of the very large amount of CCA-treated lumber in use worldwide (Beder 2003; Florida Center for Solid and Hazardous Waste Management and Florida Department of Environmental Protection 2005; Lansbury Hall and Beder n.d.-b). Disposal levels of all forms of CCA-treated waste are expected to increase, peaking around 2013 at about half maximum production levels before leveling out in 2035 at around 30 percent of maximum production (Liebowitz and Margolis 1995; Puffert 2008; Wikipedia contributors 2006). CCA-treated lumber presents difficult regulatory problems because it is a high-bulk waste stream with high potential for contamination of groundwater through leachate. In Australia, there is a specific problem in disposing of the millions of vine stakes used in the wine and horticultural industries (Perry n.d.).

Systemically, the health and safety regulation processes guaranteeing safe use of CCA-treated lumber and products are intrinsically flawed by a combination of issues in which failure can occur at any point and single errors can result in multiple failures of health and safety. For example, cutting a piece of CCA-treated lumber results in lumber pieces being without safety labels because the same label cannot easily be shared amongst multiple pieces. The problem of managing sawdust is an extension of the same problem. Both result in failures of the safety process downstream that requires users to know that the lumber is toxic. Success of the public safety awareness programs undertaken in the 1980s and 1990s depended on thousands of stores and businesses worldwide guaranteeing to provide those buying CCA-treated lumber with the necessary safety information and equipment. In parallel, appropriate health and safety information needed to be supplied to thousands of architects, designers, and contract and production managers to ensure that CCA-treated timber was specified correctly. In addition, information about the toxicity of CCA-treated timber structures needed to be provided to all who might directly or indirectly be exposed to toxic risks from them. In the case of playground equipment and structures on which children might play, this includes parents and future owners. For health and safety, it is necessary that all of these people must understand this information about managing the risks of CCA-treated lumber and act on it. This kind of process, in systemic terms, is one that is unlikely to be successful. It requires information to be passed down the line with each piece of CCA-treated lumber, its products, and its CCA-treated waste across ownership boundaries and over decades. This is a system that can break down at multiple points, and failure is especially likely because of the potential financial benefit to CCA-treatment businesses and retailers from avoiding providing safety information that might reduce sales. Taking a systemic perspective, there appears to be no obvious way to improve the current health and safety approach for CCA-treated lumber that is likely to make them intrinsically more successful.

Path Dependence and Design Issues: How CCA-Treated Lumber Became Preferred and Health and Safety Issues Were Ignored

The uptake of CCA-treated lumber can be superficially explained on the grounds that it was relatively cheap and that some organizations repressed the availability of information about the health and safety risks. This does not, however, adequately explain the complexity of the situation in which practical information about the toxicity of CCA-treatment *was* available, although intermittently, to professionals in design, manufacturing, and construction (as well as users) and in spite of this, CCA-treated lumber was widely used in ways that then and now are regarded as inappropriate. What is needed is an approach that reveals the reasons why this happened because it offers a basis for designing better health and safety regulations for this type of toxic product.

Path-dependence analysis offers an approach to understanding the complexity of why CCA-treated lumber became so popular in spite of health and safety warnings. The concept of path dependence emerged from economics (Liebowitz and Margolis 1995; Magnusson and Ottosson 1997; Puffert 2008) and is used to analyze situations such as that of CCA-treated lumber where the history of use of other products (in this case, normal wood) shapes the uptake and regulation of the new product in the ways described by, for example, Beder (2003), Steingraber (2004a), Wilson (2005), and McArdle (2002).

The concept of path dependence provides insight into how choices about technology, designed products, decisions, cultures, and human traditions strongly depend on earlier technology. For example, the early development of malleable metals (bronze and iron) facilitated the development of containers and pans in which food could be made edible or more palatable through cooking in liquid over a fire. This history of early metal development provided the path-dependent basis for the rich, complex culture of cooking technologies today.

Path dependency is particularly significant in a situation such as the introduction of CCA-treated lumber where there are positive or negative feedback loops of factors influencing the product's uptake and health and safety regulation. The following example demonstrates how path-dependence factors influence the uptake of a word-processing product.

Example: Path Dependence and Word-Processing Software

Path-dependent factors influence an individual's choice of new word-processing software. A significant path-dependent factor is the benefit to be gained from choosing a make of word-processing software that will allow easy file exchange with other people. Another path-dependent issue is guessing the software most likely to be used by others in the future. Knowing which word-processing software has been most commonly used in the past offers benefits in choosing the best technology for the future. Path-dependent factors produce strong positive feedback effects by which existing patterns of use of particular software can strongly shape consumers' choices toward a single product in the future regardless of other qualities of that product. The new product need not be the best, safest, cheapest, or whatever. It is likely to become the preferred option on the basis of the proportion of people in the past using it or something similar. In information technology this aspect of path dependence is sometimes called *network effect*.

Another, slightly bizarre, example of path dependence is the way the size of the rear quarters of horses of Roman chariots in England affected the size of the American space shuttle. The reasoning goes as follows. The width of the rear quarters of the horses dictated the width of Roman chariots. The Romans built many roads in England and chariot width determined road width. In turn, this dictated the wheel track of later carts. In time, the width of UK rail track was based on these carts because similar tooling was used. U.S. rail networks used similar track widths because they drew on the experiences of UK engineers, and this in turn influenced the dimensions of rail carriages and the diameters of U.S. rail tunnels. Now, the maximum size of space shuttle booster rockets is limited because they have to be shipped from their manufacturer, Thiokol, through rail tunnels to the launching site (Beder 2003; CPSC 2006). Thus, surprisingly, there exists a path-dependent relationship between the size of the rear quarters of early Roman military horses and the space shuttle. Perhaps if the Romans had used elephants, England's streets would not be so narrow!

In a similar path-dependent manner, the rapid uptake of CCA-treated lumber in human-built environments depended, in a complex and variegated way, on tools and technologies previously used for wood-based building construction, along with a large amount of largely tacit human knowledge, understanding, expectations, and values imbued in individuals because of their prior woodworking experiences.

In turn, the initial uptake of CCA-treated lumber in the built environment provided a path-dependent influence that shaped the designs of the built environment in ways that would be likely to use CCA-treated lumber. It did this because of the tacit and, by manufacturers and retailers, explicit associations with normal wood and the tools and techniques of wood-based construction. Path-dependency analysis suggests the decision making of designers, constructors, users, and regulators was likely to be strongly shaped by path-dependent factors in which CCA-treated lumber was seen as simply another kind of wood, in ways that overshadowed concerns about health, safety, and managing the toxic and carcinogenic issues of CCA-treated lumber because normal wood was considered safe. The knowledge, judgment, and confidence of designers, constructors, users, regulators, and decision makers is explicitly and implicitly dependent on the success and failure of prior technologies—in this case, normal, safe wood—and CCA-treated timber manufacturers and retailers strongly encouraged these groups to regard CCA-treated lumber as no different from ordinary lumber except for its functional advantages.

CCA-treated lumber is used in several ways that were all adopted ignoring its toxicity to humans. At its simplest, CCA-treated lumber *substitutes directly* in products made from normal untreated lumber where normal lumber is functionally less effective or economically more costly. This was facilitated in two ways. CCA-treated lumber is softwood, usually pine. CCA-treated softwood products also substitute for expensive hardwood lumber whose protection against attack by fungi or borers is from naturally occurring preservative factors. In this case, CCA-treated lumber substitutes for the alternative product because softwood is easier to work with than hardwoods, and because, in most cases, it is cheaper than hardwoods of an equivalent resistance to attack and deterioration. Secondly, it substitutes for other softwood products. Where costs associated with managing health and safety issues are ignored, CCA-treated softwood has been priced to be more economically viable because it does not require replacement so often.

More significantly, the uptake of CCA-treated lumber increased because the early uses of CCA-treated lumber influenced the future design of the built environment in and around homes and in public spaces to include more CCA-treated lumber via new product niches and the substitution for other products and materials. This design-based increased adoption of CCA-treated lumber into new situations was in part due to its cost advantages of simple substitution (if health and safety costs are ignored) and in part because of its path-dependent connection with traditional wood construction methods (hammers, nails, drills, bolts, chisels, screws, joints, etc.). By using CCA-treated lumber in key structural components, for example, path-dependent aspects of building construction encouraged the use of CCA-treated lumber in nearby elements because it made joining building components easier or because it used the same tools or skills as construction in normal wood. This influence on the design of nearby components is especially evident where CCA-treated lumber elements adjoin other structures. Extending the use of CCA-treated lumber across a boundary into an adjoining structure, or building connecting structures using CCA-treated timber, is often a simpler and cheaper way of solving joining problems. The examples below illustrate this in relation to fencing and other outdoor structures.

Example: Path-Dependent Aspects of the Use of CCA-Treated Lumber in Fences

The use of CCA-treated lumber for fences has substantially replaced other technologies, such as steel and concrete, which are less toxic. In post and infill forms of fence construction, the use of CCA-treated lumber for in-ground structural posts offers benefits because it is cheap and easy to cut to size on-site (typically, the toxic wood dust is allowed to blow into the nearby environment and contaminate soil). The use of CCA-treated lumber for in-ground posts encourages the use of CCA-treated lumber for infill panels because they can be easily joined to the posts and because tradepersons building fences can use the same tool set and woodworking technologies for posts and infill panels. Where CCA-treated lumber (perhaps chosen on the grounds of cost) offers advantages for the structural posts then path-dependent factors result in CCA-treated lumber almost completely displacing other fence forms, such as continuous cement fiber sheet fencing and traditional forms of nonwood fences. This occurs regardless of issues of toxicity and environmental harm because in path-dependent terms, safety-wise, CCA-treated lumber has become subconsciously regarded as normal, safe lumber.

Example: Path-Dependent Influences on the Design of Outdoor Furniture and Structures

CCA-treated lumber, as logs, has become commonly used as simple post or post-and-rail barrier fencing in public open spaces that contain informal picnic shelters, tables, and benches. Having used CCA-treated lumber for the fencing, similar path-dependent factors relating to tools and construction techniques encourage the use of CCA-treated lumber for the construction of the picnic shelters and tables. The path-dependent effects occur in the ways that the same construction team can use the same tools and construction techniques for building the fence, tables, and picnic shelters with similar technology of jointing, bolting, and trimming; using the same power tools and fasteners; and with the benefits of economies of scale—more CCA lumber can be bought at one time, thus reducing unit price. An additional path-dependent factor is this: additional use of CCA-treated lumber maintains an aesthetic tradition in that a similarity of style and appearance is maintained. This use of CCA-treated lumber for fencing and outdoor furniture is a relatively common scenario in spite of extensive warnings worldwide that CCA-treated lumber should not be used in environments associated with eating and children's play because of the high toxic and carcinogenetic risks associated with touching the lumber in situations that might involve handling food or hand-to-mouth contact. The health risks are even more serious as in many picnic areas there are no hand-washing facilities. Again, the path-dependent factors act because manufacturers and retails have encouraged others to regard CCA-treated lumber as if it were normal, safe wood, without taking into account that it is a different product with significant health and safety risks and costs.

Another way CCA-treated lumber has influenced the design of human-built environments is in situations in which other materials have been used because normal lumber would not have functioned satisfactorily. In these conditions, the poisonous footprint of CCA treatment is extended by the use of CCA-treated lumber in scenarios that otherwise would have used products and constructions made of less toxic materials such as steel, concrete, or masonry. The above fence example also shows this.

Example: CCA-Treated Lumber as the Basis for Increased Use of "Pole-House" Construction

CCA-treated lumber has enabled the economic building of "pole homes" on difficult sloping sites. Steeply sloping sites typically require major earthworks and retaining walls to provide a flat surface for building a conventional house. These are expensive but normally nontoxic construction methods. The use of CCA-treated poles and lumber offers designers and constructors opportunities for a new design approach to accommodate differences in slope and levels that reduces the cost of site works (again assuming health and safety costs are not included). In effect, CCA-treated lumber has created a new economic building construction niche. Again, the influences on designers' and builders' attitudes require that CCA-treated lumber is assumed to be similar to normal, safe wood in ways that allow them to ignore the health risks and the potential liabilities from people's exposure to arsenic from the CCA treatment of the wood.

Another path-dependent reason CCA-treated lumber has become widely used in outdoor settings is aesthetic: with its coloring, it looks like normal wood. The slight green and yellow tint of CCA-treated lumber fits aesthetically with its use in gardens and outdoor environments and gives an impression that it is environmentally friendly and nontoxic. This aesthetic association can trigger path-dependent behaviors and decision making based on earlier knowledge about normal, safe wood and leads users and less technically aware manufacturers to believe it has identical properties to ordinary wood and to behave toward CCA-treated lumber as if it were nontoxic. These path-dependent background processes result in lack of awareness of the differences in health and safety precautions and the use CCA-treated lumber in situations in which CCA-treated wood is inappropriate.

Liability Consequences

CCA-treated lumber provides a strong contemporary and well-documented example of a health and safety failure of a product of well-known toxic effects being used in a variety of products.

The scale of adverse health outcomes due to the use of CCA-treated timber is potentially of the same order as those associated with asbestos. Many of the characteristics of the CCA industry, its products, and their use replicate in structure and toxicity the asbestos debacle as described in the introduction of this volume. In terms of product development, health and safety issues, and liabilities, there are many characteristic similarities between CCA-treated lumber and asbestos (Steingraber 2004a):

- Both cause adverse health effects in their basic material form.
- Both have a primary role as constituents of other products in which their health and safety problems remain active.
- Both are problematic in health and safety terms over a long period.
- Both have significant disposal problems.

- The scale of use of both commodities is extensive and potentially affects very large numbers of people.
- Both have a substantial amount of their final production undertaken by small businesses in the relatively informal working environment at the fringe of the construction industry. These businesses are characterized by a lack of resources to enable or support sound health and safety practices in relation to CCA-treated lumber.

The history of production and use of CCA-treated lumber provides strong potential for future litigation by individuals and by class actions when it is possible to establish ill health was caused by exposure to CCA-treated lumber (Natali et al. 2003). It might be expected in time, therefore, that costs and liabilities associated with CCA-treated lumber may reflect those of current and future asbestos claims. To give an idea of the scale of the problem, in Australia, one of the manufacturers of asbestos products, James Hardie Products, on 1 December 2005, agreed to set aside $4.5 billion for future compensation (Wilson 2005).

At this stage, research in the United States has estimated a range of increased risks of bladder and lung cancer in later life for children exposed to CCA-treated playgrounds and decks. The U.S. Consumer Product Safety Commission (CPSC) estimates that children who play regularly on CCA-treated playground equipment have an increased lung or bladder cancer risk of between two and 100 times the one-in-a-million chance of cancer over a lifetime that CPSC regards as the level for regulatory action (Beder 2003; CPSC 2006). Other liabilities associated with CCA-treated timber exist for anyone having contact with the CCA components either by direct contact with the treated wood or by indirect contact via leachate, ash, smoke, sawdust, and so forth. An additional significant long-term life-cycle risk and potential liability exists because of uncertainties about disposal processes for CCA-treated timber (Clausen 2003; Lansbury Hall and Beder n.d.-b). Currently, CCA-treated lumber is exempt from a hazardous classification, although this remains a relative anomaly (Clausen 2003). This results in potential for liability through arsenic contamination of soil and groundwater via leachate.

Potentially, risk of litigation impacts on a wide range of parties (Beder 2003; McArdle 2002; Natali et al. 2003). Local governments and government and education departments responsible for public health and management of building control, especially of the use of CCA-treated timber in public spaces, may find they are subject to liability for adverse consequences where, for example, playgrounds, picnic areas, and decks open to the public were permitted to be made with CCA-treated lumber. This risk of litigation particularly applies to places where children play or food is consumed.

In the commercial arena, liability may affect shopping center shop owners and shopping center management where CCA-treated lumber has been used in ways that expose the public to risk. Public and private utilities may find themselves liable for adverse impacts where CCA-treated lumber is used in the reticulation of power and other services, and as fencing in places accessible to the public. In the housing arena, potential litigation is possible against a range of parties: those building houses, those extending and repairing houses, and constructors building garden outdoor furniture and other structures such as sheds and fences. For house owners and landowners, there is potential litigation that arises with respect to visitors and family members. For those selling property, it might be expected that the existence of CCA-treated lumber requires disclosure. Business and industry also is subject to potential claims from employees and subcontractors where full health and safety practices relating to CCA-treated lumber, including labeling, information provision, and job training, have not been maintained. Public and private refuse disposal operators may have a significant liability where it can be demonstrated that they did not manage the CCA-treated lumber refuse stream in a manner which guaranteed that CCA lumber was separated and dealt with appropriately. Clear liability exists, for example, in cases such as refuse recycling depots where CCA-treated lumber has been supplied to the public as firewood.

Underlying many of these liability pathways is the problem that an owner or manager may know that a structure is made with CCA-treated lumber but fails to inform those likely to use it. This is of particular significance in the sale of houses where the new owner should be informed of the potentially toxic risks.

In summary, the nature of the processes for healthy, safe management of CCA-treated toxic lumber is directly echoed in the liability pathways.

CCA-treated lumber is a material that requires ongoing health and safety control in all stages in its life cycle through management of its design, manufacture, and use in a range of products to its eventual disposal and remediation. Liability exists at all stages and for all involved parties.

Health and safety management strategies that rely on safety information being passed hierarchically through the supply chain or which transfer responsibility for safe use to consumers have failed. Consequently, this failure has resulted in the potential for widespread health problems, liability, and litigation.

Clearly, a different type of health and safety process and regulatory regime is needed to manage the safe use of CCA-treated lumber.

Conclusion: A New Perspective Is Needed

In summary, this chapter has:

- Described CCA-treated lumber and outlined its health and safety problems.
- Described the history of misinformation and regulation that led to the continuing use of CCA-treated lumber in ways that compromise public health.
- Used path dependence to gain insights into why CCA-treated lumber was preferred over less-toxic solutions.
- Explored the liability issues.

What emerged is a more general understanding of how CCA-treated lumber and similar killer commodity products, such as asbestos, differ from other types of killer commodities. Their complex health and safety issues emerge from their dual roles as toxic materials both in their basic form (CCA-treated lumber) and as constituents of multiple consumer products and technologies. This dual role presents problems in applying a simple approach to health and safety policies and practices across all commodity life paths, complex multiple supply chains, complex-use scenarios, and complex and difficult disposal routes. Different health and safety regimes and responsibilities may apply at different points of the life cycles of different products made from these killer commodities. More important, safe use requires that safety procedures be fully implemented at every stage.

Path-dependence analysis indicates that the prior existence of apparently similar material and technologies (in this case, natural wood and wood-based construction) creates a strong preference for the use of the killer commodity over other, less-toxic design solutions. Path-dependent factors shape the views of designers, constructors, and users so that it seems unnatural not to use CCA-treated lumber in other contexts and lead them to ignore its toxic and carcinogenic risks. Their effect has been to increase the scope of use of CCA-treated lumber beyond simple substitution of natural wood.

In addition, the systemic characteristics of the CCA-treated lumber supply chain offer many opportunities for failure of health and safety regulation, especially in terms of the tension between the duties of businesses up and down the supply chain to maximize profits for shareholders, and the reduction in their profits associated with providing health and safety information and managing health and safety risks associated with CCA-treated lumber. Consequences of these obvious systemic problems are the failures in health and safety practices found in most areas of design, manufacture, and use of CCA-treated lumber products. The scale of use of CCA-treated timber is large, and the scale of contamination is extensive and affects most individuals in developed countries in which CCA-treated lumber is or has been in widespread use.

Taken together, the above problems indicate the current approach is inappropriate because it requires serially dependent health and safety regulation processes that rely on sophisticated knowledge, high standards of ethics, and behavioral vigilance by all involved throughout the product life cycle, along with a combination of undertaking intelligent, thoughtful, and skillful action; careful choices; propagation of information of adverse affects of the product; and complex supply chains. It suggests a different perspective on this type of killer commodity is needed.

In general there are three possible strategies:

- Increased application of the precautionary principle.
- Extending the formal health and safety regulation regime into areas of use.

- Unambiguous signaling that the product is different in order to confound path-dependent assumptions.

Increased application of the precautionary principle. This may be done via a regulatory regime that only approves products for sale when there is clear knowledge that they are safe for their intended use. Most CCA-treated lumber applications would violate this, and hence it is unlikely to be satisfactory, unless as a complete ban on CCA-treated lumber.

Extending the formal health and safety regulation regime into areas of use. It is unlikely that CCA-treated timber could ever be managed in this way because of the weaknesses in binding arsenic into the wood, the high toxicity and carcinogenicity of arsenic to humans, and the systems problems. This approach is better suited to situations in which the material from which other products are made is toxic but the toxicity is fully neutralized by the time it becomes a constituent of the consumer product. This was an original aim of CCA treatment, which proved not fully effective in practice. Many health and safety regulatory frameworks tightly control the use of base materials during the manufacturing process in which they are used before they are rendered safe for use by the public. An example of this is the chemical industry, in which dangerous chemicals are tightly controlled during manufacturing, and only products that do not have safety problems and are intrinsically safe for use by untrained users are released into the public realm.

Unambiguously signaling the product is different in order to confound path-dependent assumptions. One possibility is to make CCA- treated lumber an unusual color throughout, for example, combining the preservative treatment with a strong fluorescent orange dye that could not easily be removed. This would have five helpful effects. First, it would make it clear to manufacturers, users, and others that CCA-treated lumber is a different sort of product from natural wood. Second, it would provide a ready basis to identify CCA-treated lumber and provide a means of visual connection with literature on its stringent safety requirements. Third, it would discourage inappropriate use by breaking some path-dependent associations, particularly those associated with natural wood and its safe-to-handle properties. Four, it would provide a reason to add a thick coating to CCA-treated lumber, which is a recommended means of protecting users from contact with the toxic compounds. Five, it would provide a clear indicator of when safety coatings on CCA-treated lumber are breaking down and need renewal. The latter is a weakness of current proposals to coat CCA-treated lumber used in public situations with clear varnish. Varnish degrades and falls off lumber subject to sunlight and use, and as the appearance does not change significantly, it is not obvious when recoating is needed.

The insights gained from exploring pathways of health and safety failures in managing CCA-treated lumber indicate that single-point simple regulation of the sort that has been implemented in the past is unlikely to work because of the way that health and safety information must be handed down the line and that safe practices must be implemented at every stage of the life cycle. This suggests the need for a redundant multiagency health and safety approach requiring all involved to provide safety information, undertake safe practices, and be held liable for their actions. There are at least twenty-four constituencies on which safe use of this class of toxic products depends. Each plays an important role in successful health and safety regulation:

- material manufacturers
- advertising agencies
- national health and safety agencies
- professional manufacturing associations
- professional engineering bodies
- professional design/architecture bodies
- government research organizations
- consumer product safety agencies
- national environmental protection agencies
- state and local government public health agencies
- university research organizations
- insurance providers and associations
- design and engineering organizations
- legal organizations and associations
- unions
- small business development agencies
- businesses creating products
- "do-it-yourself" constructors
- users and owners
- trade protection agencies
- national competition and consumer protection agencies
- remediation/recycling agencies
- waste disposal organizations
- urban planning and building control agencies

The health and safety roles of most of the constituencies listed above are ignored by a simplistic regulation perspective on reducing health risks for CCA-treated lumber. Acting in concert, health and safety activities undertaken by all constituencies potentially offer a more robust approach to health-risk reduction for the classes of toxic killer commodities that include CCA-treated lumber.

In summary, this chapter has laid out the history of use and health and safety failure of CCA-treated lumber, and pointed to rich document resources collated by activists and scientists. The chapter has identified that a much more complex health and safety scenario is presented by killer commodities that are materials from which other products are made. The lens of path dependence was used in this chapter to provide a deeper understanding of how a killer commodity such as CCA-treated lumber expanded its role in the built environment beyond that of simple substitution, in spite of its constituents being well-known poisons and carcinogens. The chapter concludes by suggesting that the class of killer commodities that are both products in their own right and constituents of other products be regarded as different from the outset in health and safety terms. The analyses suggest that these commodities require health and safety assessment and regulation that take into account that they form part of multiple and complex supply and life-cycle chains and by path-dependent feedback can strongly influence and extend their uptake in ways that can overrule health and safety concerns and practices. Developing successful health and safety processes is likely to require involvement of a large number of agencies in creating a health and safety culture and environment appropriate to reducing health risks.

References

ATSDR (Agency for Toxic Substances and Disease Registry)
2005 ToxFAQs for Arsenic, vol. 2006. Washington, DC: Agency for Toxic Substances and Disease Registry.
AWPA (American Wood Preservers Association)
2006 American Wood-Preservers' Association, vol. 2006. Birmingham, AL: AWPA.
Bad Developers
2005 Toxic Timber, vol. 2006. N.a.: Bad Developers.
Bancca
2004 Timeline of Efforts to Ban CCA and Arsenic in Treated Wood Products. *In* CCA Treated Wood News. Gainesville, FL: Prager.
2005 Bancca.org. Gainesville, FL: Prager.

Beder, S.
2003 Timber Leachates Prompt Preservative Review. Engineers Australia 75(6):32–34.
Canadian Forest Network
N.d. Canadian Forest Network.
Canadian Institute of Treated Wood
2006 Canadian Institute of Treated Wood.
Clausen, C. A.
2003 Reusing Remediated CCA-Treated Wood. *In* Managing the Treated Wood Resource II. Allen M. Kenderes, ed. Madison: USDA Forest Products Laboratory.
Cookson, L.
2005 Safety of Timber Treated with CCA Preservative, vol. 2006. CSIRO.
Cooper, P. A.
1999 Future of Wood Preservation in Canada: Disposal Issues. *In* Proceedings of the 20th Annual Canadian Wood Preservation Association Conference, October 25–26. Vancouver, BC.
CPSC (Consumer Product Safety Commission)
2003 Fact Sheet. Chromated Copper Arsenate (CCA)-Treated Wood Used in Playground Equipment Part 1. Bethesda, MD: Consumer Product Safety Commission.
2006 Consumer Safety, vol. 2006. Bethesda, MD: Consumer Product Safety Commission.
Environmental Research Foundation
2006 Environmental Research Foundation, vol. 2006. New Brunswick, NJ: Environmental Research Foundation.
EPA (Environmental Protection Agency)
2005 Chromated Copper Arsenate (CCA): Consumer Safety Information Sheet: Inorganic Arsenical Pressure-Treated Wood. Washington, DC: U.S. Environmental Protection Agency.
2006a Chromated Copper Arsenate (CCA), vol. 2006. Washington, DC: Environmental Protection Agency.
2006b Chromated Copper Arsenate (CCA): Consumer Safety Information Sheet: Inorganic Arsenical Pressure-Treated Wood, vol. 2006. Washington, DC: Environmental Protection Agency.
Florida Center for Solid and Hazardous Waste Management, and Florida Department of Environmental Protection
2005 Guidance for the Management and Disposal of CCA-Treated Wood, vol. 2006. Tallahassee, FL: Florida Center for Solid and Hazardous Waste Management and Florida Department of Environmental Protection with assistance from the University of Florida

College of Engineering and University of Miami College of Engineering.

Freeman, M. H., T. F. Shupe, R. P. Vlosky, and H. M. Barnes
2003 Past, Present, and Future of the Wood Preservation Industry. Forest Products Journal 53(10):8–15.

HBN (Healthy Building Network)
2001a Fact Sheet. Arsenic Wood: Hazards and Alternatives. Washington, DC: Healthy Building Network.
2001b Pressure-Treated Wood. Washington, DC: Healthy Building Network.

Lansbury Hall, N., and S. Beder
2005 Treated Timber: Ticking Time-Bomb. The Need for a Precautionary Approach in the Use of Copper Chrome Arsenic (CCA) as a Timber Preservative, vol. 2006. Wollongong, New South Wales, Australia: University of Wollongong.
N.d.-a Treated Timber: Consumer Information, vol. 2006. Wollongong, New South Wales, Australia: S. Beder.
N.d.-b Waste Options, vol. 2006. Wollongong, New South Wales, Australia: S. Beder.

Lewis, P., and S. Heeringa
2003 FIFRA Scientific Advisory Panel meeting at the Sheraton Crystal City Hotel, Arlington, Virginia. December 3–5, 2003. A Set of Scientific Issues Being Considered by the Environmental Protection Agency Regarding: Draft Preliminary Probabilistic Exposure and Risk Assessment for Children Who Contact CCA-Treated Wood on Playsets and Decks and CCA-Containing Soil around These Structures, vol. 2006. Washington, DC: FIFRA SAP.

Liebowitz, S. J., and S. E. Margolis
1995 Path Dependence, Lock-In, and History. Journal of Law, Economics and Organization 11(1):205–226.

Magnusson, L., and J. Ottosson, eds.
1997 Evolutionary Economics and Path Dependence. Cheltenham: Elgar.

McArdle, Elaine
2002 Arsenic: Treated Lumber May Be Next Wave of Litigation. Three Class Actions, Other Suits Pending. LawyersUSA, October 14.

Natali, A. L., L. A. Chiafullo, and R. J. Valladares
2003 CCA-Treated Wood Litigation and Insurance Coverage Issues, vol. 2006. Eagan, MN: Thomson FindLaw.

Nico, Peter S., Scott E. Fendorf, Yvette W. Lowney, Stewart E. Holm, and Michael V. Ruby
2005 Chemical Structure of Arsenic and Chromium in Chromated Copper Arsenate (CCA) Treated Wood. Stanford, CA: SSRL.

Perry, P.
N.d. Getting Stuck in the Standards Rut. http://www.paulperry.net/notes/standard_guage.asp.

Prager, J.
2003 Treated Wood's "Smoking Gun": 1977 Memos from an Industry Insider Reveal CCA Wood Toxicity, vol. 2006. Gainesville, FL: Bancca.org.

Puffert, D.
2008 "Path Dependence." EH.Net Encyclopedia, edited by Robert Whaples. February 10. http://eh.net/encyclopedia/article/puffert.path.dependence

Rahman, F. A., D. L. Allan, C. J. Rosen, and M. J. Sadowsky
2004 Heavy Metals in the Environment. Arsenic Availability from Chromated Copper Arsenate (CCA)–Treated Wood. Journal of Environmental Quality (33):173–180.

Rebstock, P.
2006 6th Annual Competition Law and Regulation Review 2006 Wellington, vol. 2006. Auckland: Commerce Commission.

Sharp, R., B. Walker, R. Wiles, J. Houlihan, and S. Gray
2001 The Poisonwood Rivals. The Dangers of Touching Arsenic Treated Wood. Washington, DC: Environmental Working Group and Healthy Building Network.

Sharp, R., and B. Walker
2001 Poisoned Playgrounds. Arsenic in Pressure-Treated Wood, vol. 2006. Washington, DC: EWG.

Steingraber, Sandra
2004a Late Lessons from Pressure-Treated Wood, Part 1. February 5, 2004. *In* Rachel's Environment and Health News. New Brunswick, NJ: Environmental Research Foundation.
2004b Late Lessons from Pressure-Treated Wood, Part 2. February 5, 2004. *In* Rachel's Environment and Health News. New Brunswick, NJ: Environmental Research Foundation.

TPAA (Timber Preservers Association of Australia)
2006 Timber Preservation: Conserving the Nation's Heritage, vol. 2006. Brighton, VIC: TPAA.

WEI-IEO (Western European Institute for Wood Preservation)
2006 Western European Institute for Wood Preservation, vol. 2006. Brussels: WEI-IEO.

Wikipedia
2006 Path Dependence. Wikipedia, the Free Encyclopedia.

Wilson, I.
2005 Unions Welcome Signing of James Hardie Asbestos Compensation Deal. Melbourne, VIC: ACTU.

Part Two
MEDICAL AND PHARMACEUTICAL COMMODITIES

CHAPTER SEVEN

U.S. HEALTH CARE

Commodification Kills

Martha Livingston

Health care, a killer commodity? Health care heals people; it doesn't kill them—right? Well, not always. In this chapter, we will take a look at one instance in which health care can be seen as a killer commodity. First, though, here's what this chapter *isn't* about.

It *isn't* an exposé of drugs and treatments that kill, although nearly a hundred thousand people die each year in the United States from medical errors (Kohn, Corrigan, and Donaldson 2000), and anywhere from 76,000 to 137,000 suffer from bad drug reactions (Lazarou, Pomeranz, and Corey 1998).

It *isn't* a look at the way the Food and Drug Administration has in recent years colluded with the pharmaceutical industry to rush new drugs onto the market without adequate study of the attendant problems. Readers will be familiar with several recent cases: Rezulin for diabetes, introduced in the late 1990s, turned out to be toxic to livers, and by the time it was removed, 63 people had died. Vioxx and other COX-2 inhibitors were found to increase the likelihood of heart attack (Wolfe et al. 2005).

It *isn't* a look at the underreporting of medical malpractice. Thousands of patients are injured or killed each year not only from medical mistakes—doctors, like the rest of us, are human and make mistakes—but also by medical malpractice, that is, mistakes that should not have occurred; that involved negligence, carelessness, or physician impairment; and that lacked systems to control these situations (see, for example,

Morris 2006). We've all heard about cases in which the wrong limb was amputated. Now, patients are asked to autograph the body part that is slated for surgery. During the 2004 presidential election, because then-vice-presidential candidate John Edwards was a trial lawyer specializing in malpractice suits, Americans heard a lot of chatter about greedy malpractice ambulance chasers costing the health-care system billions through the overfiling of meritless lawsuits. In fact, only about two or three of every hundred *legitimate* malpractice suits—cases in which actual malpractice has occurred, with serious consequences to the patient—are ever actually filed, and very little of the enormous U.S. health-care outlay—perhaps 1 or 2 percent—has anything to do with malpractice suits. It turns out that malpractice insurance premiums vary not with claims or settlements, but with how well insurance companies' investments are doing (Americans for Insurance Reform 2002); when insurers need to improve the bottom line, they raise premiums, which can be a tremendous burden on medical practices. Nor have malpractice premiums actually increased as a percentage of doctors' practice fees; in fact, they have declined slightly in the past 20 years (Rodwin, Chang, and Clausen 2006).

No, this chapter *isn't* about any of these critically important issues. We're not going to detail how poor-quality health care can kill or injure. We're not going to look at the content or quality of health care at all. Rather, what we *will* examine is the commodification of health care in the United States, with the result that millions of us are not able to get health care when we need it. Commodification—transforming health care from a necessary service to a commodity available only to those who can afford it; when it is a product we buy, not a service we receive when we need it—kills.

According to the most conservative estimate (Institute of Medicine 2002), 18,000 Americans die each year of treatable conditions simply because they are unable to get timely care. Consider the case of Tracy Pierce, an Indiana man who recently died of kidney cancer at age 37 (*Times of Frankfort* 2006). Pierce was fully insured. When his cancer was diagnosed, his doctors proposed a treatment plan which they submitted to his insurance company, First-Health Coventry. The insurer denied the treatment repeatedly on the basis that it was either "unnecessary" or "experimental." As Pierce lay dying, untreated, less than two years later, the insurer even denied coverage for oral morphine.

Everywhere else in the rich, industrialized world, except in the United States, health care is considered a right. In one form or another, throughout Europe, from Japan to Australia and Canada, all other wealthy countries provide access for all to world-class care. The way each country organizes and pays for health care varies based on each country's history, culture, and politics, from public insurance and private delivery of care, as in Canada, to the national health service program in the United Kingdom, in which the government organizes the health-care system in addition to paying the bill. Strictly speaking, socialized medicine—that famous bogeyman of the U.S. health-care debate—doesn't exist in capitalist countries, according to Roemer (1991). (For more discussion of social*ized* and social*ist* health care, see, e.g., Sigerist 1937; Navarro 1986; and Singer and Baer 1989.) If we accept Roemer's definition, that socialized medicine happens only in socialist countries, then for the purposes of our discussion, in which we compare the United States only to other *rich* industrialized nations, socialized medicine is not part of the discussion—because there is no rich socialist nation on the planet today. (According to the World Bank [2007], "high income" is defined as $10,726 per capita income or more.) In fact, even though it isn't considered fair in comparative health policy to compare the health status of rich nations with that of poorer nations, some far poorer nations—defined by the World Bank as having a per-capita income of $876 to $3,465—do a better job of using what resources they have to maximize the health status of their people. Cuba, with a per-capita income of $3,166 (WHO 2006), exports doctors worldwide, trains doctors from many nations including the United States, and maintains the best health indicators in Latin America. Cuba's infant mortality statistics are in fact better than those of the United States (CDC 2006).

The United States spends more money on health care than any other nation on Earth: over $2 trillion this year, or more than 16 percent of gross domestic product (GDP), which is to say almost one out of every six dollars we spend in our economy, or about $7,000 for every man, woman, and child in the country (Borger et al. 2006). This is about twice as much as the next most-expensive health-care systems in the world, those of Switzerland, Germany, and Canada. Among the rich nations, health-care spending of about 8 to 10 percent of GDP is the norm. Remarkably, more than half the money in our health-care system is public money—for

Medicare, Medicaid, and uninsured care covered by some states. In other words, we actually already spend more *public* money than all of those countries with universal health care systems; as Woolhandler and Himmelstein (2002) say, we're paying for national health insurance—and not getting it.

And yet close to 47 million Americans, or about 16 percent of our 300 million people, had no health care coverage either public or private over the last two years (DeNavas-Walt, Proctor, and Lee 2005). This number seriously underestimates the problem, however. About 40 million more people weren't covered for some of those 24 months, and the majority of them were uninsured for more than six months. Combine them with the always uninsured, and close to 80 million Americans are without coverage at any given moment. Even these numbers underestimate the problem, because many millions more of us are underinsured. That is, we think we're insured, but—like those flimsy hospital gowns—we turn out to be covered for some things, but that crucial part, the condition we actually have, remains uncovered. For example, an estimated five million women of childbearing age have insurance that doesn't include maternity care. Many with preexisting conditions—health conditions they had before they became insured by the current insurer—find those conditions excluded. Millions more are stuck at jobs they'd rather leave simply because they or a family member have a preexisting condition which would not be covered under a new insurer; this is called "insurance indenture," or "job lock." Using a tactic known as the "hassle factor," insurance companies routinely deny claims on the first round, knowing that many of us will find it too much of a hassle to resubmit claims or appeal denial of coverage. In Terry Pierce's case, his doctors repeatedly requested coverage for his cancer treatment, and were repeatedly denied. Or consider the case (Barlett and Steele 2004:27–32) of 51-year-old New Jersey high-school teacher Lynn Oldham, who was unfortunate enough to develop a rare, life-threatening side effect from the chemotherapy she was given for breast cancer. She came close to dying, spent six months in the hospital, left unable to walk, and had visual and other impairments. She used up her many sick days, and coworkers donated some of theirs so that she could remain insured while fighting for her life and health. Eventually, she ran out of sick days, and was forced to buy her insurance through a COBRA plan, at $750 a month. Colleagues raised funds to cover her insurance. After a year, her insurer, Blue Cross of New Jersey, started questioning every bill, and she and her husband wound up fighting the hospital, collection agencies, and the insurance company. Lynn said, "You have to fight every single bill. . . . And not everyone is capable of doing that when they're emotionally disabled by grief or illness. . . . It demands letter-writing skills. What about the people who can't do that?"

More than half of the two million Americans declaring bankruptcy, both uninsured and insured, list medical expenses as a major contributor; remarkably, 75 percent of them are insured (Himmelstein, Warren, Thorne, and Woolhandler 2005). First, you get sick; then, you face financial disaster at the same time you're trying to combat illness. Close to 15 years of New York City emergency medical technician Joy Kallio's life were lost to illness as a result of our health-care system, as she recounted at a 2005 congressional health-care hearing. One day, at age 32, she

> woke up stricken with severe low back pain, pain like I had never felt before. I couldn't get out of bed. It was diagnosed by MRI as several herniated discs and spinal stenosis. At that time I had top-of-the-line health insurance with all the bells and whistles that Blue Cross/Blue Shield offered; there was no better to be had. I had always been healthy, and in ten years had not made a single claim. After my first claim for coverage of conservative treatment for my back pain, BC/BS tripled my premiums.
>
> The treatment didn't help. My symptoms worsened, and I could no longer work. For a self-employed person that meant no income. . . . My savings lasted two years, and when they were exhausted I lost my apartment, health insurance, and all my doctors. I applied for welfare . . . and I got $351.00 per month to live on and Medicaid. I moved into a 6' × 10' room in a single room occupancy hotel on the upper west side of Manhattan.
>
> Eventually I started bleeding, and developing pelvic infections. It took a year to get an appointment with a gynecology clinic at the community health center to examine the cause. By then I was bleeding continuously. That's when they found the necrotic tumor in my uterus. I was very ill, weighing only 86 pounds. They removed the tumor. . . . My bleeding and internal infections continued. I went to 5 major hospitals in Manhattan and kept asking doctors if endometriosis could be the cause of my severe pain and illness. They said "no" and refused to perform the expensive diagnostic laparoscopy required to establish the diagnosis. . . .

> Finally I was so swollen and inflamed that I was unable to urinate, my kidneys were backing up, and I was able to convince a doctor to do the diagnostic laparoscopy necessary to determine the cause. While inside she found my entire abdominal cavity was covered with stage 4 endometriosis lesions, and the disease had invaded many of my organs. She said, "You must have been in agony, for so long." My insides were so fibrotic they were like "saddle leather, very, very difficult to cut through." My extensive endometriosis required a specialized surgical treatment to remove it, and no endometriosis surgeons would operate on a Medicaid patient, so even after my diagnosis I could not get treatment. . . . I was placed in a program for chronic incurable pain and given daily morphine with which to endure my disease. Taking morphine took the edge off my pain and allowed me to be able to think more clearly again. (Kallio 2005)

Kallio then did an enormous favor for an anesthesiologist, tutoring him for months so that he could pass his licensing board examination. His wife

> was so grateful to me for helping her husband that she made a few phone calls for me, and [a prominent specialist] agreed to do my surgery. When I woke up from the operation I was in much less pain than I had been in for 15 years. Not all of it was operable, because it had advanced too far, but I was able to sit, stand, and walk again. I was able to think of something besides pain again. I started to gain some weight and people told me it was like watching a phoenix rising from the ashes. (Kallio 2005)

Who are the uninsured? The majority are full-time, low-wage workers, or workers for small employers who can't afford the yearly double-digit increases in the cost of private insurance, or self-employed people and their families. Increasingly, even those employed by large firms are uninsured, either because the employer can no longer afford health insurance or because the worker cannot afford the employee portion of the premium. In 2005, the average premium for private family coverage ($10,880) surpassed the amount a full-time worker made at a minimum-wage job ($10,712) (Gabel, Claxton, and Gil 2005). Forty-one percent of Americans earning from $20,000 to $40,000 were uninsured for some portion of 2005, an increase from 28 percent in 2001 (Collins et al. 2006). For those earning below $20,000, that figure rises to 53 percent. When people have no insurance, they delay care; millions are walking around with undiagnosed diabetes and hypertension, perhaps discovered only years later, when they turn up in emergency rooms with strokes and heart attacks and other long-term consequences of these silent killers. Millions of Americans live with uncorrected visual impairment (Vitale, Cotch, and Sperduto 2006). Of the 18,000 Americans who die each year of treatable conditions, some are women who die of cervical cancer (Grady 2005), a very preventable and treatable disease, either because they are uninsured or because their insurance does not include routine gynecological screening. (Some doctors "game" the system by creating a diagnosis when they are doing preventive screenings; no doubt a future medical anthropologist will wonder, for example, at the epidemic of "nonspecific vaginitis" among American women being given Pap smears!) Prospective patients are typically confronted with the question, "what kind of insurance do you have?" If we flunk the test—if we have, as they say, a negative wallet biopsy—the likelihood of our getting timely, appropriate care is greatly reduced. Even insured Americans have relatively little to say about choosing caregivers and treatments, since most are covered by one single plan, including a limited panel of doctors. When employers change plans from year to year based on cost considerations, because double-digit insurance premium increases have become problematic even for major corporations, patients are required to find new providers, sacrificing continuity of care. For all of us, but especially for groups who have traditionally had a hard time finding respectful health-care practitioners (poor people, Americans of color, and many women), the lack of choice of provider can result in dramatically reduced quality of care.

Doctors, too, are commonly frustrated at their inability to provide timely, appropriate care. They spend an enormous amount of time haggling with insurance companies and managed-care plans to get their patients the care they need, arguing with claims personnel who have no medical background. Their office staff works full-time processing mountains of paperwork and making endless calls. There are more than 1,200 insurance companies writing health insurance policies, and within each there are numerous insurance "products," so the task of keeping up with who's covered for what and at what rate of reimbursement is enormous. The "hassle factor" for doctors results in their choosing their battles, a demoralizing activity: which patient most urgently needs me to fight? Insurance companies hold all the cards in negotiations with doctors; after all, if doctors cost them too much—have too many sick patients, use too much care—they can be dropped from the insurance company's panel of participating doctors. Benjamin Brewer (2006), a doctor in private practice, reported that a single-payer national health-insurance system would enable him to reduce his four office staff, most of whom spend most of their time on insurance-related paperwork, to one. Fighting with insurance companies for claims reimbursement has become so difficult a chore for many doctors that a new industry, "denials management," has developed; for a percentage of the returns, these firms will recover claims that have been denied (Fuhrmans 2007). The website of one, Athena Health, says on its home page: "Run a practice, not an obstacle course [www.athenahealth.com]." The continuity of care issue affects doctors as well as patients in less satisfying practices with ever-changing patients, determined not by their or their patients' wishes but by insurance companies' bottom lines. Overall, the system compromises and deforms the relationship between providers and patients.

As we have seen, health care in the United States costs a great deal more than health care anywhere else on the planet. Where's all that money going? We often hear that, well, Americans simply demand, and get, more health care than others. Not so: in fact, by comparison with the other rich nations, Americans have a relatively low or average number of both doctor visits and hospital stays (OECD 2005). We hear, too, that the United States really carries the ball on medical research; again, the amount of medical research performed in the United States is about average (Hefler, Tempfer, and Kainz 1999; Rosselli 1998; Woolhandler, personal communication). We also hear that we have more high-tech equipment in the United States, but in fact Italy and Japan each have more MRI machines per million population, and Germany, Denmark, and Japan each have more CT scanners than we have (OECD 2005). And the United States lags behind the rest of the wealthy nations in health-information technology (Anderson, Frogner, Johns, and Reinhardt 2006). It's not malpractice, either, though Americans *are* more likely to sue for damages in malpractice. But that's because, without a national health-insurance system, injured patients have to sue in order to get their future medical expenses covered—not a problem for people in other countries with national health-care programs.

Is it that our health care is simply superior, and therefore more costly? A look at health outcomes says not; our life expectancy is relatively low compared to the other rich nations (OECD 2005) and our infant mortality, now at 28th (CDC 2006) worldwide, is behind Cuba's. Save the Children reports (2006) that the United States lags far behind in neonatal mortality, 32nd of 33 countries, ahead only of Latvia. Of course, health outcomes are not only about access to timely care. Countries with greater income inequality and poorer social programs have worse health outcomes, and income inequality is higher in the United States than anywhere else in the industrialized world.

If greater use, superior quality and outcomes, or more research output don't explain the enormous amount of money being spent in a health-care system which leaves a large proportion of Americans unable to access timely care, what does? For one, administrative costs. Contrary to the national mantra "the government can't do anything right; the private sector can't do anything wrong," our Medicare program spends less than 4 percent, and Medicaid 5 to 6 percent, on administration; the private sector spends anywhere from 15 to 33 percent. Woolhandler, Campbell, and Himmelstein (2004), for example, found that the United States spends about 31 percent of its health-care dollars on administration, compared to Canada's 16.7 percent, or $1,059 per capita versus $307, and concluded that the money saved by moving to a single-payer system similar to Canada's—over $200 billion—would be enough to cover all uninsured Americans, and improve coverage for all, without our having to add any new money into the system. Denying care, and processing endless paper, does not only kill people—it's very expensive. Consider this: from 1970 to the present, the number of doctors and nurses has increased about 100 percent, that is, we've doubled the number of doctors and nurses. During the same period, the number of health-care administrators has increased by 2900 percent (Woolhandler and Himmelstein 2005).

Where else is the money going? Well, of course, to profit—some of it enormous. Dr. Linda Peeno worked briefly as medical director for the for-profit insurer Humana and was told, when she started, that "it costs us about 10 percent of every health care premium dollar to run this company. Your job is to help us keep as much as possible of the rest." That is, her job was to deny as much health care as possible (Peeno 1996). Insurers refer to the amount of the health-care premium dollar that is actually spent on health care as the "medical-loss ratio," or "medical-cost ratio." Peeno describes coming to see the million-dollar artworks on corporate headquarters walls as representing care denied to patients. For-profit corporations' primary responsibility is to make profits for their shareholders; that's what corporations do—and in health care, they're getting better at it all the time. According to Bethely (2006), "whereas 10 years ago many plans had medical-cost ratios in the high 80s or 90s, now the highest percentage among large, publicly traded health insurers is Health Net, at 83.9 percent. Aetna, which had a medical-cost ratio well into the 90s when CEO John Rowe, MD, took over in 2000, recorded a ratio of 76.9 percent in 2005, Dr. Rowe's final full year before his retirement. That was the lowest medical-cost ratio for the nation's largest publicly traded plans."

The pharmaceutical industry (Big Pharma) is the single most profitable industry in the United States, with close to 20 percent net profit in recent years (e.g., Angell 2004). Contrary to Big Pharma's claim that these profits are necessary in order to support their research program, in fact this is net profit—after all expenditures, including research and development costs. This figure contrasts with an average corporate profit rate of 5 to 6 percent.

In addition to the bottom line, there is the matter of what is politely called "executive compensation." Freed (2006) revealed that UnitedHealth Group Inc.'s chairman and CEO William McGuire was awarded $1.6 billion in unexercised stock options for 2005. As Don McCanne (2006a) comments, "UnitedHealth Group's medical loss ratio for 2005 was 78.6 percent. That means that UnitedHealth retained for its own intrinsic uses, including profits, 21.4 percent of premiums paid. Profit for 2005 was $3.3 billion. For that performance, CEO McGuire receives $1.6 billion in unexercised stock options."

In this era of corporate scandal, health-care corporate executives are no exception. Readers will be familiar with the case of Richard Scrushy, CEO of HealthSouth, who was recently tried and acquitted on charges of fraud and money laundering (Johnson 2005), though other HealthSouth executives landed behind bars for fraudulent accounting that Barlett and Steele (2004:84) call "a Ponzi scheme of sorts." Another interesting case is that of doctor and former Senate Majority Leader Bill Frist, whose family owns Healthcare Corporation of America (HCA), the largest for-profit hospital chain in the United States. When Frist joined the Senate, we were told that he had placed his holdings in the family business in a "blind trust." The country was surprised to learn, therefore, that Frist had sold off his holdings in HCA in the spring of 2005, just before the stock's price took a nosedive. (Barlett and Steele [2004:22] claim that HCA's billing practices to uninsured patients are especially vicious.)

For-profit health care is not only more expensive; much research has also documented that its outcomes are worse than those in nonprofit or publicly delivered care (e.g., Schlesinger and Gray 2006; Harrington et al. 2001; Thomas, Orav, and Brennan 2000; Tu and Reschovsky 2002). In the 1990s, for example, for-profit dialysis corporations were found to be skimping on costs by reusing tubing kits designed for single use, leading to increased risk of infection (Garg, Frick, Diener-West, and Powe 1999:1653). When profits are primary, care is necessarily worse, and results in worse outcomes.

By now, almost everyone agrees that our system is broken; there are sharp differences, however, about how to fix it. Many Americans understand that the solution has to involve getting rid of the profiteers and moving to a "Medicare for all" system similar to Canada's. Physicians for a National Health Program (www.pnhp.org), a national organization of doctors, other health care professionals, and activists, has advocated for a single-payer solution and done groundbreaking research on our health-care mess since the late 1980s. But there are huge, powerful forces within both business and government that oppose such a system, arguing that government must not be the solution to any social problems, including health care. President George W. Bush's health-care adviser, Allan Hubbard (2006), explicitly describes the two approaches to fixing the system, rejecting the Medicare for all single-payer approach in favor of "consumer-directed" health care, based on the view that if Americans shopped more wisely for health care, all our problems would be solved: "Health care is expensive because the vast majority of Americans consume it as if it were free. Health insurance policies with low deductibles insulate people from the cost of the medical care they use. . . . To control health care costs, we must give consumers an incentive to spend money wisely." Hubbard admitted, at the World Health Congress in April 2006, that this plan does not work for the chronically ill: "But, I want to be perfectly frank, the chronically ill is a problem that is very difficult to solve." He further admitted, at the same session, that emergency care also did not fit his model.

This prompted Don McCanne (2006b) to comment: "Why would the administration support a reform proposal that they quite frankly concede will not work? It's because they recognize that the status quo is not sustainable, and the only other realistic option is a single payer system. . . . Their real reason for opposing single payer is that their anti-government ideology overrides all other considerations and trumps reform that they know will work, merely because it is a government solution."

Health care, as a for-profit industry in the United States, is a killer commodity. Worse yet, the export of neoliberal ideology in the health-care sector, and the consequent privatization of the previously public asset of parts of health-care systems, is leading to its transformation into a killer commodity around the world. (Neoliberalism, this generation's version of laissez-faire economics, holds that the market should determine everything; government's role is seen as simply providing those services, such as stabilizing currency, balancing budgets, and providing security forces, which support the operation of a "free" market. All other government services, including social services, health care, even access to safe water, are seen as interfering with the operation of the market and are to be minimized and privatized [see, for example, Harvey 2005 and Chomsky 2002]). Canadians, geographically, economically, and ideologically closer to and therefore most susceptible to this infection, have confronted a nonstop barrage of pro-privatization rhetoric, and have had to fight against numerous attempts to chip away at the public system (see, for example, Armstrong and Armstrong 2002; Armstrong et al. 1994; Fuller 1998; Rachlis 2005; and Canadian Health Services Research Foundation 2000–2006). Europe's national health programs have been under increasing attack. Pollock (2006) reports that in the UK, the National Health Service is now spending money on paperwork, advertising, and competition that was unheard of until very recently and turning more and more public money over to private, for-profit corporations, including some from the United States. Koivusalo (2005) finds this ideological infection throughout Europe. Waitzkin and others (e.g., Iriart and Waitzkin, 2006; Iriart, Merhy, and Waitzkin 2001; Stocker, Waitzkin, and Iriart 1999) warn about the killer effects of export of the U.S. health-care "model" in Latin America. The prior Howard government in Australia was an especially enthusiastic proponent of privatizating social services, including the health-care system (see, for example, Gray 2004 and Gardner and Barraclough 2002). From the other side, Atlas (2006:A15), a Hoover Institution senior fellow, recently wrote urging the Chinese government to adopt the market-based "consumer-directed health care" model in China, avoiding what he called the "mistakes of the West . . . which include sheltering patients from direct payment of health costs, overregulating health insurance," and so forth, in a direct echo of Hubbard's proposal for the United States.

In 1969, reports Barbara Ehrenreich (2004:115–116), she described to economists Paul Sweezy and Harry Magdoff what a mess the U.S. health-care system was and how it didn't work:

> Paul's quiet response was, in so many words: Oh, but it is a system; it's just a system for doing something else. Then for the first time I could see the parts fitting together, the gears of the huge jerry-rigged structure finally meshing, the machine working just fine—grinding out profits. . . . Health care is just a by-product of the health system.

Because of the political and ideological hegemony of the United States, we owe it not only to the people of the United States but also to the people of the world to fight for the de-commodification of the killer commodity that is the U.S. health-care system. As this is written, more and more Americans—from uninsured workers to corporate CEOs—are discovering what Sweezy knew 37 years ago: that our health-care system is designed not to bring health care to people, but profits to corporations. With nearly a sixth of the U.S. economy involved in health care, it is no wonder that opponents of national health insurance have fiercely resisted change for a century. We need to wrest U.S. health care from the profiteers, and create a system of health care for people, not for profit.

How? The system has dramatically worsened since the Clinton health-care reform debacle of the early 1990s; former president Bill Clinton, himself the perpetrator of a cumbersome, corporate-centered plan, recently warned against other nations adopting the for-profit U.S. health-care model. Calling the system "insane" and a "colossal waste of money," Clinton (Moore 2006:A14) urged Canadians seeking to solve wait-list problems to "conduct a public set of hearings on every other advanced health-care system and see who solved that problem best. Surely there's somebody who has figured out how to solve this problem. . . . Don't do anything that will lead to increased administration costs and letting the financing tail wag the health-care dog."

The movement for a rational national health-care program has been around for more than 100 years, waxing and waning with the political tides. Terris (1999) called this history "National Health Insurance in the United States: A Drama in Too Many Acts." In past decades, activists urged the creation of a national health-service system similar to the UK's, arguing that "merely" paying the bills, as in a national health insurance system, does little to fix the many problems associated with privately delivered, fee-for-service health care. The Medicare and Medicaid programs were a compromise growing out of the call for a national health service in the 1960s. In recent decades, however, health-care activism has focused primarily on financing, demanding that government create a publicly financed national health insurance system while leaving in place the private delivery of care—actually a relatively modest demand.

As the current system becomes less and less sustainable, the movement to overhaul health-care financing now includes a broader coalition of forces than ever. Since the majority of privately insured Americans get their health care through employment, unions have for many years regarded health benefits as a major service they can deliver to their members as well as, often, a source of funding for other union activity. But in recent years unions have had an increasingly difficult time maintaining these benefits, and many strikes have been waged principally over health benefits (Nealis 2006). Since 2005, over 250 unions, union locals, and central labor councils have signed on to support Congressman John Conyers's single-payer "Medicare for All" national health insurance bill, HR 676. The bill has provided an organizing vehicle for Americans demanding change, urging legislators to sign on as cosponsors, and organizing congressional hearings.

In 2007 with a new balance of power in Congress, polls show that the majority of Americans want the government to fix the broken health-care system, even if it means paying more taxes (e.g., CNN Poll/Opinion Research Corp., 9 May 2007, *New York Times*/CBS News Poll, 23–27 February 2007). Health-care reform is consistently characterized as the leading domestic policy issue on the minds of Americans. Michael Moore's 2007 movie, *Sicko*, created a buzz about the contrast between availability of health care in other countries and the horrors, for *insured* Americans, of the current system.

Two major stumbling blocks stand in the way of success for this vital social movement: power and imagination. Power? That's the easy part; we know who's got it. Those in the for-profit health-care industry, along with the politicians they support with enormous lobbying efforts (who, as we have seen before, are sometimes one and the same, as in the case of former Senate Majority Leader Bill Frist), will continue to fight to preserve their large slice of the profitable American health-care system: two trillion dollars is a lot to fight for. Imagination? That's harder. Too many working Americans, after 25 years of neoliberal attack, have been persuaded that they can't fight city hall, that even though our health-care system is killing and injuring them, and even though all other rich, industrialized nations—and many poorer ones—provide health care to all of their people, it's "politically impossible" in the United States, that, in the words of former UK prime minister Margaret Thatcher, "there is no alternative." We need to learn from popular antiglobalization struggles around the world—from the successful fight in Bolivia against water privatization to movements to forgive third-world debt—and to remind ourselves that in the United States ordinary, powerless people have made enormous social change too. A humane U.S. health-care system is necessary, possible, and worth fighting for.

Acknowledgments

Many thanks to Bill Livant; Len Rodberg; Joy Kallio; the staff of Food for Thought Books, Amherst, Massachusetts; and the library staff at SUNY College at Old Westbury.

References

Americans for Insurance Reform
2002 Medical Malpractice Insurance: Stable Losses/Unstable Rates. New York: Americans for Insurance Reform.
Anderson, Gerard F., Bianca K. Frogner, Roger A. Johns, and Uwe E. Reinhardt
2006 Health Care Spending and Use of Information Technology in OECD Countries. Health Affairs 25(3): 819–831.

Angell, Marcia
2004 The Truth about the Drug Companies: How They Deceive Us and What to Do about It. New York: Random House.

Armstrong, Pat, and Hugh Armstrong
2002 Wasting Away: The Undermining of Canadian Health Care. Toronto: Oxford University Press.

Armstrong, Pat, Hugh Armstrong, Jacqueline Choiniere, Gina Feldberg, and Jerry White
1994 Take Care: Warning Signals for Canada's Health System. Toronto: Garamond Press.

Atlas, Scott W.
2006 Health Care for 1.3 Billion People? Leave It to the Market. Wall Street Journal, May 1: A15.

Barlett, Donald L., and James B. Steele
2004 Critical Condition: How Health Care in America Became Big Business and Bad Medicine. New York: Doubleday.

Bethely, Jonathan G.
2006 Health Plans Make More, Spend Less in 2005; Insurers' Medical-Cost Ratios Are Lower Than Ever. American Medical News, March 6. http://www.ama-assn.org/amednews/2006/03/06/bisd0306.htm.

Borger, Christine, Sheila Smith, Christopher Truffer, Sean Keehan, Andrea Sisko, John Poisal, and M. Kent Clemens
2006 Health Spending Projections through 2015: Changes on the Horizon. Health Affairs Web Exclusive 25(2):w61–w73.

Brewer, Benjamin
2006 Government-Funded Care Is the Best Health Solution. Wall Street Journal Online, April 18. http://online.wsj.com/article/SB114528925682927634.html.

Canadian Health Services Research Foundation
2000–2006 Mythbusters. Series of 20 monographs. www.chsrf.ca.

CDC (Centers for Disease Control and Prevention)
2006 Eliminate Disparities in Infant Mortality. CDC Fact sheet. Electronic document, www.cdc.gov/omh/AMH/factsheets/infant/htm.

Chomsky, Noam
2002 Understanding Power: The Indispensable Chomsky. New York: New Press, ed. Peter R. Mitchell and John Schoeffel.

Collins, Sara R., Karen Davis, Michelle M. Doty, Jennifer L. Kriss, and Alyssa L. Holmgren
2006 Gaps in Health Insurance: An All-American Problem. Findings from the Commonwealth Fund Biennial Health Insurance Survey. New York: Commonwealth Fund.

DeNavas-Walt, Carmen, Bernadette D. Proctor, and Cheryl Hill Lee
2005 U.S. Census Bureau Current Population Reports: P 60–229: Income, Poverty, and Health Insurance Coverage in the United States: 2004. Washington, DC: U.S. Government Printing Office.
Ehrenreich, Barbara
2004 Remembering Paul. Monthly Review 56(5):115–116.
Freed, Joshua
2006 UnitedHealth Panel May Face Scrutiny. SFgate.com, April 23.
Fuhrmans, Vanessa
2007 Billing Battle: Fights over Health Claims Spawn a New Arms Race. Wall Street Journal, February 14: 1.
Fuller, Colleen
1998 Caring for Profit: How Corporations Are Taking Over Canada's Health Care System. Vancouver, BC: New Star Books/Canadian Centre for Policy Alternatives.
Gabel, Jon, Gary Claxton, Isadora Gil, Jeremy Pickreign, Heidi Whitmore, Benjamin Finder, Samantha Hawkins, and Diane Rowland
2005 Health Benefits in 2005: Premium Increases Slow Down, Coverage Continues to Erode. Health Affairs 24(5):1273–1280.
Gardner, Heather, and Simon Barraclough
2002 Health Policy in Australia, 2nd ed. South Melbourne, Victoria, Australia: Oxford University Press.
Garg, Pushkal P., Kevin D. Frick, Marie Diener-West, and Neil R. Powe
1999 Effect of the Ownership of Dialysis Facilities on Patients' Survival and Referral for Transplantation. New England Journal of Medicine 341(22):1653–1660.
Grady, Denise
2005 2 New Approaches May Reduce Cervical Cancer Deaths for Poor. New York Times, November 2.
Gray, Gwendolyn
2004 The Politics of Medicare. Sydney, New South Wales, Australia: University of New South Wales Press.
Harrington, Charlene, Steffie Woolhandler, Joseph Mullan, Helen Carrillo, and David U. Himmelstein
2001 Does Investor Ownership of Nursing Homes Compromise the Quality of Care? American Journal of Public Health 91(9):1452–1455.
Harvey, David
2005 A Brief History of Neoliberalism. Oxford: Oxford University Press.
Hefler, Lukas, Clemens Tempfer, and Christian Kainz
1999 Geography of Biomedical Publications in the European Union, 1990–98. Lancet 353(9167):1856.

Himmelstein, David, Elizabeth Warren, Deborah Thorne, and Steffie Woolhandler
2005 MarketWatch: Illness and Injury as Contributors to Bankruptcy. Health Affairs Web Exclusive, February 2. http://content.healthaffairs.org/cgi/content/full/hlthaff.w5.63/DC1.

Hubbard, Allan
2006 The Health of a Nation. New York Times, April 3.

Institute of Medicine, Committee on the Consequences of Uninsurance
2002 Care without Coverage: Too Little, Too Late: 163. Washington, DC: National Academies Press.

Iriart, Celia, Emerson Elias Merhy, and Howard Waitzkin
2001 Managed Care in Latin America: The New Common Sense in Health Policy Reform. Social Science and Medicine 52:1243–1253.

Iriart, Celia, and Howard Waitzkin
2006 Argentina: No Lesson Learned. International Journal of Health Services 36:177–196.

Johnson, Carrie
2005 Jury Acquits HealthSouth Founder of All Charges. Washington Post, June 29: A01.

Kallio, Joy
2005 Testimony, Citizens' Congressional Hearing. New York Times, May 14.

Kohn, Linda T., Janet M. Corrigan, and Molla S. Donaldson, eds.
2000 To Err Is Human: Building a Safer Health System. Washington, DC: National Academies Press.

Koivusalo, Meri Tuulikki
2005 The Future of European Health Policies. International Journal of Health Services 35(2):325–342.

Lazarou, Jason, Bruce H. Pomeranz, and Paul N. Corey
1998 Incidence of Adverse Drug Reactions in Hospitalized Patients: A Meta-Analysis of Prospective Studies. Journal of the American Medical Association 279(15):1200–1205.

McCanne, Don
2006a $1.6 billion for UnitedHealth's McGuire. Quote of the Day, April 25. http://www.pnhp.org/news/2006/april/16_billion_for_uni.php.
2006b Allan Hubbard Explains the President's Health Reform Plan. Quote of the Day, April 21. http://www.pnhp.org/news/2006/april/allan_hubbard_explai.php.

Moore, Oliver
2006 Avoid U.S. Health Model: Clinton. Globe and Mail (Toronto), May 16: A14.

Morris, Charles R.
2006 Apart at the Seams: The Collapse of Private Pension and Health Care Protections: A Century Foundation Report. New York: Century Foundation Press.

Navarro, V.
1986 What Is Socialist Medicine? Monthly Review 38(3):61–73.

Nealis, Wayne
2006 Building a Movement for Health Care: Key to Organizing the Unorganized? WorkingUSA: The Journal of Labor and Society 9:79–97.

OECD
2005 Health data. Retrieved June 2006: www.oecd.org/topicstatsportal/0,3398,en_2825_495642_1_1_1_1_1,00.html.

Peeno, Linda
1996 Managed Care Ethics: The Close View. Prepared for the U.S. House of Representatives Committee on Commerce, Subcommittee on Health and Environment, May 30.

Pollock, Allyson
2006 The Politics Column. New Statesman, May 1.

Rachlis, Michael
2005 Public Solutions to Health Care Wait Lists. Ottawa: Canadian Centre for Policy Alternatives.

Rodwin, Marc A., Hak J. Chang, and Jeffrey Clausen
2006 Malpractice Premiums and Physicians' Income: Perceptions of a Crisis Conflict with Empirical Evidence. Health Affairs 25(3):750–758.

Roemer, Milton
1991 National Health Care Systems of the World, vol. 1. Oxford: Oxford University Press.

Rosselli, Diego
1998 Latin American Biomedical Publications, the Case of Colombia in Medline. Medical Education 32:274–277.

Save the Children
2006 State of the World's Mothers 2006: Saving the Lives of Mothers and Newborns. Westport, CT: Save the Children.

Schlesinger, Mark, and Bradford H. Gray
2006 How Nonprofits Matter in American Medicine and What to Do About It. Health Affairs 25(4):287–303.

Sigerist, Henry E.
1937 Socialized Medicine in the Soviet Union. New York: Norton.

Singer, Merrill, and Hans A. Baer
1989 Toward an Understanding of Capitalist and Socialist Health. Medical Anthropology 11:97–107.

Stocker, Karen, Howard Waitzkin, and Celia Iriart
1999 The Exportation of Managed Care to Latin America. New England Journal of Medicine 340(14):1131–1136.
Terris, Milton
1999 National Health Insurance in the United States: A Drama in Too Many Acts. Journal of Public Health Policy 20(1):13–35.
Thomas, Eric J., E. John Orav, and Troyen A. Brennan
2000 Hospital Ownership and Preventable Adverse Events. Journal of General Internal Medicine 15(4):211–219.
Times of Frankfort
2006 Man Dies after Insurance Co. Refuses to Cover Treatment. Times of Frankfort (Indiana), February 11.
Tu, Ha T., and James D. Reschovsky
2002 Assessments of Medical Care by Enrollees in For-Profit and Nonprofit Health Maintenance Organizations. New England Journal of Medicine 346(17):1288–1293.
Vitale, Susan, Mary Frances Cotch, and Robert D. Sperduto
2006 Prevalence of Visual Impairment in the United States. Journal of the American Medical Association 295(18):2158–2163.
Wolfe, Sidney, Larry Sasich, Peter Lurie, Rose-Ellen Hope, Elizabeth Barbehenn, Deanne E. Knapp, Amer Ardati, Sherri Shubin, Diana B. Ku, and Public Citizen's Health Research Group
2005 Worst Pills, Best Pills. New York: Pocket Books.
WHO (World Health Organization)
2006 www.who.int/countries/cub/en.
Woolhandler, Steffie, Terry Campbell, and David U. Himmelstein
2004 Health Care Administration in the United States and Canada: Micromanagement, Macro Costs. International Journal of Health Services 34(1):65–78.
Woolhandler, Steffie, and David U. Himmelstein
2002 Paying for National Health Insurance—and Not Getting It. Health Affairs 21(4):88–98.
2005 Unpublished Analysis of CPS (Current Population Survey) and BLS (Bureau of Labor Statistics) Data, presented in PNHP slide show. Chicago: PNHP.
World Bank
2007 http://go.worldbank.org/K2CKM78CC0.

CHAPTER EIGHT

SILICONE SEDUCTION

Are Cosmetic Breast Implants Killer Commodities?

Pamela I. Erickson and Ann M. Cheney

In 1992, the Food and Drug Administration (FDA) imposed a ban on the sale of silicone gel breast implants for cosmetic purposes after reports that they might be related to autoimmune diseases and evidence that some early models may have leaked excessively (FDA 2004), raising serious questions about their long-term safety. The ban was the result of a heated decade of debate between women's health advocates who opposed them, and plastic surgeons, implant manufacturers (Dow Corning, Mentor, and Inamed), and consumers who wanted them to remain on the market. The decision to ban silicone gel implants was based on the FDA's determination that there was insufficient scientific evidence to deem them safe. As a result, silicone gel implants were banned for cosmetic reasons pending research supporting their safety, although they could still be sold under compassionate need exemptions (e.g., for breast reconstructions) or the investigational device exemption (IDE) for research purposes in clinical studies (FDA 2004; Kessler 1992a; National Research Center for Women & Families 2006).

Thirteen years later, the two top silicone implant manufacturers, Mentor and Inamed Corporation, submitted premarket approval applications (PMAs) to the FDA that included the results of the studies they had been conducting under the IDE exemption in order to prove their product safe and bring it back on the consumer market. On July 28, 2005, the National Women's Health Network (NWHN 2005) sent a news alert to all subscribed members relaying the message that the FDA had informed Mentor Corporation that their products were approvable (FDA 2005a). Two months later, the FDA advised Inamed Corporation that their products were also approvable if certain conditions were met (FDA 2005b). This approvability announcement set off another round of heated public debates over the safety of silicone gel implants.

At the time of the approvability announcements, it was estimated that the financial impact of the reintroduction of silicone implants to the U.S. consumer market would be considerable. In the first year alone, the market for silicone implants was projected to double. Silicone implants are preferred by women and surgeons over saline implants, and they cost twice as much. The gross income to the manufacturer alone was estimated to reach somewhere near $700 million dollars. According to CNN's Aaron Smith, Mentor's stock price (the only supplier of silicone implants in the United States) jumped about 60 percent in the six months following the FDA's approvability announcement, while Inamed's stock remained flat (Smith 2005).

On November 17, 2006, over a year after notice of approvable status and well after the most vocal public opposition had died down, the FDA lifted its 14-year ban on silicone gel breast implants, approving those manufactured by Mentor and Allergan (formerly Inamed) for breast reconstruction and cosmetic purposes, but limited cosmetic use to women over age 21 and required that all patients be advised that regular (three years after insertion and every two years thereafter) magnetic resonance imaging (MRI) screening was required for early detection of implant rupture. The FDA also required each company to conduct post-approval studies that would follow 40,000 women for ten years to further establish the safety of the devices. On November 20, 2006, the price of stock surged by 8 percent for Allergan and 11 percent for Mentor.

The controversy over silicone gel breast implants is a long-standing debate over their safety and effectiveness. The major constituencies in this debate are plastic surgeons, breast implant manufacturers, female consumers, and women's health advocates, all of whom tried to influence the regulatory decisions of the FDA. Plastic surgeons and breast implant manufacturers urged FDA approval, while women's health organizations and many advocates supported a continued ban. Women who have implants, potential consumers, and women in general have long been divided on the safety of implants. Women with a history of adverse health consequences that they associate with silicone implants fought vehemently against their approval, but many other women encouraged it. The lifting of the ban has not quelled opposition from health advocates who see the approval of silicone gel implants as an enormous setback for women's health. After the approval, Dr. Sidney Wolfe, director of Public Citizen's Health Research Group, a nonprofit public interest organization, said: "In terms of adverse safety and health information known at the time of approval . . . *silicone gel breast implants are the most defective medical device ever approved by the FDA* [emphasis added]" (Public Citizen 2006).

In this chapter we try to answer the fundamental question of whether FDA approval of silicone breast implants sacrificed women's health for the economic interests of the manufacturers of implants and the surgeons who implant them into women's bodies.

Why Do Women Want Silicone Implants: Medicalization and the Female Breast

Beginning in the 1930s, American attitudes about the primary function of the female breast began to shift from lactation to sexual pleasure. The large, eroticized breast became particularly popular around World War II and remains so today. This transition coincided with other changes, including the displacement of breastfeeding by bottle-feeding and changes in attitudes toward small breasts from "unfortunate but functional" to pathological (Latteier 1998). As large breasts became the ideal, women availed themselves of various, although experimental, methods to augment their breasts, including insertion of rubber sponges into the breasts and injections of estrogen, beeswax, petroleum jelly, vegetable oils, and finally silicone itself, and this was believed to improve their marriages, their lives, and most importantly the beauty of their bodies (Angell 1996; Haiken 1997). The first silicone gel breast implant surgery was performed in 1962, and plastic surgeons, psychologists, and psychiatrists quickly identified several diseases for which breast augmentation was the treatment (Jacobson 2000). Thus began a new trend in which patients could be surgically altered to achieve their beauty ideal, and plastic surgeons could claim, as do many satisfied consumers, that both medical and cosmetic breast surgeries increase self-esteem and improve the lives of American women.

In combination with improved surgical techniques, television, our most popular medium, has emphasized that women's breasts should be considered primarily for their aesthetic and sexual pleasures. Postmillennium television series actively promote the normalization of surgical alteration and have even made it a form of entertainment, beginning with *Nip/Tuck* in 2002, an award-winning medical drama about two plastic surgeons. By 2003, reality TV shows like *Extreme Makeovers*, *I Want a Famous Face*, and *The Swan*, allowed the public to watch weekly as participants transformed themselves through cosmetic and surgical means (Turner 2004). During *Extreme Makeover*'s 2004–2005 season, Mentor Corporation advertised its saline breast implants at least once a week with a 30-second commercial aimed at delivering more than 61 million impressions to women aged 18 to 49. According to Mentor, their purpose was to educate women interested in breast augmentation, to help them find a plastic surgeon, and to direct "patients" toward the best available products (McGuire 2004; New York Stock Exchange 2004). According to Mentor's president and CEO, Joshua H. Levine, "*Extreme Makeover* has had a tremendous positive impact on the growth of breast augmentation and other cosmetic procedures, and we are pleased to be in this innovative relationship with them" (New York Stock Exchange 2004). The increasing medicalization of the lack of attractiveness in American society (Clarke et al. 2003; Dworkin 2001) has undoubtedly contributed to both the plastic surgery and media industries.

In 2006, American consumers spent more than $11.4 billion on surgical and nonsurgical cosmetic procedures and almost $1.2 billion on breast augmentation, which ranked first among the top five surgical cosmetic procedures (breast, liposuction, nose, eyelid, tummy tuck) (ASPS 2007). According to statistics from the American Society of Plastic Surgeons (ASPS), the vast majority of breast augmentations (85 percent) are done for cosmetic rather than reconstructive or medical reasons (ASPS 2007), and business is booming.

White women from economically advantaged backgrounds in their early thirties are the modal recipients of breast implants (Bondurant et al. 2000; Goin and Goin 1981; Sarwer et al. 2000), but it is also among the top three most common cosmetic surgery procedures for Latina and Asian American women (ASPS 2007). Most (65 percent) of the women who received implants in 2006 were age 20 to 39; 32 percent were 40 or older;

and only 3 percent were 18 to 19 years old (ASPS 2007). Although the FDA recommends that women under age 19 should not have breast augmentation, there was an 8 percent increase in teenagers who received implants between 2000 and 2004 (Ault 2005; ASAPS 2006a). Although this trend decreased from 2005 to 2006, it is estimated that 45 percent of implant procedures among teenagers are done solely for cosmetic reasons (Ault 2005).

The technology of silicone breast implants has evolved steadily since the first implant surgery in 1962 in response to the problems encountered with different designs and materials. A polyurethane foam coating was introduced in the 1970s to reduce the degree to which the body produced fibrous tissue as a protective lining around the implant. This model was discontinued in 1991 because the coating disintegrated quickly and led to complications. In the 1980s a double-lumen implant, with two cavities and two shells, was developed. In 1995 the "trilucent" implant, filled with fat from soybean oil, was introduced in Europe but removed from the market in 1999 because the filler was toxic. Today, implants come in a variety of styles—smooth versus textured, round versus anatomically shaped, single lumen versus double lumen, and fixed volume versus inflatable—and the shells containing the silicone have become thinner and seamless. With all these improvements, breast implants seemed to be the answer to distress over small breasts.

The linking of breast size and appearance with sexuality and self-esteem has made breast augmentation the number-one cosmetic surgery in the United States. The American idealization of an unrealistically slender, yet buxom, young female body (Boodman 2004; Turner 2004) and the medicalization of unattractiveness sustain its use, enriching the medical profession, the medical device manufacturers, and the pharmaceutical companies, but are they safe?

The Safety of Silicone Implants Questioned

Beginning in the late 1970s and early 1980s reports began to surface about health problems associated with the leakage of silicone into the body that resulted from the permeability and rupture of silicone implants (Uretsky et al. 1979). In addition, evidence began to accumulate that the polyurethane coating could degrade within the body and produce toxic, carcinogenic substances. Other research found that free-floating silicone could affect women's breast milk and breast-fed infants (Guidoin et al. 1992; Zimmerman 1998).

Despite this initial evidence that silicone implants had the potential to cause serious health problems in women, they remained on the consumer market as unregulated products throughout the 1970s and 1980s. Even in 1976, when Congress granted the FDA the authority to regulate medical devices, silicone breast implants were granted Class II status (requiring some controls such as performance standards, user education, and postmarket surveillance studies) but were absolved from the more rigorous premarket approval (Class III) regulatory process since they had already been on the market for 15 years (ASAPS 2006a). With its new authority to regulate medical devices, the FDA considered breast implants, then still rather rare, a low priority compared to other devices like heart valves that were potentially lifesaving (Zuckerman 2001). Since the beginning in the early 1960s, then, the manufacturers of implants had the liberty to change the content and consistency of their implants without meeting any requirements for safety and without significant FDA oversight. Plastic surgeons continued to insert silicone implants despite mounting evidence of their compromised safety record (Zimmerman 1998).

By the 1980s breast augmentation surgery was one of the most common procedures in plastic surgery, yet most of the women who had the surgery were neither told nor were they aware that their implants had not been proven safe by the FDA (National Research Center for Women & Families 2006). Women began to assert publicly that they were experiencing illnesses that they attributed to the silicone that was migrating throughout their bodies after their implants ruptured. They complained of symptoms such as fatigue, pain, joint problems, and other symptoms that are commonly associated with connective tissue or autoimmune diseases. According to Zimmerman (1998) many of the women she interviewed felt they had not received enough information to make an informed decision about the long-term risks of implants. They also felt deceived not only by their doctors but also by the government into thinking that implants were safe. Most had not received any information about the potential harm from implants aside from cautions about the complications of surgery itself. They were not told about other possible complications like capsular contraction, pain, dissatisfaction with cosmetic result (e.g., wrinkling, shifting, scarring, uneven size), hematoma, reduced sensation in the breast, wound-healing problems, interference with mammography, and many others. Neither were they informed that their implants could leak or rupture or that they might need repeat surgery. Despite testimonies about symptoms and ill health, medical professionals tended to dismiss their patients' experience as anecdotal or as part of the normal risks of implant surgery, and implants remained on the consumer market, although both physicians and manufacturers were aware of the leakage and rupture problems (National Research Center for Women & Families 2006).

In 1984 the first product liability case concerning implants was brought against the Dow Corning Corporation (*Stern v. Dow Corning*), which was then the largest of the silicone gel implant manufacturers. The case alleged a connection between implant failure and the systemic illnesses that women were reporting to their physicians (Angell 1996; Zimmerman 1998; Jacobson 2000). The case attracted a great deal of media attention and forced the issue of the safety of breast augmentation into the public arena. Many other individual lawsuits against Dow Corning (a total of 12,359 by 1993) and other manufacturers resulted in multimillion-dollar punitive fines against breast implant manufacturers. The juries in these cases based their decisions on the determination that safety information was withheld from patients (National Research Center for Women & Families 2006). In December 1992 Dow Corning withdrew its products from the market (FDA 2004) before the major victory was won. The 1994 class-action lawsuit/global settlement against breast implant manufacturers resulted in a $4.2 billion settlement that was set aside for women with breast implants, $3.2 billion of which was to be paid by Dow Corning. The company filed for bankruptcy in 1995, however, leaving women little hope of receiving monetary compensation (Sims and Lundberg 2001). The company later recovered but when Dow Corning filed only $80 million dollars in damages had been awarded (Frontline 2006; Sims and Lundberg 2001; Zimmerman 1998). Throughout the litigation process, the manufacturers continued to assert that the scientific evidence did not support an association between silicone implants and autoimmune disease.

Although scientists had begun to express concerns about the safety of silicone implants beginning in the late 1970s, and the FDA heard these concerns at a 1978 advisory committee meeting, the FDA ignored the need to regulate implants for 10 years (House Government Operations Committee 1992), despite the fact that by the early 1980s most of the risks that eventually led to the removal of the implants from the market were already known or suspected (National Research Center for Women & Families 2006). In 1988 the FDA classified silicone gel implants as Class III devices, which required the manufacturers to submit premarket approval (PMA) along with data that supported a reasonable assurance of safety and efficacy.

Between 1976 and 1992, the FDA allowed the manufacturers of implants and plastic surgeons to assess the safety and effectiveness of silicone breast implant devices. As Jacobson (2000) points out, deregulation was a hallmark of the Reagan-Bush era (1981–1993), and the power and authority of the FDA had been greatly weakened during that time. The push to regulate silicone implants came from then FDA chief, David Kessler (appointed by George H. W. Bush), who promoted greater scientific rigor in the regulatory function of the FDA. Kessler's goal was to assess the safety and effectiveness of silicone implants using a risk/benefit model grounded in scientific data and expert knowledge (Kent 2003).

This FDA push for evidence-based medicine was counterbalanced by the lobbying efforts of industry and the medical profession to keep silicone implants on the market. The months before the November 1991 meeting of the FDA advisory panel provided the manufacturers and plastic surgeons with the opportunity to lobby the FDA and Congress on behalf of their product (House Government Operations Committee 1992). The Health Industry Manufacturers Association hired James Benson, former director of the FDA's Center for Devices and Radiological Health, as a lobbyist for their interests. The American Society of Plastic and Reconstructive Surgeons (ASPRS) hired three lobbying firms that placed lobbyists in Washington in October 1991 and organized a cadre of "satisfied consumers," who stormed Washington to support the return of silicone implants to market. One of the lobbyists hired by the ASPRS was Mark Heller, who had testified only a year earlier on behalf of the FDA's Office of General Counsel in a December 1990 breast implant hearing. Such examples of the revolving door between the FDA and the biomedical technoscience industry create conflicts of interest that call into question the FDA's ability to provide unbiased judgments based on scientific evidence. (House Government Operations Committee 1992).

After more than a decade of controversy about the negative health consequences of silicone gel breast implants, the FDA finally convened to discuss the safety of the devices in November 1991. The FDA General and Plastic Surgery Devices Panel voted unanimously to advise the FDA that implants filled "a public health need for breast reconstruction and revision for medical or surgical reasons and that the implants should continue to be available while the companies collected additional data" despite the recognition that the data presented by the companies were insufficient (FDA 2004). A few months later, in January 1992, the FDA called for a voluntary moratorium on the use of silicone implants pending a more thorough review of the health risks. Finally, David Kessler, FDA commissioner at the time, restricted the use of silicone breast devices to controlled clinical studies for reconstruction after mastectomy, correction of congenital deformities, or replacement of ruptured silicone gel-filled implants due to medical or surgical reasons (FDA 2005a, 2005b).

When Kessler imposed the ban on silicone implants, he indicated that after 30 years of use, there were a series of questions that had not yet been and needed to be answered before the FDA could approve them: 1) How often do implants leak and what materials are getting into the body? 2) How often do implants break and how long do they last? 3) How often do women with implants suffer adverse effects? 4) To what extent do implants interfere with mammography examinations? 5) Can implants increase a woman's risk of developing cancer? and 6) Is failure of the devices related to autoimmune and connective tissue diseases? (Kessler 1992b). In 1992, the FDA sided with the scientists, physicians, women's health advocates, and victims who believed that there was not enough evidence to determine that silicone implants were safe and that the risks outweighed the benefits even though the certainty of risk could not be determined from the data then available (Jacobson 2000; Kent 2003).

After the ban was instituted, the only way for women to get silicone implants for cosmetic purposes in the United States was to participate in the IDE studies as part of the premarket approval process (Duenwald 2005). Although saline breast implants manufactured by both Mentor and Inamed remained on the market, they have less desirable cosmetic effects than silicone implants, and this is the main reason for the continued seduction of American women by silicone gel implants. Women who wanted silicone either enrolled in IDE trials stateside or left the country to get them. Silicone implants are legally sold, widely used, and available in Europe, Latin America, and Australia, and during the ban, many American women had surgery abroad. Prior to November 2006, Europe, South America, and Mexico were the major destinations for American women who wanted the natural feel of silicone implants despite the cost of the trip, the fact that silicone implants cost twice as much as saline implants, and the accessibility and availability of already approved saline devices stateside (Duenwald 2005).

Because of the lack of scientific data to settle the controversy surrounding the safety of silicone breast implants, in 1997 the Department of Health and Human Services (DHHS) asked the Institute of Medicine (IOM) to conduct an independent review of all past and ongoing scientific research regarding the safety of silicone breast implants. A committee of experts was assembled to assess the evidence related to the primary problems that had surfaced in association with implants: systemic disease (asserted by women with implants), the biological and immunological effects of silicone and other chemical components found in implants, the impact of breast implants on offspring, and interference with mammography results (FDA 2004). This report was released in 1999 (see Bondurant et al. 2000).

Assessing the Risks of Implants

The risks of breast implant procedures are related to both the risks of surgery under general anesthesia and to the adverse health effects of the insertion of implants into the human body. We discuss these risks below.

Surgery and General Anesthesia

There are different approaches to breast augmentation surgery that usually involve one of three kinds of entry incisions: a small incision underneath the breast (inframammary fold), near the nipple (circum or periaerolar position), or within the armpit (axillary fold). The implant is placed subcutaneously behind the breast tissue, on top of the chest muscle or submuscularly, under the pectoral muscle. The type of operation reflects consideration of patient's desires, the surgeon's suggestions, the type of implant device used, and differences in individual patients' fat and body tissue (ASAPS 2006a; Bondurant et al. 2000). The surgery is an outpatient procedure that takes about one to two hours under general anesthesia and usually entails a one- to two-week recovery. Risks of undergoing general anesthesia depend on the patient's general health and the experience of the anesthesiologist. Rare but serious risks include cardiac arrhythmias, dangerous increases or decreases in blood pressure, rapid increase in body temperature, difficulty breathing, collapse of blood vessels because of low blood pressure, heart attack or stroke, and death due to cardiac arrest or to complications such as changes in heartbeat, blood pressure, body temperature, or breathing (WebMD 2006).

Local and Perioperative Complications

The FDA brochure mandated for patients lists 26 potential complications of implant surgery, including asymmetry, breast pain, breast tissue atrophy, calcification/calcium deposits, capsular contracture, chest wall deformity, delayed wound healing, extrusion, galactorrhea (milky discharge from nipple), granuloma, hematoma, iatrogenic injury or damage, infection, inflammation or irritation, malposition or displacement of implants, necrosis, nipple or breast changes, palpability or visibility, ptosis (drooping), redness or bruising, rupture or deflation, scarring, seroma (collection of fluid under the skin), unsatisfactory style or size, and wrinkling or rippling (FDA 2004). The most common of these health consequences are capsular contraction, tissue hardening, rashes, implant rupture, and infection (FDA 2004; Bondurant et al. 2000:124; Marwick 1999). Capsular contracture involves the formation of scar tissue that squeezes the implant and can cause pain and discomfort. Many surgeons suggest that capsular contraction is a normal result of implant surgery that all women will experience to some degree. In severe cases, resurgery is required (Bondurant et al. 2000).

Implant Rupture and Silicone Migration

Breast implants do not last forever, and most will rupture within ten years (FDA 2004).

The rate of rupture varies by manufacturer, by implant type, and by method of insertion (i.e., subglandular or submuscular), but a detected rupture requires the removal of the implant and, if desired, its replacement. Before rupture rates were studied, ruptures were thought to be rare, but rupture rates are actually quite high, estimated at 4 percent within three years of implantation, but 50 to 75 percent after ten years (Brown et al. 2000). The majority of implanted women experienced rupture within a ten-year time frame and rupture rates significantly increased with age of the implant (Brown et al. 2000; Zuckerman et al. 2005). Rupture of silicone implants can be caused by the normal aging of the implant, damage from surgical instruments, too much handling during surgery, damage during procedures to the breast for other reasons (e.g., biopsy, fluid drainage), compression during mammogram, trauma, capsular contracture, and umbilical placement of implants (FDA 2004). Thus, most women who have implants will require resurgery, perhaps as many as four or five resurgeries, over the course of their lives.

When implants rupture, silicone gel can migrate outside of the scar tissue capsule that forms around the implant into surrounding body tissues, the circulatory system, and lymph nodes. Migrated silicone can cause lumps (granulomas) in the breast, chest wall, armpit, arm, or abdomen (FDA 2004), but ruptures can also be asymptomatic and, thus, difficult to detect (Brown et al. 2000; Brown et al. 2001). Silicone implant ruptures are more likely than saline implant ruptures to be "silent" (i.e., not as easily visible as deflation of ruptured saline implants) and undetected for long periods (Sarwer et al. 2000; Nash 2003). The FDA recommends MRI for evaluation of patients with suspected rupture or leakage of silicone gel implants (FDA 2004). The degree to which silicone leaks adversely affect the body has been the major controversy in the debate over the safety and effectiveness of silicone implants. It has been hypothesized that migrated silicone could be linked to serious diseases, such as connective tissue disorders and cancer, as discussed below.

Removal and replacement of implants requires resurgery with its attendant risks. The FDA consumer brochure (FDA 2004) clearly states that women with implants are likely to need one or more resurgeries over their lifetime due to local complications and that multiple operations can result in unsatisfactory cosmetic outcomes.

The potential risks associated with rupture are the source of FDA-mandated product labeling instructions and recommendations for "best care" practices that include regular MRI screening every two years, beginning three years after insertion and removal or replacement of ruptured implants. The cost-preventive MRI screening (currently about $1,000 to $2,200) over a woman's lifetime will probably exceed the original cost of the implant surgery, which is currently about $4,500 to $10,000 depending on the state in which it is done. These costs are not likely to be covered by health insurance (New York Times 2007).

Systemic Diseases: Autoimmune Diseases and Connective Tissue Disease

The biggest debate about the long-term effects of implant rupture concerns whether or not silicone leakage is associated with systemic diseases such as cancer, connective tissue disease (CTD), and autoimmune disease. CTDs include both those with autoimmune characteristics (e.g., lupus, rheumatoid arthritis, and scleroderma) and those without autoimmune characteristics (e.g., fibromyalgia, chronic fatigue syndrome). The cause of CTDs is not known. The IOM report reviewed over 3,300 articles as well as testimony from manufacturers, researchers, and women with silicone implants and concluded that there was insufficient evidence to validate a connection between silicone gel implants and systemic diseases in women.

Prominent epidemiological studies such as the Mayo Clinic Study (Gabriel et al. 1994), the Nurses Health Study (Sánchez-Guerrero et al. 1995), and two studies of Danish (Friis et al. 1997) and Swedish (Nyrén 1998) women all concluded that silicone implants were not related to systemic disease. Conversely, the Women's Health Cohort Study (Hennekens et al. 1996), which had the largest sample of all these studies, did find a significant risk of connective-tissue disease, but these results have been criticized because they relied on unverified self-reports of disease (Bondurant et al. 2000). A meta-analysis of extant research concluded that "from a public health perspective, breast implants appear to have a minimal effect on the number of women in whom connective diseases develop, and elimination of implants would be unlikely to reduce the incidence of connective tissue diseases" (Janowsky et al. 2000:789).

One study published after the IOM report concluded that breast implant rupture and silicone migration outside the scar capsule was related to fibromyalgia, a syndrome characterized by widespread pain, fatigue, and sleep disturbance whose cause is unknown (Brown et al. 2001; Brown et al. 2000). This study used MRI to identify the prevalence of implant rupture and extracapsular silicone gel in a cohort of 344 women who said they were satisfied with their silicone gel breast implants. Through MRI, radiologists discovered that over half of the 687 (55 percent, $N = 378$) breast implant devices scanned were ruptured and an additional 7 percent were suspected of rupture. Notably, 77 percent of the women had at least one implant that was classified as ruptured or indeterminate. MRI findings indicated that silicone had migrated outside of both the device and the fibrous scar capsules in 21 percent ($N = 73$) of the women in the study (Brown et al. 2000). Furthermore, women whose MRIs displayed silicone gel outside the fibrous scar tissue reported higher rates of fibromyalgia (Brown et al. 2001). These researchers concluded that there was an association between implant rupture, silicone leakage, and fibromyalgia. However, this finding was not repeated in a similar study of Danish women (Holmich et al. 2003).

Taken together, the studies to date have not confirmed a strong link between silicone implants and systemic diseases. The FDA consumer brochure indicates that the risk is low, but that studies have not been large enough or long enough to resolve the issue (FDA 2004).

Breast Cancer and Mammography

The weight of the evidence to date suggests that there is no relationship between silicone gel implants and breast cancer. However, both the IOM report (Bondurant et al. 2000) and a more recent study (Miglioretti et al. 2004) suggest that silicone gel implants can interfere with mammography screening by obscuring breast tissue, thereby delaying diagnosis of breast cancer. However, neither study suggested that there was an increased risk of mortality due to delayed diagnosis for this reason.

Other Cancers

Studies funded by the National Cancer Institute (NCI) concluded that silicone implants increase a woman's overall risk of cancer by 21 percent with an excess risk of brain and respiratory cancers (Brinton et al. 2001; Flynn and Zuckerman 2006). Other cancers that have been higher in women with implants in more than one study include cancers of the cervix, vulva, lung, and stomach (Brinton et al. 2001; FDA 2004; McLaughlin et al. 2004).

Breast-feeding and Child Health

At least one study reported an association between infants who have been breast-fed by silicone gel–implanted mothers and sclerodermalike esophageal disease (Flick 1994). The IOM (Bondurant et al. 2000) report found no evidence for such a link, but they did find that breast implants can interfere with a woman's ability to lactate in 28 to 64 percent of implanted women and can cause inadequate milk supply. Thus, while not directly causing disease in children, implants can interfere with breast-feeding, which confers significant immune system advantages to a breast-fed infant (Bondurant et al. 2000).

The IOM Report and Subsequent Studies

The IOM report is the most prestigious and widely cited study of the risks of silicone implants to date. The expert scientific panel concluded that there was a lack of evidence to support any relationship between silicone gel implants and the most serious threats to women's health that had been raised by researchers and the public that had led to the lawsuits in the 1990s and the eventual ban on cosmetic use of silicone implants in 1992—autoimmune and connective tissue diseases, breast cancer, and diseases among breast-fed infants of women with implants. Furthermore, the IOM asserted that since there are over 1.5 million women with silicone breast implants, statistically some of these women would be expected to develop such diseases but no excess burden of these diseases was found in women with implants. On the basis of this report, the FDA approved silicone gel implants for cosmetic purposes. Studies conducted subsequent to the IOM report have shown mixed results regarding CTDs and at least two studies suggest a relationship between silicone implants and cancers of the brain, lung, cervix, vulva, and stomach. Although association is not evidence of cause, these results signal that further research is needed to determine the reason for the elevated risk of these cancers in women with silicone implants. In addition, the numerous criticisms of extant studies point to the need for better-designed prospective studies with larger samples and longer-term follow-up in order to be certain of the long-term safety of silicone gel implants with respect to serious chronic diseases.

The bad news from these studies of implants, however, is that they interfere with breast-feeding and detection of breast cancer by mammography, and they have high rates of local complications, rupture and leakage of implants, and potentially high lifetime costs for resurgery and preventive screening. The national average for surgeon's fees in 2006 was $3,600 for breast augmentation, and the total cost of breast augmentation now ranges between $4,500 and $10,000 depending on the state in which it is done (ASPS 2006). Total expenditures on breast augmentation in the United States already exceed one billion dollars, more than expenditures for any other kind of plastic surgery (ASPS 2007). It is easy to see that the breast augmentation industry is an important income generator for plastic surgeons and the manufacturers of implants. In the face of all the risks, we must ask ourselves whether the physical and monetary costs of breast augmentation are worth it when the only benefit to women is psychological.

Psychological Benefits of Breast Augmentation

Research suggests that women seek breast implants because they experience depression and low self-esteem due to dissatisfaction with the appearance of their breasts (Goin and Goin 1981). Sarwer et al. (2000) have analyzed past studies that included preoperative psychological evaluations of breast augmentation patients. Their results suggest that women who seek cosmetic surgery experience symptoms of depression, have low self-esteem, and may also display other psychopathologies. Several recent studies have found a higher rate of suicide among women with implants that may be due to underlying psychological problems or to increased distress because of implant complications (FDA 2004; McLaughlin et al. 2004). There is evidence for both prior conditions (Pukkala et al. 2003; Joiner 2003) and postimplantation distress (Zuckerman 2003). Brinton et al. (2001) found that suicide among women with silicone implants was four times greater than that of women having other kinds of cosmetic surgery and two to three times greater than that of women of the same age in the general population.

Body Image Dissatisfaction

Susan Bordo (1993) asserts that women suffer from dissatisfaction with their physical appearance because they do not have the culturally idealized body type, which they can change through diet, exercise, and/or cosmetic surgery. According to Sarwer et al. (1998), body image dissatisfaction is an important psychological construct for understanding women's desire for breast enhancement. In particular, breast augmentation surgery appears to improve self-esteem and overall psychological well-being for the women who have it. Indeed, increased self-esteem and an improved sex life are the major benefits of breast augmentation surgery cited by the American Society for Aesthetic Plastic Surgery on their website (ASAPS 2006b):

> Women who undergo common elective cosmetic surgery procedures not only feel better about their bodies, but also have higher degrees of satisfaction with their sex lives, including ability to orgasm . . . *the greatest benefits were seen in women who had breast augmentation/breast lift and/or body contouring procedures* [emphasis added].

In an effort to bolster their self-esteem, however, women may disregard, overlook, or be misinformed about the potential health consequences and long-term costs of silicone breast implants. One of the major problems in the entire breast implant controversy is the failure of governmental regulation to recognize the relationship between the plastic surgery and breast implant industries and women's increased dissatisfaction with their bodies (Eggertson 2006).

FDA Approval and Oversight

The FDA did stipulate stringent conditions for approval that included requirements for full disclosure of the risks and complications of the surgery itself, the expected shelf life and rupture and leakage rates of the implants, the probable necessity for resurgery in the future, and the potential complications women might experience with breast-feeding and mammography. Thus, the final FDA decision took seriously its obligation to fully inform prospective patients of the many non-life-threatening complications of breast implants. In addition, the postapproval studies mandated by the FDA required Mentor and Allergan to follow all implant recipients for ten years to assess the safety of their products with respect to local complications and rupture rates; the rates, signs, and symptoms of both connective tissue disorders and neurological diseases; effects on offspring, reproduction, lactation, and interference with mammography; rates of suicide and cancer; and compliance with MRI screening guidelines (Peck 2006).

One of the major concerns regarding approval that was voiced early on, however, was the fact that once the implants reached the market, the FDA would no longer have the authority to enforce research and informed consent (Zuckerman 2003). The specific conditions for approval of the devices (i.e., informed consent, best practices recommendations, follow-up studies) were set to remedy this problem, but it is too early to determine the extent to which FDA recommendations have been or will be implemented by manufacturers and surgeons.

Despite the FDA's intention of protecting women by recommending periodic MRI screening, it is becoming increasingly evident that many plastic surgeons (as many as 99 percent according to Dr. Scott L. Spear, chairman of plastic surgery at Georgetown University Hospital) think there are problems with the recommendations to physicians and patients concerning MRI follow-up: "They bring a lot of red tape and expense" (New York Times 2007). The two largest plastic surgery associations (the ASPS and ASAPS) advise their members to adhere to the FDA guidelines, but compliance cannot be enforced by the FDA, since only product labeling is mandated by law. Thus, there is no way to ensure that physicians will comply with the MRI follow-up protocol even though they might recommend it to their patients. Similarly, there is no way to ensure that patients will adhere to the costly follow-up recommendations of their physicians. Although the FDA and the manufacturers will be monitoring compliance with MRI screening, silicone implants are now on the market as consumer products, and the FDA has no teeth with which to enforce compliance.

Interest Groups and Financial Gain

According to Angell (1996:19–20), it was a coalition of "advocates of tough government regulation, women who believed breast implants had caused them to become ill, and feminists who thought it was about time someone put a stop to women being pressured to conform to male fantasies" that orchestrated the 1992 FDA ban breast implants. There was as well, however, an FDA that wanted to use the impartiality of scientific evidence to make a decision about implants, an opposing coalition of consumers who wanted implants, and surgeons and manufacturers who had very much to gain financially from their approval.

Plastic surgeons have long supported the approval of silicone implants. ASPS surgeons predicted that they would perform up to 25 percent more breast augmentations in 2007 and that they expected about 40 percent of their patients to choose silicone implants (PlasticSurgery.org 2007). Plastic surgeons are also uniquely qualified to assess health risks and benefits of implants because of their extensive knowledge and clinical experience. One of the panel members of the FDA premarket approval deliberations was a plastic surgeon whose research was supported by Inamed but stated that his personal financial interest would not interfere with his decision about approval (Steinbrook 2005). We must ask whether the opinions of expert plastic surgeons were completely impartial (Jacobson 2000).

The manufacturers of implants also stood to make a lot of money after approval, and many were accused of underreporting or covering up problems with their products during IDE studies. There were several instances of whistle-blowing during the 12-year ban. The full account of these incidents is difficult to trace, but manufacturers were accused of underreporting and suppressing negative study outcomes and using contaminated materials in manufacturing. The 1998 investigation of allegations that Mentor used contaminated silicone in its manufacturing process is one example. No charges were filed against Mentor, but the company signed a consent decree promising to manufacture its implants in compliance with the FDA's Quality System Regulation practices. It is certainly easy to see why the manufacturers would want to present their products in the best light because the financial incentive is so great.

The women's health advocates who lost this last round of deliberations over silicone seduction still advise caution, continue to contest the conclusion that silicone implants are safe on the grounds that the studies were flawed, and decry the lack of attention given to the lived experience of so many women who believe their implants have made them ill. They call the approval of silicone breast implants for cosmetic reasons a travesty.

The contesting claims that implants are safe and improve women's self-esteem and that they cause misery, health problems, and even death are found in the research, in the media, and on the many websites that advocate or oppose silicone implants. Both Mentor and Allergan now have products that are approved as safe and effective by the FDA. All the elements of a good plot line—subjective suffering, objective scientific rationality, and the corrupting influence of greed justified by the alleviation of subjective suffering—will continue to make this story that has not ended and will be followed for many years to come.

Discussion

The breast implant controversy is no longer about whether or not silicone implants heighten women's risk of breast cancer and autoimmune disease. The weight of the existing evidence suggests no greater risk for these specific diseases among women with implants than among those who have undergone other kinds of plastic surgery or those in the general population. The research does suggest, however, that the rupture rates of silicone gel implants are quite high and that silicone can migrate outside these devices into the body where it may cause health problems. In addition, several studies suggest higher rates of brain, lung, cervical, vulva, and stomach cancer and elevated rates of suicide.

Most of the studies assessing the health risks of silicone implants had samples that were too small and women with far fewer years of exposure to their implants than required according to many scientists. Thus, most researchers have qualified their conclusions about implant safety with statements like this: "Our results, therefore, cannot be considered definitive proof of the absence of an association between breast implants and connective-tissue disease." (Gabriel et al. 1994:1700). The FDA consumer handbook itself says "these studies have not been large enough to resolve the question of whether or not breast implants slightly increase the risk of CTDs or related disorders" (FDA 2004). In sum, the major criticism of past studies that examined the relationship between silicone gel implants, autoimmune and connective tissue diseases, and cancer is that they relied on small sample sizes of participants without a long history of implants and an insufficient follow-up period to detect dose response relationships. As Diana Zuckerman (2003:2), president of the National Center for Policy Research for Women and Families, points out, "almost all the studies in the Institute of Medicine report suffered from the same shortcomings . . . too small, and too short."

While scientific evidence of safety is the meaningful measure for physicians and surgeons, it does not take into account the misery many women have experienced because of their implants, and thus it erases the personal, lived experience of individuals. The standards for safety and efficacy do not deny that some people will experience problems, only that the devices do not appear to be associated with elevated risk of the problems women suffer. Thus the FDA, as the protector of the public's health, studies the safety of products, approves them if they meet scientific standards, and increases the confidence of the consumer in the drugs and devices it approves (Jacobson 2000). The FDA has now concluded that silicone implants are safe and effective, but this finding is still contested.

What we find most notable about the history of FDA decisions about silicone implants is that both the ban in 1992 and approval of Mentor's and Allergan's products in 2006 were made despite the lack of solid, long-term evidence that supports the long-term safety and effectiveness of these devices. Moreover, both decisions relegated the non–life threatening, but potentially serious medical complications associated with their use to the category of expected side effects. Both decisions were made in response to political pressure from the stakeholders and under conditions of conflicting and contested scientific evidence. While women's health advocates won the day in 1992 perhaps because there was so little good research at the time, the biomedical industry won in 2006 based on research whose interpretation is contested. Thus, it was largely the absence of the serious, life-threatening health risks that women's health advocates proposed (CTDs, autoimmune diseases, cancer), albeit based on flawed studies, that tipped the victory to industry, plastic surgeons, and the many

American women who feel they need to alter their bodies with surgically implanted bags of silicone gel.

The continuing question of the possible longer-term effects of silicone leaked into women's bodies undermines the confidence of many in the scientific community in the FDA decision. The FDA itself, even after approving the implants, requires continued study by the manufacturers. What is the American consumer who wants silicone implants because their cosmetic effect is superior to that of saline implants to believe?

The drama of the breast implant controversy is about the safety of silicone breast implants with little discussion of why so many women feel the "need" for breast implants. It is eminently understandable that women who have had breast cancer or women who have severe congenital breast abnormalities would want to avail themselves of plastic surgery to normalize their ravaged bodies and that this would have tremendous psychological benefit to them. But in 2006, only 15 percent of breast augmentation surgeries were done for medical or reconstructive reasons. Eighty-five percent were for cosmetic purposes (ASPS 2007).

American women have long been taught to improve their appearance by using the many health and beauty products on the market, but this seems no longer enough. Breast implant manufacturers such as Mentor and Allergan as well as the surgeons who install their products in women's bodies feed off the growing trend for women to use extraordinary means in the pursuit of beauty, acceptance, and sexual power. As one plastic surgeon asserted: "Patients sometimes misunderstand the nature of cosmetic surgery. It's not a shortcut for diet or exercise. *It's a way to override the genetic code* [emphasis added]" (Morgan 2003:168). Thus, surgery can remake every woman into an ideal that is only rarely seen in nature, and, in doing so, makes the normal abnormal. Indeed, we have pathologized the normal and medicalized perceived unattractiveness. In the brave new world of technologically created perfect bodies, women can lose their health and their wealth in the pursuit of the ideal breasts.

Women have breast augmentation surgery to give them power in a male-dominated world. But, implanted breasts can also cause a lifetime of health and medical problems, and they can provide only a simulation of real power that stems from a very different base. Even if long-term studies ultimately exonerate implants, what force of culture can be so strong as to make women subject themselves to the knife and to the many "acceptable" injuries and complications associated with breast implants and pay a lot of money for their morbidity?

Is breast augmentation in the West significantly different from female genital cutting (FGC) in Africa and the Middle East? Both are surgeries. Both have complications. Both make women more appealing to men. Both seem necessary and normal in cultural context. It is, perhaps, the ultimate irony that American mothers who would protest FGC have given breast augmentation surgery to their teenage daughters (Kreimer 2004), perpetuating, as it were, the same female-to-female ritual system involved in FGC. Perhaps we should use a new term to cover all female surgical alterations (FSAs) that will allow us to think about and theorize the cross-cultural implications of the new biotechnology that medicalizes female unattractiveness and shapes and sculpts the female body to the reigning cultural images of beauty.

If this story tells us anything, it tells us that there is a significant need for strong, judicious, evidence-based oversight of the capitalist marketing of medical devices. Silicone breast implants are not without tremendous risk and cost. Both of these issues have been played down by the Biomedical TechnoService Complex that stands to make a great deal of money from the silicone breast implant industry. Are silicone implants killer commodities? After wading through all the data, we conclude that the evidence is not yet in and await the results of the larger and longer-term studies that even the FDA suggests are necessary to establish safety and efficacy. What is clear from the studies to date is that implants cause a great deal of morbidity and will likely need to be replaced at least once during a woman's lifetime. Thus, there is profit to be made at the physical and fiscal expense of the American women who will choose cosmetic breast augmentation with silicone implants.

Women are now free to "choose" silicone breast implants. The need for patient education, informed consent, continued federal regulation of the devices, and further research is now more urgent than ever, as is the need to problematize the medicalization and commodification of women's bodies under the neoliberal influence of the free-market economy and the Biomedical TechnoService Complex, which aggressively markets silicone gel implants to women who have been convinced that their natural bodies need unnatural improvement.

References

Angell, Marcia

1996 Science on Trial: The Clash of Medical Evidence and the Law in the Breast Implant Case. New York: Norton.

ASAPS (American Society of Aesthetic Plastic Surgeons)

2006a 2005 ASAPS Statistics. Electronic document, www.surgery.org/press/procedurefacts-asqf.php.

2006b Women's Self-Image and Sexual Satisfaction Increase after Cosmetic Surgery. Electronic document, http://surgery.org/public/news-release.php?iid=427§ion=.

ASPS (American Society of Plastic Surgeons)

2006 2005 Statistics. Electronic document, www.plasticsurgery.org/public_education/2005Statistics.cfm.

2007 2000/2005/2006 National Plastic Surgery Statistics. Electronic document, www.plasticsurgery.org/media/Press_Kits/Procedural-Statistics-Press-Kit-Index.cfm.

Ault, Alicia

2005 Caution Urged as More Teens Seek Breast Implants. OB/GYN News, March 1. Electronic document, www.findarticles.com/p/articles/mi_m0CYD/is_5_40/ai_n13472441.

Bondurant, Stuart, Virginia Ernster, and Roger Herdman, eds.

2000 The Safety of Silicone Breast Implants. Institute of Medicine. Washington, DC: National Academy Press.

Boodman, Sandra G.

2004 For More Teenage Girls, Adult Plastic Surgery. Rise in Breast Implants, Other Procedures Raises Doubts about Long-Term Effects. Washington Post, October 26: A01. Electronic document, www.washingtonpost.com/ac2/wp-dyn/A62540-2004Oct25?language=printer.

Bordo, Susan

1993 Unbearable Weight: Feminism, Western Culture and the Body. Berkeley: University of California Press.

Brinton, Louise A., Jay H. Lubin, Mary Cay Burich, Theodore Colton, S. Lori Brown, and Robert N. Hoover

2001 Cancer Risk at Sites Other Than the Breast Following Augmentation Mammoplasty. Annals of Epidemiology 11(4): 248–256.

Brown, Lori S., Michael S. Middleton, Wendie A. Berg, Mary Scott Soo, and Gene Pennello

2000 Prevalence of Rupture of Silicone Gel Breast Implants Revealed on MRI Imaging in a Population of Women in Birmingham, Alabama. American Journal of Roentgenology 173:1057–1064.

Brown, Lori S., Gene Pennello, Wendie A. Berg, Mary Scott Soo, and Michael S. Middleton
2001 Silicone Gel Breast Implant Rupture, Extracapsular Silicone, and Health Status in a Population of Women. Journal of Rheumatology 28(5):996–1003.
Clarke, Adele E., Janet K. Shim, Laura Mamo, Jennifer Ruth Fosket, and Jennifer R. Fishman
2003 Biomedicalization: Technoscientific Transformations of Health, Illness, and U.S. Biomedicine. American Sociological Review 68(2):161–194.
Duenwald, Mary
2005 Despite Ban, a Gray Market in Silicone Implant Thrives. New York Times, April 21. Electronic document, www.nytimes.com/2005/04/21/fashion/thursdaystyles/21implant.html?ex=1149566400&en=06fe383c7e690649&ei=5070.
Dworkin, Ronald W.
2001 The Medicalization of Unhappiness. Public Interest 144:85–99.
Eggertson, Laura
2006 Breast Implant Advisory Panel: More Study on Silicone Leakage. Canadian Medical Association Journal 174(4):443.
FDA (Food and Drug Administration)
2004 FDA Breast Implant Consumer Handbook 2004. Electronic document, www.fda.gov/cdrh/breastimplants/handbook2004/indexbip.html.
2005a FDA Statement on Approvable Letter to Mentor Corporation. Electronic document, www.fda.gov/bbs/topics/NEWS/2005/NEW01233.html.
2005b FDA Statement on Approvable Letter to Inamed Corporation. FDA Statement. Electronic document, www.fda.gov/bbs/topics/news/2005/new01213.html.
Flynn, Rachael, and Diana Zuckerman
2006 Ruptured Silicone Breast Implants Linked to Debilitating Diseases. BreastImplantinfo.org. Electronic document, www.center4research.org/implantfibro.html.
Flick, John A.
1994 Silicone Implants and Esophageal Dysmotility: Are Breast-fed Infants at Risk? Journal of the American Medical Association 271(3):240–241.
Friis, Søren, Lane Mellemkjaer, Joseph K. McLaughlin, Vibeke Breiting, Susanne Krüger, William Blot, and Jörgen Olsen
1997 Connective Tissue Disease and Other Rheumatic Conditions Following Breast Implants in Denmark. Annals of Plastic Surgery 39:1–8.

Frontline
2006 Breast Implants on Trial: Chronology of Silicone Breast Implants. Electronic document, http://www2.pbs.org/wgbh/pages/frontline/implants/cron.html.

Gabriel, Sherine E., W. Michael O'Fallon, Leonard T. Kurland, C. Mary Beard, John E. Woods, and L. Joseph Melton
1994 Risk of Connective-Tissue Diseases and Other Disorders after Breast Implantation. New England Journal of Medicine 330(24):1697–1702.

Goin, John M., and Marcia Kraft Goin
1981 Changing the Body: Psychological Effects of Plastic Surgery. Baltimore: Williams & Wilkins.

Guidoin, Robert, Marc Therrien, Catherine Rolland, M. King, J. L. Grandmaison, Serge Kaliaguine, Pierre Blais, Hooshang Pakdel, and Christian Roy
1992 The Polyurethane Foam Covering the Meme Breast Prosthesis: A Biomedical Breakthrough or a Biomaterial Tar Baby? Annals of Plastic Surgery 28(4):342–353.

Haiken, Elizabeth
1997 Venus Envy: A History of Cosmetic Surgery. Baltimore: Johns Hopkins University Press.

Hennekens, Charles H., I-Min Lee, Nancy R. Cook, Patricia R. Hebert, Elizabeth W. Karlson, Fran LaMotte, JoAnn E. Manson, and Julie E. Buring
1996 Self-Reported Breast Implants and Connective-Tissue Diseases in Female Health Professionals. A Retrospective Cohort Study. Journal of the American Medical Association 275(8):616–621.

Holmich, Lisbet R., Kim Kjoller, John P. Fryzek, Mimi Hoier-Madsen, Ilse Vejborg, Carsten Conrad, Susanne Sletting, Joseph K. McLaughlin, Vibeke Breiting, and Søren Friis
2003 Self-Reported Diseases and Symptoms by Rupture Status among Unselected Danish Women with Cosmetic Silicone Breast Implants. Plastic and Reconstructive Surgery 111(2):723–732.

House Government Operations Committee
1992 The FDA's Regulation of Silicone Breast Implants: A Staff Report Prepared by the Human Resources and Intergovernmental Relations Subcommittee of the House Government Operations Committee. December. Electronic document, www.info-implants.com/BC/0028.html.

Jacobson, Nora
2000 Cleavage: Technology, Controversy, and the Ironies of the Man-Made Breast. New Brunswick, NJ: Rutgers University Press.

Janowsky, Esther C., Lawrence L. Kupper, and Barbara S. Hulka
2000 Meta-Analyses of the Relation between Silicone Breast Implants and the Risk of Connective Tissue Diseases. Massachusetts Medical Society 342(11):781–790.

Joiner, Thomas E., Jr.
2003 Does Breast Augmentation Confer Risk of or Protection from Suicide? Aesthetic Surgery Journal 23(5):370–375.

Kent, Julie
2003 Lay Experts and the Politics of Breast Implants. Public Understanding of Science 12(4):403–421.

Kessler, David
1992a The Basis of the FDA's Decision on Breast Implants. New England Journal of Medicine 326(23):1713–1715.
1992b Statement on Silicone Gel Breast Implants. Electronic document, www.fda.gov/bbs/topics/speech/spe00012.htm.

Kreimer, Susan
2004 Teens Getting Breast Implants for Graduation. Women's News, June 6. Electronic document, www.womensenews.org/article.cfm/dyn/aid/1861/context/archive.

Latteier, Carolyn
1998 Breasts: The Women's Perspective on an American Obsession. New York: Haworth Press.

Marwick, Charles
1999 Are They Real? IOM Report on Breast Implant Problems. Journal of the American Medical Association 281(4):314–315.

McGuire, Stephen
2004 Ads for Implants to Debut on Reality TV. Medical Marketing and Media 39(9):30.

McLaughlin, Joseph K., Thomas N. Wise, and Loren Lipworth
2004 Increased Risk of Suicide among Patients with Breast Implants: Do the Epidemiologic Data Support Psychiatric Consultation? Psychosomatics 45(4):277–280.

Miglioretti, Diana L., Carolyn M. Rutter, Berta M.Geller, Gary Cutter, William E. Barland, Robert Rosenberg, Ronald K. Weaver, Stephen H. Taplin, Rachel Bullard-Barbash, Patricia A. Carney, Bonnie C. Yakaslas, and Karla Lerlikowske
2004 Effects of Breast Augmentation on the Accuracy of Mammography and Cancer Characteristics. Journal of the American Medical Association 291:442–450.

Morgan, Kathryn Pauly
2003 Women and the Knife. Cosmetic Surgery and the Colonization of Women's Bodies. *In* The Politics of Women's Bodies. Sexuality,

Appearance, and Behavior, 2nd ed. Rose Weitz ed. Pp. 164–183. New York: Oxford University Press.

Nash, Karen
2003 Surgeons Ponder Using Silicone. Cosmetic Surgery Times, November 1. Electronic document, www.cosmeticsurgerytimes.com/cosmeticsurgerytimes/article/articleDetail.jsp?id=75207.

National Research Center for Women & Families Implant Information Project
2006 The FDA's Regulation of Silicone Breast Implants. Electronic document, www.breastimplantinfo.org/what_know_3-FDA1992.html.

New York Stock Exchange
2004 News release. July 29. Electronic document, http://ccbn.compuserve.com/releasetext.asp?ticker=mnt&coid=76343&client=compuserve&release=614733.

New York Times
2007 Implants Are Back, and So Is Debate. New York Times, May 24. Electronic document, www.nytimes.com/2007/05/24/fashion/24skin.html?_r=1&oref=slogin.

NWHN (National Women's Health Network)
2005 Silicone Gel Breast Implant News. National Women's Health Network, July 28. Electronic document, www.nwhn.org/alerts/alerts_details.php?aid=43.

Nyrén, Olof, Li Yin, Staffan Josefsson, Joseph K. McLaughlin, William J. Blot, Martin Engqvist, Lars Hakelius, John D. Boica Jr., and Hans-Olof Adami
1998 Risk of Connective Tissue Disease and Related Disorders among Women with Breast Implants: A Nation-wide, Retrospective Study in Sweden. British Medical Journal 316:417–422.

Peck, Peggy
2006 FDA Allows Return of Silicone-Gel Breast Implants. Medpage Today, November 20. Electronic document, http://medpagetoday.com/Surgery/PlasticSurgery/tb/4557.

PlasticSurgery.org
2007 Plastic Surgeons Analyze Impact of Silicone. Press release. May 25. Electronic document, www.plasticsurgery.org/media/press_releases/Plastic-Surgeons-Analyze-the-Impact-of-Silicone.cfm.

Public Citizen, The Health Research Group
2006 Statement of Dr. Sidney Wolfe, Director of Public Citizen's Health Research Group. Nov. 17—Silicone Gel Breast Implants Most Defective Medical Device Ever Approved by the FDA. November 17. Electronic document, www.citizen.org/hot_issues/issue.cfm?ID=1477, accessed April 27, 2007.

Pukkala, Eero, Ilona Kulmala, Sirpa-Liisa Hovi, Elena Hemminki, Ilmo Keskimaki, Loren Lipworth, John D. Boice, and Joseph K. McLaughlin
2003 Causes of Death among Finnish Women with Cosmetic Breast Implants, 1971–2001. Annals of Plastic Surgery 51:339–342.
Sánchez-Guerrero, Jorge, Graham A. Colditz, Elizabeth W. Carlson, David J. Hunter, Frank E. Speizer, and Matthew H. Liang
1995 Silicone Breast Implants and the Risk of Connective-Tissue Diseases and Symptoms. New England Journal of Medicine 332:1666–1670.
Sarwer, David B., Jodi E. Nordmann, and James D. Herbert
2000 Cosmetic Breast Augmentation Surgery: A Critical Overview. Journal of Women's Health and Gender-Based Medicine 9:843–856.
Sarwer, David B., Thomas A. Wadden, Michael J. Pertschuck, and Linton A. Whitaker
1998 The Psychology of Cosmetic Surgery: A Review and Reconceptualization. Clinical Psychology Review 18(1):1–22.
Sims, Suzanne, and George D. Lundberg
2001 Maybe Now Is the Time to Lift the Ban on Silicone Breast Implants. Medscape General Medicine 3(2). Electronic document, www.medscape.com/viewarticle/408121.
Smith, Aaron
2005 A Better Breast Implant: Next Generation of Silicone Implants Could Grow Sales. CNN Money, August 25. Electronic document, http://money.cnn.com/2005/08/25/news/midcaps/implants/index.htm.
Steinbrook, Robert
2005 Financial Conflicts of Interest and the Food and Drug Administration's Advisory Committees. New England Journal of Medicine 353(2):116–118.
Turner, Leigh
2004 Cosmetic Surgery: The New Face of Reality TV. British Medical Journal 328:1208. Electronic document, http://bmj.bmjjournals.com/cgi/content/full/328/7449/1208.
Uretsky, Barry F., Jennifer J. O'Brien, Eugene H. Courtiss, and Mathias D. Becker
1979 Augmentation Mammoplasty Associated with Severe Systemic Illness. Annals of Plastic Surgery 3(5):445–447.
WebMD
2006 Risks of General Anesthesia. WebMD. Electronic document, www.webmd.com/hw/health_guide_atoz/tr5871.asp.

Zimmerman, Susan M.
1998 Silicone Survivors: Women's Experiences with Breast Implants. Philadelphia: Temple University Press.
Zuckerman, Diana
2001 Commentary. Are Breast Implants Safe? Medscape General Medicine 3(4). Electronic document, www.medscape.com/viewarticle/408187.
2003 Statement of Diana Zuckerman, PhD, president, National Center for Policy Research for Women & Families. Electronic document, www.breastimplantinfo.org/what_know/dz_fda_test_oct03.html.
Zuckerman, Diana, Elizabeth Nagelin-Anderson, and Elizabeth Santoro
2005 What You Need to Know about Breast Implants. Issue Brief: National Research Center for Women & Families. Electronic document, www.center4research.org/implantfacts.html.

CHAPTER NINE

SELLING SICKNESS/CREATING DEMAND

Direct-to-Consumer Advertising of Prescription Drugs

Joan E. Paluzzi

Since 1997 when the FDA removed many of the regulatory restrictions that had prohibited direct-to-consumer advertising (DTCA) of prescription drugs in the United States, we have been bombarded daily by an ever-growing storm of the multimedia promotion of drugs. Open a magazine (especially a magazine whose targeted demographic is middle-aged women); turn on the television (network morning and evening news broadcasts, sports coverage, and some PBS programs are particularly popular programs for drug sponsors); or log on to commercial Internet sites and the chances are very good that at any given moment, you will encounter advertisements for prescription drugs. There are ads for drugs for the treatment or prevention of depression, insomnia, allergies, ADHD, the side effects of cancer chemotherapy, Alzheimer's disease, overactive bladders, erectile dysfunction, acid reflux, rheumatoid arthritis, strokes, diabetes, heart attacks, high cholesterol, restless legs syndrome, and so on. On one end of this spectrum there are serious diseases known to have a negative impact on the quality and, at times, the length of life. For individuals with these major illnesses, the advances of modern scientific research have extended life spans and improved quality of life, often literally making the difference between life and death. On the other end of the spectrum exist variable constellations of physical and emotional manifestations that occur in otherwise healthy people either for known behavioral or environmental reasons which are only mildly or occasionally evidenced.

For these individuals, making the decision to assume the risks of taking medicines (because there are always risks) should be a strategy that entails careful and deliberate consultation with their physician. A study published in *JAMA* in 2006 conducted national surveillance of emergency room visits over a two-year period by individuals experiencing adverse drug reactions. The weighted annual estimate for the United States was 701,547 individuals, with 3,487 requiring hospitalization. Older individuals (over 65 years of age) were more likely to present with adverse reactions and were also more likely to require hospitalization (Budnitz et al. 2006). Successfully marketing drugs to essentially healthy people requires more than convincing people to choose one brand over another; it often first requires convincing them that they may not be as healthy as they assume they are.

Beneath the incessant advertising hype there is a disturbing subtext that repeatedly delivers the message that whatever your problem is, it is a potentially serious problem and, most importantly, there is a pill that will "fix" it. Concerns and issues that these practices and the market context in which they are situated raise include:

1. Commodification of the products that are at times essential to the maintenance of health such as medicines ultimately results in the commodification of health itself by creating differential access to essential resources driven by the dynamics of the market rather than human need. First and foremost, health is a basic human right, perhaps the most fundamental of all universal human rights. Health encompasses a broad range of human experience, ranging from access to potable water and sanitary facilities to adequate nutrition, health services, and medicines. Good health serves as the foundation from which all other human rights arise; without it, nothing else is achievable or sustainable. It is not possible to meaningfully endorse health as a human right while at the same time supporting its commodification. The unequal distribution of access to medicines (and health care), not only between the developed countries and developing countries but also within developed and developing countries, raises the issue of ownership of scientific advancements. With large parts of the research necessary for

the development of new medicines conducted within tax-supported institutions by scientists who receive their training within publicly funded universities and with the reliance on public participation for the completion of drug trials, it is argued that this public investment in the common good should result in the benefits achieved by this investment bypassing the market-driven economic model through the development of a more equitable model of outcome and advantage distribution.

2. Over the last 50 years, the pharmaceutical industry[1] has consistently justified the high costs of medicines by attribution to the high costs of research and development necessary to bring a drug through the long research and development process (R&D). However many, if not the majority of "new" drugs in recent years are "me-too" products (variations with only minor adjustments of existing medicines or existing drugs whose use is extended to a previously unspecified condition). The slight variations rarely result in any significant increased benefit but enable companies to extend existing patents or obtain new patents while bypassing much of the cost and effort required to research and develop truly innovative, beneficial compounds (Angell 2005; Goozner 2004). Average investment in R&D by pharmaceutical companies is a fraction of their investment in promotion and marketing (Angell 2005; Ismail 2005). Many of these "new" drugs show little actual improvement in outcomes over older drugs that are available in reputable generic forms at a fraction of the cost to the patient. It is a logical extension of the market-based model that the same industry responsible for the promotion of patented medicines would also work assiduously (albeit at times more surreptitiously) to discredit the use and prescription of any generics by challenging the safety and efficacy of all generic medicines.

3. Despite ongoing attempts to do so, it is becoming virtually impossible to unequivocally identify the instances of conflict of interest surrounding the practices and profits of the drug industry. Politicians on every level of the political system as well

as the agencies they oversee are the targets of multimillion-dollar, coordinated lobbying efforts; physicians continue to receive grants, gifts, honorariums, conference opportunities, and positions on the "speaking bureaus" of large pharmaceutical companies; and media outlets receive billions of dollars in advertising revenue from the industry. And it is precisely because the public must rely upon these very same groups to assure adequate oversight of development, safe release, and long-term use of new medicines; prescription of the most cost-efficient, efficacious treatment; and widely disseminated reporting of adverse side effects and interactions that this is so alarming.

4. All medications carry a risk of adverse side effects, allergic reactions, and potentially harmful interactions with other medicines, food, and alcohol. By law, the industry is required to provide this information to patients. But dire warnings are not compatible with effective advertising. Whether they are related by a voice-over narrator whose tone changes and speech speeds up in order to quickly provide the information or the entire patient advisory information brochure is reproduced in minuscule typeface on the reverse side of print advertisements, the most critically important information is delivered in a manner that almost assures it will not receive the focused attention it deserves. Many of the health problems for which medicines are sought by patients and prescribed by physicians today could be managed or eliminated with basic lifestyle changes involving modification of diet, exercise practices, and the reduction of known risks such as smoking and alcohol consumption. The financial success of the billion-dollar drug industry attests to the large-scale conditioning of the American public and their physicians to accept that any disruption in physical, mental, or emotional equilibrium requires some form of medication and further, that only the most recently introduced compounds will be effective. Direct-to-consumer advertising increasingly is the mechanism by which this message is delivered and reinforced.

Selling Symptoms and Diseases along with Their Treatments

From 1955 through 1976, the U.S. Senate Antitrust and Monopoly Subcommittee investigated practices within a wide range of different U.S. industries. The pharmaceutical industry had grown rapidly during this time and issues concerning administered pricing (prices fixed by the industry rather than driven by market dynamics), promotional activities, ownership of pharmaceutical businesses, and U.S. drug company operations in Latin America were among the practices that came under the scrutiny of the subcommittee, particularly during the chairmanship tenure of Senator Estes Kefauver of Tennessee (1957–1963).

During an April 1960 session, Dr. Arthur Dale Console, the former research director for a large pharmaceutical company, testified on the prices and medicinal value of the drugs being marketed across the entire research-based industry. In this earlier era, direct-to-consumer advertising of prescription drugs was virtually nonexistent, so the marketing practices under investigation were almost exclusively targeted at physicians and pharmacies. Stressing that he was speaking about the industry as a whole, Dr. Console stated:

> The incidence of disease cannot be manipulated and so increased sales volume must depend at least in part on the use of drugs unrelated to their real utility or need, or in other words, improperly prescribed. Human frailty can be manipulated and exploited and this is fertile ground for anyone who wishes to increase profit. (Library of Congress 1960:10369)

This simple summary of the presumptive supply-and-demand dynamic inherent in the commodification of prescription medicines changed dramatically in 1997 when the U.S. Food and Drug Administration (FDA) relaxed the regulations restricting direct-to-consumer promotional activity. Medicines had been promoted to a small extent in popular media since the 1980s but because the FDA required full disclosure of all potential side effects and harmful interactions, the ads were prohibitively long and, in terms of television airtime, prohibitively expensive. The pharmaceutical industry began to push the limits, for example, running "reminder ads" that mentioned a drug by name but did not elaborate on any use or side effects, encouraging the viewers to "ask your doctor." With effective lobbying as well as assertions that "commercial speech" was a protected First Amendment right, the FDA relaxed the constraints and opened the floodgates. Now, the manufacturers are required to report only the most common or dangerous side effects (Hawthorne 2005; NIHP 2003). During the 1990s, a user-fee system was also initiated within the FDA. The result is that "more than half of the FDA's drug review work is now funded directly by the pharmaceutical industry" (Moynihan and Cassels 2005:19). All of this in turn has arguably resulted in what Dr. Console and his contemporaries had reasonably assumed was virtually impossible: the manipulation of disease incidence.

Case Study: Restless Legs Syndrome

> There's a name for why millions can't relax tonight: Restless Legs Syndrome. Restless Legs Syndrome (RLS) is a recognized medical condition. One that's shared by nearly 1 in 10 US adults.
>
> —Drug advertisement print ad, 2006

Restless legs syndrome (RLS) is described as "an urge to move the legs with or without paresthesia [tingling, numbness], worsening symptoms at rest, and transient improvements with activity, and worsening of symptoms in the evening and night" (Ondo 2005:1165). Although primary RLS (the presence of uncomfortable leg sensations without clear association to underlying, chronic disease) has been described, it is a poorly understood constellation of neurological complaints that is believed at times to have a strong genetic component. Secondary RLS has been demonstrated to strongly correlate with other chronic conditions such as iron deficiency, uremia, and diabetic neuropathy. In other words, it is most often a condition that is idiopathic or part of a constellation of possible expressions of some underlying physiological disease or altered state, not a disease in and of itself. For the small number of individuals with constant, severe RLS symptoms, treatment is necessary to promote uninterrupted sleep and to relieve the significant physical and emotional discomfort they experience.

The following illustrates the manner in which DTCA is often as much about marketing a "disease" as it is about marketing a drug. It is also a succinct illustration of the concerns that have emerged about conflict-of-interest behaviors (particularly between the pharmaceutical industry and nonprofit organizations) and the convoluted relationships that characterize the current commodified health milieu.

In 2003, British-based pharmaceutical giant GlaxoSmithKline (GSK) noted in their annual report that application to the regulatory authorities in the EU and United States had been completed for a new use of the drug Requip (ropinirole HCL) for treatment of primary RLS (GSK 2003). Requip is one of a group of drugs referred to as dopamine agonists and has been on the market for years as a treatment of Parkinson's disease. By 2004 GSK had approval to market Requip in the EU for the treatment of RLS and in May 2005, the FDA approved the same use in the United States (GSK 2004; MNT 2005). The task before them in preparation for the launch of Requip as a treatment for RLS was to move this poorly understood and highly variable constellation of leg sensations into the public consciousness as an accepted "syndrome."

Perhaps the most focused source of information about RLS can be found at the Restless Legs Syndrome Foundation and on its website. The foundation is an advocacy, research, and education organization founded solely to promote public awareness and scientific research of RLS. It was founded in 1990 with a small but committed group of supporters, many of whom themselves suffered from particularly severe and debilitating forms of the condition. In 1997 the foundation awarded $10,000 for targeted research; by 2005 they were able to award $226,670 (RLSF 2006). Annual reports for the foundation are available online for years 2003, 2004, and 2005. The largest donors in 2003 ($250,000 or more) to the foundation were GSK (manufacturers of Requip), Boehringer Ingelheim (manufacturers of another dopamine agonist, called Mirapex [pramipexole dihydrochloride]), and Pfizer (which at the time had an agonist compound called sumanirole in development for treatment of both Parkinson's disease and RLS). In 2004, only GSK was listed as a "gold corporate partner" ($250,000 or more), with Pfizer now designated as a "bronze partner" (at least $50,000). In July 2004, Pfizer announced they were discontinuing further development of sumanirole. In 2005 Pfizer was no longer listed as a donor at any level; only one gold corporate partner remained: GSK. Also in 2005 Boehringer Ingelheim Pharmaceuticals and GSK-USA were reported as "Leaders" at $10,000 plus. The Merck Employee Giving Campaign (Merck manufactures Sinemet [levodopa/carbidopa], long used for the treatment of Parkinson's and used by some practitioners for treatment of severe RLS) came in as a "Sponsor" with a donation somewhere between $1,000 and $4,999 (RLSF 2003).

In 2005, the RLS Foundation, in conjunction with the Society for Women's Health Research (SWHR), released findings from a survey of 1,000 U.S. adults that concluded that RLS is "largely under-recognized and poorly understood" and that much more effort is needed to educate the public (RLSF 2005a). The SWHR lists over 20 pharmaceutical companies, including GSK, Wyeth, and Pfizer as members of their Corporate Advisory Council (SWHR 2006).

Another nonprofit organization, the National Sleep Foundation (which refers to itself as NSF^2) contracts marketing companies to perform annual phone surveys titled "Sleep in America Poll." Among the donors listed in their annual reports for 2003 and 2004 (the only reports currently available online) are a number of large pharmaceutical companies, including GlaxoSmithKline (specific amounts of donations are not specified or ranked). Each of the five summaries of polls available online (2002 to 2006) devotes considerable attention to detailing the presence of restless leg movements in respondents. The 2005 phone survey conducted by the NSF polled a random, representativc sample of 1,506 adults in the United States. The survey reports that 15 percent of the surveyed population reported symptoms of RLS (leg discomfort "at least a few nights a week that is worse at night") and concluded that 10 percent are actually "at risk" for the development of restless legs syndrome (NSF 2005).

The 2003 NSF survey was devoted to the theme of older Americans and focused a great deal of attention on the elaboration of reports of any abnormal sensations in the legs and their correlation to diseases. The complaints of "unpleasant" sensations in the legs were substantially higher among seniors who also reported the existence of one or more chronic conditions such as heart disease and diabetes. The survey concluded, therefore, that the likelihood that individuals would be *at risk* (emphasis in the original) for RLS rose dramatically in the presence of chronic diseases such as arthritis, heart disease, and diabetes. The survey also reports that about 5 to 7 percent of older adults have actually been diagnosed with RLS (NSF 2003).

In that same year, the brief biographies of the large board of directors of the NSF included that of immediate past president Ronald L. Krall, who in 2003 was senior vice president of worldwide development and research and development for GlaxoSmithKline (NSF 2003). In 2005, Dr. Krall became the first recipient of the Restless Legs Syndrome Foundation Science Award for "his outstanding support of research that has advanced the understanding of restless legs syndrome." The press release announcing the award concluded with: "Disclosure statement: GlaxoSmithKline is a Gold Level Sponsor with an unrestricted educational grant to the RLS Foundation. The decision to select Dr. Krall for the Restless Legs Syndrome Foundation Science Award was made independently of any corporate relationship" (RLSF 2005b).

Although the consensus among researchers is that RLS is a condition much more common in aging populations, the NSF annual polls that addressed sleep patterns among children and adolescents also included multiple questions about leg movements (although they refrained from using the actual term *restless legs* in the poll that focused on children, instead asking their caretakers about "uncomfortable feelings in legs"). The 2006 poll focused on adolescents and it reported the following:

> Two questions were asked in order to examine what percentage of adolescents who may be at risk for restless legs syndrome. First, adolescents were asked if they have had unpleasant feelings in their legs, like creepy, crawly, or tingly feelings at night with an urge to move when they laid down to sleep in the past two weeks. Next, those that had these feelings at least a few nights a week were asked if moving their legs or feet makes them feel better. *Those adolescents who said that moving their legs always or sometimes makes them feel better are considered at risk for restless legs syndrome.* (emphasis added; NSF 2006:39)

Side Effects and Precautions

The obligatory informational section on the reverse side of magazine advertisements for Requip is printed in a smaller type font and asks, "What are the possible side effects of REQUIP?" Conveniently, the ad answers its own question: "Most people who take REQUIP tolerate it well" and then proceeds to caution about the possibility of "nausea, vomiting, dizziness and drowsiness." There is also a description of possible postural hypertension (a sudden drop in blood pressure when going from sitting or reclining to a standing position). Also: "It is possible that you could fall asleep while doing normal activities such as driving a car, doing physical tasks or using hazardous machinery. . . . Hallucinations are another reported side effect although more common in patients who take Requip for Parkinson's." "Other Information" includes reports of increased risk of melanoma in people with Parkinson's disease: "It is not known if this problem is associated with Parkinson's disease or the medicines used to treat Parkinson's disease." And finally, "A small number of patients taking medicines to treat Parkinson's disease, including Requip, have developed a problem with gambling. It is not known if this problem is directly related to the medicines."

These and other ads are remarkably adept at instilling anxiety and alarm over the mere possibility of disease or illness while at the same time minimizing the very real risks associated with the medicines they are trying to sell. Apparently, if you are a pharmaceutical company, you can have your cake and eat it too.

At this time, only Requip has been specifically approved by the FDA for treatment of primary RLS, although other neuroactive drugs (including Requip) have been used for the treatment of severe RLS symptoms for years (a practice called "off-label prescribing"). The DTCA campaign by GSK for the treatment of restless legs syndrome with Requip hit both the airwaves and print media sources in 2005 and began the process of introducing a new "syndrome" to people who had never heard of it.

Originally set to expire in 2002, Requip's patent will now expire in two years and this begs the question of why GSK is making the large investment now. Several factors could potentially be at play here, starting with the most apparent: the enormous potential for profits from focused campaigns publicizing the symptoms of RLS and Requip's status as the only drug officially approved for treatment. By establishing name recognition with consumers before the release of generic versions of the drug, GSK can also assure brand loyalty among consumers who have been convinced that generic versions of any drugs are dangerous or ineffective. Finally, and as another variant on the latter theme where brand recognition can be extremely profitable, there is always the possibility that there are plans to seek approval for over-the-counter (OTC) sales of the drug in the future.

In their 2005 annual report, GSK reports that sales of Requip rose 34 percent to £156 million (around 290 million in U.S. dollars). How responsive to all of this have U.S. physicians been? By the first quarter of 2006, weekly prescriptions for Requip in the United States had quadrupled since its release as a specific treatment for RLS in the spring of 2005 (GSK 2005).

Redefining Health

In recent years highly publicized cases such as the controversy over the uses of hormone replacement therapy (HRT) have revealed tangled webs of collaboration between the pharmaceutical industry, research institutions, nonprofit organizations, funding agencies, and the media industries. Restless legs syndrome is not the only once-obscure or relatively rare constellation of physical manifestations that have been organized into a disease or syndrome as the focus of drug-selling campaigns geared to the general public (Moynihan and Cassels 2005). Irritable bowel syndrome, premenstrual dystrophic disorder (and PMS), social anxiety disorder, irritable bladder, and erectile dysfunction have all been essentially commodified in the same manner. There are individuals who suffer from these or related disorders and benefit from medical interventions that may or may not include pharmacological agents. However, in many cases individuals with mild or vague symptoms are demanding treatment for symptoms that often, left to the discretion of their physicians, would be managed without drugs.

How responsive are physicians to patient demands for medications they have learned about through DTCA? The short answer is, very responsive. One study compared patient populations between the United States and Canada. The prescribing rate was higher overall in Sacramento (where DTCA is thriving) than in Vancouver, Canada (where DTCA is still restricted as it is in most of the world). Patients requesting medicines they had seen in DTCA were 16.9 times likely to receive prescriptions for the drugs they requested, or alternatives. The pharmaceutical industry claims that because medicines must be prescribed by a physician, there is an inherent "safety net" in the system. The authors assert that this does not provide adequate protection. For example, it is flawed protection if physicians are ordering drugs they would not normally have ordered because of patient demand. They add that the ads in no way provide sufficient information to the patient in terms of risk/benefit estimations and side effects (Mintzes et al. 2003).

Another study published in the *Journal of the American Medical Association* utilized "standardized patients" who were randomly assigned to make 298 visits to physicians who were not previously familiar with them. Patients presented reporting symptoms of either major depression or adjustment disorder with one of three request types made during the visit: brand-specific drugs, general requests for nonspecified medicines, or no medicine request. For patients who presented with symptoms of depression, physicians prescribed antidepressants for 76 percent of those who requested nonspecific medications; 53 percent of those who requested specific medicines linked to DTCA; and 31 percent who did not request any medications were given a prescription. In the case of adjustment disorder, there were significantly less prescriptions dispensed but in this case 55 percent of the patients requesting a brand name were given the requested prescription, 39 percent of the general requests were met, and only 10 percent were prescribed medicines even though they had not requested them. The authors concluded that the impact of patient requests for antidepressants was "profound" (Kravitz et al. 2005:1995).

An increase in prescribing new, expensive drugs inevitably increases health care across the board. It also inevitably leads to increases in adverse effects whether they are known side effects, interactions with other prescription or nonprescription drugs, or new, unforeseen side effects that become evident only after long-term use. The widely publicized case of Merck's arthritis drug, Vioxx, is the most obvious recent example. Following are brief descriptions of some of the specific concerns and side effects that have recently arisen associated with the use of specific drugs for the treatment of indigestion, erectile dysfunction, and osteoporosis.

The High Cost of Burritos

Drugs either prescribed (or now available OTC) to control the amount of acid produced in the upper digestive tract have been and continue to be among the consistently best-selling medicines in the United States. H2 receptor antagonists (H2 blockers) include the enormously popular drugs Pepcid (famotidine), Tagamet (cimetidine), Zantac (ranitidine), and Axid (nizatidine). The proton pump inhibitors (PPIs) that were developed more recently include Prilosec (omeprazole), Prevacid (lansoprazole), and Nexium (esomeprazole). Both of these popular, highly profitable classes of drugs are used for the treatment of gastric reflux (a.k.a. heartburn) and a more serious variant, gastroesophageal reflux disease (GERD). With the exception of omeprazole, the PPIs are relatively new drugs that remain available by prescription only.

Cimetidine, the first of the H2 blockers introduced in the United States in 1977, went off patent in 1994 and became available without prescription in 1995. The move to OTC was expected to improve dramatically falling profits on the drug that had followed the expiration of the patent and the concurrent introduction of cheaper generic versions of cimetidine (New York Times 1995). The first "me-too" drug, ranitidine (Zantac), followed relatively quickly and did offer improvements by decreasing some of the drug interaction issues associated with cimetidine. Subsequent iterations of H2 blockers have been virtually indistinguishable from each other in terms of efficacy, and with the exception of nizatidine (Axid) are all available OTC and still promoted vigorously in print and video media ads. Unlike the prescription drug ads where obviously anxious patients report that they didn't realize they were seriously damaging the lining of their esophagus, the OTC drug ads tend to take a decidedly less dramatic approach, emphasizing their effectiveness in treating heartburn and essentially promoting the idea that one should eat whatever one likes even when personal experience has demonstrated that a particular food is known to cause indigestion. For example, there is an ad that shows a man at an airport preparing to bite into a large, messy burrito with his comically panicked family racing across the room to prevent him from taking that first bite. He tells them to "relax" because he has taken a pill in anticipation of his dietary indiscretion. Everyone smiles in relief as they head for the plane.

People now routinely use these drugs to self-medicate for gastric upset and heartburn. This raises concerns on two levels: on the one hand, specific drugs and their potential side effects and on the other, the promotion of the entire category of "acid reducers." In 2001 the FDA issued a strong advisory that OTC famotidine should be taken in substantially reduced dosage levels by individuals with impaired renal function. Adverse effects listed in the announcement of the advisory included central nervous system side effects such as psychiatric disturbances, insomnia, somnolence, anxiety, and depression (CMAJ 2001). This is of particular concern in elderly patients who may be unaware of gradually declining renal function and in whom these potential side effects may be attributed to what some individuals still consider to be a normal, negative decline associated with aging. Print and Internet ads for the drug continue to promote it enthusiastically and, as usual, include side effects and cautions at the bottom or on the back of pages, in much smaller print. Warnings, including the advice that use should be supervised by a physician in people with impaired renal function, can be found only with careful reading of all of the small print, arguably something that the folks most at risk for this complication (older individuals with declining health) are unlikely to do (or are unable to do . . . the print can be exceptionally small).

Of much broader concern is the fact that these drugs mask or suppress gastrointestinal symptoms and when taken over a long period of time may delay the seeking of treatment for what could be potentially serious diseases such as gastric and esophageal malignancies. Esophageal cancer (adenocarcinoma) is one of the most rapidly increasing malignancies in this country; it has a very high mortality rate and early detection is absolutely essential for slowing or curing the cancer. During the 2004 annual Digestive Disease Week conference held in 2004 in New Orleans, a paper from a research team from India headed by Dr. Mohandas Mallath was presented that purported to draw a correlation between increased carbonated beverage consumption in the United States and increases in adenocarcinoma of the esophagus (Harby 2004). The popular media immediately began repeating the information, despite the fact that Dr. Mallath himself had commented that, while essential, "these kinds of epidemiological studies are not a very good level of evidence" (Harby 2004). By 2006, follow-up investigations of the connection between soda intake and increasing esophageal cancer included a multicenter, population-based case-control study by a large team headed by Yale researcher Susan T. Mayne. Their findings concluded that there is an *inverse* relationship between carbonated drinks and the incidence of adenocarcinoma (Mayne et al. 2006).

Eliminating increased soda consumption as a potential causative factor requires us to look elsewhere for possible correlations to account for the increases in esophageal adenocarcinoma over the past 20 years. Usually related to a failure of an anatomical sphincter to prevent backflow of contents from the stomach to the esophagus, chronic and severe acid reflux (now referred to as GERD) can, over a period of many years, cause changes in the tissue of the distal esophagus. This in turn is referred to as Barrett's esophagus and, left untreated, individuals with this condition are thought to be many times more likely to develop adenocarcinoma of the esophagus. One study reported that individuals with long-standing (more than 20 years) and severe reflux had an odds ratio of 43.5 for contracting adenocarcinoma of the esophagus (Lagergren et al. 1999). Factors such as smoking, excessive alcohol consumption, genetic factors, and increasing obesity in this country (excessive abdominal fat accumulation constitutes a risk factor because of the intraabdominal pressure it generates and the presumptive ingestion of high-fat foods) have been among the factors discussed as related features of the increase in this type of cancer. PPI drugs are usually first-line treatment for Barrett's esophagus. However, Peter Belafsky (2005:6), who maintains that patients need to have careful monitoring before initiating and while taking these drugs, writes:

> PPIs are not benign. . . . Some of the more common side effects of PPIs include headache, nausea, diarrhea, constipation, flatulence, abdominal pain, and dry mouth. Some less frequent but more serious side effects include anaphylactic shock, Stevens-Johnson syndrome, pancreatitis, interstitial nephritis, and fatal toxic epidermal necrolysis.

Another serious concern is that with the availability and vigorous marketing of OTC PPIs and H2 blockers, people with severe GERD and/or Barrett's esophagus will self-medicate just enough to stay relatively symptom free and comfortable (and away from their doctor's office) but not enough to prevent the formation of cellular dysplasia that can over the long term lead to cancer. On October 20, 2000, the Nonprescription Drugs and Gastrointestinal Advisory Committees of the Food and Drug Administration met in Gaithersburg, Maryland, to evaluate the application made by pharma companies AstraZeneca and Procter & Gamble to allow Prilosec to be made available without a prescription. Although most of the H2 blockers had been OTC for several years, this was the first request for a PPI drug. It was noted in a brief report of the meeting that although the manufacturers' recommendation was to limit the use of the drug to a maximum of ten days for either prevention or treatment of heartburn, in actual-use studies, 65 percent of the subjects using it as prevention and 19 to 22 percent of those using it to treat actual symptoms of heartburn exceeded these recommendations (FDA 2000). It was not, however, considered to be sufficient reason for denying the request to market the drug OTC.

Raising the Bar

Some of the most pervasive advertising of prescription drugs is to promote the use of medications to enhance male sexual performance. There are now several drugs (phosphodiesterase type 5 inhibitors) available that are advertised as treatment for male sexual dysfunction (referred to as erectile dysfunction or ED), including Viagra (sildenafil citrate), Levitra (vardenafil), and Cialis (tadalafil). Medical conditions such as spinal cord injuries, hypogonadism, diabetes mellitus, and some medications to treat these and other diseases such as hypertension and heart disease can impede the ability of a man to develop and satisfactorily maintain an erection. For these men, ED drugs often permit significantly improved sexual functioning. However, it is also generally accepted that the use of these drugs is seen by some men as a way to enhance normal sexual performance. For example, urologists who are the specialists in treatment of this disease only accounted for 25 percent of Viagra prescriptions in 1999 (NKUDIC 2005).

A recent television ad for one of the drugs shows a speaker standing in a large, empty stadium where he solemnly intones that "more than half of the men over the age of 40 suffer from ED (erectile dysfunction) . . . enough to fill this stadium many times over." Many times over indeed. Half of the men over the age of 40, according to the 2000 U.S. census, would require a stadium capable of holding around 26,793,521 men (Census 2000). Aside from the problematic issue of how erectile dysfunction is defined in this context (a single or rare occurrence? chronic problems?), the numbers are inflated. It is also deceptive to imply that all men over 40 are at equal risk. The National Institute of Diabetes and Digestive and Kidney Diseases at the National Institutes of Health (NIH) estimates that only about 5 percent of 40-year-old men and 15 to 20 percent of 65-year-old-men experience erectile dysfunction but assert that "it is not an inevitable part of aging." Another NIH agency estimates a year 2000 prevalence of erectile dysfunction for men between the ages of 40 to 69 to be between 20 to 46 percent (8,962,410 to 20,613,543) (NKUDIC 2005).

Concerns have arisen about potential correlation between the use of ED drugs and a rare condition that can adversely affect vision. In July 2005, the FDA issued an advisory for all three of the major ED drugs reporting that a small number of men have lost eyesight in one or both eyes some time after taking either Viagra, Cialis, or Levitra. Resulting from a blockage of blood flow to the optic nerve, this type of vision loss is called nonarteritic anterior ischemic optic neuropathy (NAION) (FDA 2005). At that time the FDA also instructed the companies to include an advisory within the drug labeling. However, reports of the possible link between NAION and ED drug use had been known within the FDA at least as early as January 2004 when an agency drug safety reviewer had recommended that a warning be required on the drugs' labels (ASHP 2005). In a letter to the acting commissioner of the FDA dated June 24, 2005, Senator Charles E. Grassley of Iowa demanded immediate action on labeling changes. He also expressed concern that because the physicians most likely to treat the eye condition (ophthalmologists) may not be aware that the men they are treating have been taking ED drugs and that the physicians prescribing the drug (e.g., urologists) might remain unaware of the frequency in which this blindness is occurring, there may actually be serious underreporting of the dangerous side effect (Grassley 2005).

Annie Potts et al. (2006) critique the excessive use of these drugs from a sociocultural perspective. They challenge the assumptions inherent in "sexuopharmaceutical solutions" to changes in erectile experience as men age. Through the use of narratives of older men, they present another vision of male sexual pleasure that emerges from experience and maturity but that has become increasingly marginalized in the era of aggressive promotion of ED drugs with suggestive, sexy ads that privilege long-lasting erections as the standard of normal sexual behavior regardless of age (Potts, Grace, Vares, and Gavey 2006).

The Return of Phossy Jaw

Another widely promoted group of drugs are the bisphosphonates used to treat osteoporosis in women. These drugs in both oral and injectable forms were initially (and continue to be) used in the treatment of women suffering from multiple myeloma and metastatic breast cancer to prevent a specific kind of bone resorption. They have served to increase the quality of life for many of these women. However, they are powerful drugs with potentially serious gastrointestinal/esophageal side effects and patients with decreased renal function need to be closely monitored when taking these drugs.

Prior to receiving approval from the FDA for Fosamax in 1995 for the treatment of osteoporosis (the first of the bisphosphonates approved for this use in the United States), Merck began launching what an article in the *Wall Street Journal* described as an "aggressive campaign" to educate both physicians and patients about osteoporosis. Their tactics included cosponsoring a media campaign with the nonprofit National Osteoporosis Foundation strongly encouraging women to seek (expensive) screening for osteoporosis. They also helped to finance increased production of osteoporosis diagnostic equipment by two manufacturers (Tanouye 1995).

The DTCA for these medicines is aimed at menopausal and postmenopausal women and clearly conveys the message that significant and potentially pathological bone loss is virtually a given with the aging process. In the United States, the two drugs targeted with DTCA for the treatment of osteoporosis are Fosamax (alendronate sodium) and Boniva (ibandronic acid). In addition to potentially dangerous side effects in women with decreased renal function and in all women who take the drug due to the possibility of upper gastrointestinal/esophageal injury, another potentially serious side effect, osteonecrosis of the jaw, has recently been linked to the use of bisphosphonates. This is related to a physical deformity (referred to as phossy jaw) observed among 19th century match factory employees who had chronic and prolonged exposure to white phosphorus during the manufacturing process (Cope 2005). Osteonecrosis or avascular necrosis of the jaw is a serious condition caused by a temporary or permanent interruption in the blood supply to the jaw ultimately resulting in collapse and destruction of bone (Cope 2005). The link between bisphosphonates and this alarming side effect was made as early as

2003 in an article that appeared in the September edition of the *Journal of Oral Maxillofacial Surgery* titled "Pamidronate (Aredia) and Zoledronate (Zometa) Induced Avascular Necrosis of the Jaws: A Growing Epidemic," by R. E. Marx. Both drugs are in the bisphosphonate class of medicines but used in cancer therapies and neither was marketed for the treatment of osteoporosis. The Aredia website now contains the following message: "Aredia is no longer promoted by Novartis Pharmaceuticals Corporation." It then redirects interested browsers to another similar drug (Zometa). Both the old Aredia site and the current Zometa site include disclosures about the possible occurrence of osteonecrosis, something that cannot be found as of May 5, 2006, on the Merck Fosamax home page nor on the Roche/GSK Boniva site. From 2004 onward, there have been an increasing number of articles appearing in the medical, surgical, and dental journals linking this class of drugs and osteonecrosis of the jaw (see, for example, Ruggiero et al. 2004; Farrugia et al. 2006; Woo et al. 2006). The aggressive DTCA continues for both of these drugs, including an ad that shows a series of physicians (or actors posing as physicians, impossible to know which with any certainty) promoting the use of the drug and advising the listeners to "ask me" about osteoporosis treatments.

The first class-action suit against Merck over Fosamax was filed in the fall of 2005. The only action taken by the FDA appears to be a request that Merck amend its package labeling of Fosamax, which they did in July 2005 by inserting two additional paragraphs in the precautionary statements targeted to prescribing physicians (while still publicly maintaining that there is absolutely no evidence of a link between Fosamax and osteonecrosis of the jaw) (Carreyrou 2006).

The issues and problems that have arisen with the drugs discussed here merely represent a sampling of issues and problems that have arisen in the promotion and use of these specific classes of drugs. Beyond this small sample lie all of the problems surrounding other classes of drugs that have entered the market in the last 15 to 20 years for the treatment of conditions such as high cholesterol, coronary artery disease, diabetes, obesity, and so forth. Recent history has shown the current limits of existing regulatory agencies. With an ever-increasing number of DTCA campaigns over which the FDA is charged with oversight, budget and personnel shortages have created an impossible backlog of incomplete or delayed inspections and regulatory processes.

The Bigger Picture

The concerns generated by industry practices in the United States are concerns that, for many of us, are conditioned by affluence, choice, and a passive relinquishment of responsibility for our own physical and emotional well-being. It does not in any way exonerate the industry for questionable or unsafe practices nor the FDA for slow response to concerns nor physicians for using anything except sound medical evidence in making their therapeutic recommendations, but at some point in this equation, individuals who are able to do so must also take responsibility for asking the questions that need to be asked and challenging the hegemony inherent in mass media advertising. That being said, we must also acknowledge a large segment of the population in this country who, by virtue of age, poor health, and/or low socioeconomic status, may also be among the most vulnerable and will continue to require the enactment and enforcement of safeguards to prevent abuses and to remove failures and flaws in the system.

Beneath the controversies, discussions, and attempts to make sense of the current promotion and use of medicines must be the understanding that medicines have become one of the most consistently profitable commodities in history. From this comes the realization that the sale and distribution of pharmaceutical products will be governed by the same market dynamics as other commodities and those dynamics require the unceasing expansion of markets. One way to assure this expansion is, as demonstrated here, to continue to manipulate public understanding of the features that constitute health and sickness through the use of DTCA. The United States and other high-income countries, the places where the profits on medicines are the highest, have finite populations. To continue to generate demand requires that the companies must develop strategies that will expand the perceived need for medication within those populations. For example, in the United States, as the baby-boomer juggernaut ages, the companies have effectively created "life-stage" demands that tap into the desire to maintain a youthful appearance and function.

The discussion to this point has centered on marketing and promotional practices within the United States. However, the companies within the pharmaceutical industry serve as exemplars of multinational corporations, and the consequences and impact of their practices play a particularly important role in the current international health environment. The profits gained (driven by DTCA) in this country are the fuel that drives the power and influence these companies have throughout the world. The mandated restrictions on DTCA in most other countries of the world are a negligible advantage in the poorest countries where it is offset by markedly less access to even the most essential medicines coupled with failing or absent regulatory infrastructures (Leach et al. 2005). The disparity between countries where millions of dollars are spent on drugs for illnesses that may or may not actually require them (or for that matter, actually exist) and the majority of the world where people die daily from curable, treatable diseases such as TB, malaria, and HIV for want of the most basic (but unprofitable) medicines continues to grow and will long remain as an indictment of greed and misplaced priorities.

Within the last two years there have been an unprecedented number of critical books, editorials, and articles about the research pharmaceutical industry detailing the issues surrounding not only their use of direct-to-consumer advertising but their pricing practices, conflicts of interest, relationships to doctors and regulatory agencies, and their high profits (e.g., Angell 2005; Hawthorne 2005; Kassirer 2005; Moynihan and Cassels 2005; and Goozner 2004). The sales and profits within the industry have become a ubiquitous part of this society-wide discussion of industry practices but some figures are worth repeating for the sake of emphasis:

- The CDC reports that in the United States, retail spending on prescription medicines more than tripled from 1992 (48.2 billion dollars) to 2002 (162.4 billion). In per capita terms, it estimates an increase from $64 in 1982 to $569 in 2002 (Goulding 2005).
- The top research pharmaceutical company in the world, Pfizer Inc., posted global pharmaceutical sales of 50.9 billion dollars in 2004 (with a profit for that year estimated to be 11.3 billion). It is estimated that Pfizer spent 16.9 billion on marketing and promotion and 7.68 billion on research and development (Ismail 2005). Overall, roughly 30 to 35 percent of the industry's

resources go into the promotion and marketing of drugs, while research and development receives 15 to 17 percent.

- The combined sales of the top 20 research pharmaceutical companies for 2004 is estimated at $332.5 billion, with combined spending for marketing and promotion by the top 11 within that group projected to be around 100 billion dollars (Ismail 2005). To provide some sorely needed global perspective, the combined GDP of five of the poorest sub-Saharan countries: Mali, Burkina Faso, Ghana, Central African Republic, and Zambia (total population of over 63 million people) is around 25 billion dollars, a quarter of the resources spent on advertising and promotion by the top 11 pharmaceutical companies (WDIO 2004).
- In 2004, the industry spent 123 million dollars lobbying the U.S. government (the House, the Senate, the FDA, the Department of Health and Human Services and other offices).[3] This protects interests not only in the United States but also has continued to influence U.S. trade policies, evidenced by strict regulation against price controls, prohibition of price negotiation, and the imposition of equally rigid intellectual property protection clauses that are a regular feature of U.S. bilateral trade agreements.
- In addition to an investment of $675 million in lobbying since 1998, the industry has contributed $133 million in state and federal election campaigns.
- Six of the top 11 pharmaceutical companies are U.S.-based firms. In 2005 the annual salaries (including stock options and stock-option grants) of their CEOs ranged from $1,972,596 to $16,419,270, with an average of $9,009,911 and a median salary between $11,298,642 and $12,236,522 (AFL-CIO 2006). The top-paid executive in this group receives only 2 million dollars less than the entire public health budget for the Central African Republic (WDIO 2003).

Conclusion

There are neither quick nor easy solutions for the many problems in the current global situation of grossly disproportionate access to medicines and the failure of regulatory agencies to adequately protect the public. Direct-to-consumer advertising has been released from its Pandora's box in the United States and become a multibillion-dollar industry in its own right. It would require an unprecedented display of political will to wrestle it back in. As the FDA and other federal agencies continue to be overwhelmed by the sheer amount of information requiring oversight and regulation, we can expect to see more incidents where action to regulate drugs that exhibit harmful side effects will be delayed.

In addition to the power and influence that money can buy, the industry's hegemony also emerges from their role in the development of new drugs. As long as the pharmaceutical companies maintain control over the process of drug research and development, we will continue to see drugs created because of their potential for large profits rather than as a response to critical human need. And we may continue to stand by helplessly (haplessly) as they justify their exorbitant prices and restrictive policies with unverifiable claims of cost (e.g., "800 million dollars" for the development of a new drug) by holding us hostage to their threats of research on new compounds "grinding to a halt" if enforcement of patents, even in the poorest countries, is not rigidly enforced. Alternative, nonprivatized models of R&D are sorely needed to begin the de-commodification of medicines. We could begin with enforced transparency across a wide spectrum of related experiences. For example, routine and verifiable reporting of actual R&D costs; full and open disclosure of the connections between the industry, nonprofit sectors, the institutions that fund university research, and the researchers themselves; and open admission of the ties that exist between physicians and the pharmaceutical companies. The FDA should be staffed and funded in a manner sufficient to the growing needs of effective oversight. We can make our elected officials aware of our outrage over the growing global inequalities in access to medicine (we may first have to elect a more responsive government). Finally, we can refuse to allow a 30-second television commercial to define the quality of our health.

Notes

1. Throughout this chapter, references to the pharmaceutical industry refer exclusively to research-based companies (as opposed to the generic industry).

2. The National Sleep Foundation uses the acronym NSF but is not related to the National Science Foundation, which is also widely referred to as the NSF. This caused some initial confusion for me (and I suspect for others) when I found an Internet site detailing recent findings from the "NSF-sponsored sleep survey."

3. Evidence of the success of this investment in lobbying effort can be seen (as one example) in the final form of the drug plan to assist seniors with the cost of their medicines (Medicare D). The most cost-effective, administratively simple plan would have been a single-payer plan that mandates the use of generic drugs when available. Instead, seniors must wade through a bureaucratic maze of the numerous private companies who administer the plan, forcing them to seek advice, in many cases, from people who will profit from their enrollment.

References

AFL-CIO
2006b Executive PayWatch Data Base. Electronic document, www.aflcio.org/corporatewatch/paywatch/ceou/database.cfm.

Angell, M.
2005 The Truth about the Drug Companies: How They Deceive Us and What to Do about It. New York: Random House.

ASHP
2005 American Society of Health-System Pharmacists. Under Scrutiny, FDA Calls for Labeling Changes on ED Drugs. Press release. Electronic document, www.ashp.org/news/ShowArticle.cfm?id=11635.

Belafsky, P.
2005 Pro: Empiric Treatment with PPIs Is Not Appropriate without Testing. American Journal of Gastroenterology 101(1):6–11.

Budnitz, D. S., D. A. Pollack, K. N. Weidenbach, A. B. Mendelsohn, T. J. Schroeder, and J. L. Annest
2006 National Surveillance of Emergency Department Visits for Outpatient Adverse Drug Events. Journal of the American Medical Association 296(15):1858–1866.

Carreyrou, J.
2006 Fosamax Drug Could Become Next Merck Woe. Wall Street Journal, April 12: B1.

Census
2000 Detailed Tables. Electronic document, http://factfinder.census.gov/servlet/DTTable?_bm=y&-geo_id=01000US&-ds_name=DEC_2000_SF1_U&-mt_name=DEC_2000_SF1_U_PCT012.

Cope, D.
2005 Clinical Update: A Non-Healing Fractured Mandible. Clinical Journal of Oncology Nursing 9(6):685–687.

CMAJ (Canadian Medical Association Journal)
2001 Drug advisory: Famotidine (Pepcid). Electronic document, www.cmaj.ca/cgi/content/full/165/4/462-a.

Farrugia, M. C., D. J. Summerlin, E. Krowiak, T. Huntley, S. Freeman, R. Borrowdale, and C. Tomich
2006 Osteonecrosis of the Mandible or Maxilla Associated with the Use of New Generation Bisphosphonates. Laryngoscope 116(1):115–120.

FDA
2000 Joint Meeting of the Nonprescription Drugs and Gastrointestinal Advisory Committees. October 20. Electronic document, www.fda.gov/OHRMS/DOCKETS/AC/cder00.htm#Gastrointestinal.
2005 FDA Alert. NAION. Electronic document, www.fda.gov/cder/consumerinfo/Viagra.

Goozner, M.
2004 The $800 Million Pill. Berkeley: University of California Press.

Goulding, M.
2005 Trends in Prescribed Medicine Use and Spending by Older Americans 1992–2001. Aging Trends 5, February 2005. Electronic document, www.cdc.gov/search.do?sort=&subset=nchs&action=search&queryText=Trends+in+Health+and+Aging+No.+5&restrict=true&x=10&y=10.

Grassley, C. E.
2005 Letter from the chairman of the U.S. Senate Committee on Finance to the Acting Commissioner of the FDA. Electronic document, www.senate.gov/~finance/press/Gpress/2005/prg113005lett3.pdf.

GSK (GlaxoSmithKline)
2003 Improving Performance Every Day. Annual report, GlaxoSmith Kline. Electronic document, www.gsk.com/financial/reps03/annual_report2003.pdf.
2004 New Challenge, New Thinking. Annual report, GlaxoSmithKline. Electronic document, www.gsk.com/investors/reps04/annual-report-2004.pdf.
2005 Human Being. Annual report, GlaxoSmithKline. Electronic document, www.gsk.com/investors/annual-reports.htm.

Harby, K.
2004 Esophageal Adenocarcinoma Appears to Be Affected by Common Beverages. Medscape Medical News Online. Electronic document, www.medscape.com/viewarticle/478184.

Hawthorne, F.
2005 Inside the FDA: The Business and Politics behind the Drugs We Take and the Food We Eat. Hoboken, NJ: Wiley.

Ismail, M. A.
2005 Drug Lobby Second to None: How the Pharmaceutical Industry Gets Its Way in Washington. Special report, Center for Public Integrity. Electronic document, www.publicintegrity.org/rx/report.aspx?aid=723.

Kassirer, J. P.
2005 On the Take: How Medicine's Complicity with Big Business Can Endanger Your Health. Oxford: Oxford University Press.

Kravitz, R. L., R. Epstein, M. D. Feldman, C. E. Franz, R. Azari, M. S. Wilkes, L. Hinton, and P. Franks
2005 Influence of Patients' Requests for Direct-to-Consumer Advertised Antidepressants: A Randomized Controlled Study. Journal of the American Medical Association 293(16):1195–2002.

Lagergren, J., R. Bergström, A. Lindgren, and O. Nyrén
1999 Symptomatic Gastrointestinal Reflux as a Risk Factor for Esophageal Adenocarcinoma. New England Journal of Medicine 340:825–831.

Leach, B., J. E. Paluzzi, and P. Mundari
2005 UN Millennium Project Task Force V Final Report: Access to Essential Medicines Working Group. Prescription for Healthy Development: Increasing Access to Medicines. London: Earthscan.

Library of Congress
1960 Administered Prices in the Drug Industry: Hearings before the Subcommittee on Antitrust and Monopoly of the Senate Committee on the Judiciary, 86th Congress, 2nd Session: 10369 (1960) (statement of Dr. A. Dale Console).

Mayne, S. T., H. A. Risch, R. Dubrow, W. H. Chow, M. D. Gammon, T. L. Vaughan, L. Borchardt, J. B. Schoenberg, J. L. Stanford, A. B. West, H. Rotterdam, W. J. Blot, and J. F. Fraumeni Jr.
2006 Carbonated Soft Drink Consumption and Risk of Esophageal Adenocarcinoma. Journal of the National Cancer Institute 98(1):72.

Mintzes, B., M. L. Barer, R. L. Kravitz, K. Bassett, J. Lexchin, A. Kazanjian, R. G. Evans, R. Pan, and S. A. Marion
2003 How Does Direct-to-Consumer Advertising (DTCA) Affect Prescribing? A Survey in Primary Care Environments with and without Legal DTCA. Canadian Medical Association Journal 169(5):405–412.

Moynihan, R., and A. Cassels
2005 Selling Sickness: How the World's Biggest Pharmaceutical Companies Are Turning Us All Into Patients. New York: Nation Books.
MNT
2005 Medical News Today: Restless Leg Syndrome Drug, Requip, Approved by FDA. Electronic document, www.medicalnewstoday .comprinterfriendlynews.php?newsid=23995.
New York Times
1995 SmithKline Can Sell Tagamet as Nonprescription Drug in the U.S. New York Times, June 20.
NIHP (National Institute of Health Policy)
2003 The Food and Drug Administration: Where Has It Been? Where Is It Going? Issue brief, National Institute of Health Policy. Electronic document, www.nihp.org/Issue%20Briefs/Issue-Brief-2-28-03.htm.
NKUDIC (National Kidney and Urological Disease Clearinghouse)
2005 National Kidney and Urological Disease Clearinghouse: A Service of the National Institute of Diabetes and Digestive and Kidney Diseases (NIH). Electronic document, http://kidney.niddk.nih.gov/kudiseases/pubs/impotence.
NSF (National Sleep Foundation)
2003 Annual report, National Sleep Foundation. Electronic document, www.sleepfoundation.org/about/index.php?secid=&id=135 2004 annual report.
2005 2005 Sleep in America Poll. Summary findings, National Sleep Foundation. Electronic document, www.sleepfoundation.org/hottopics/index.php?secid=16&id=392.
2006 2006 Sleep in America Poll. Summary findings, National Sleep Foundation. Electronic document, www.sleepfoundation.org/hottopics/index.php?secid=16&id=392.
Ondo, W. G.
2005 Restless Legs Syndrome. Neurologic Clinics 23(4):1165–1185.
Phillips, H., W. Hening, P. Britz, and D. Mannino
2006 Prevalence and Correlates of Restless Legs Syndrome: Results from the 2005 National Sleep Foundation Poll. Chest 129(1):76–80.
Potts, A., V. M. Grace, T. Vares, and N. Gavey
2006 "Sex for Life"? Men's Counter-Stories on "Erectile Dysfunction," Male Sexuality and Aging. Sociology of Health and Illness 28(3):306–329.
RLSF (Restless Legs Syndrome Foundation)
2003 Restless Legs Syndrome Annual Report 2003. Electronic document, www.rls.org/NetCommunity/Document.Doc?&id=140.

2005a New National Survey Shows Restless Legs Syndrome (RLS) Is Largely Under-Recognized and Poorly Understood by U.S. Adults. Press release. November 10, 2005. Electronic document, www.rls.org/NetCommunity/Document.Doc?&id=68.

2005b RLS Foundation Presents First Science Award to Dr. Ronald Krall. Press release. November 15, 2005. Electronic document, http://www.rls.org/NetCommunity/Document.Doc?&id=72.

2006 Grant Awards Graph. Electronic document, www.rls.org/NetCommunity/Page.aspx?&pid=239&srcid=178.

Ruggiero, S. L., B. Mehrotra, T. J. Rosenberg, and S. L. Engroff

2004 Osteonecrosis of the Jaw Associated with the Use of Bisphosphonates: A Review of 63 Cases. Journal of Oral Maxillofacial Surgery 62(5):527–534.

SWHR (Society for Women's Health Research)

2006 www.womenshealthresearch.org/about/cac.htm.

Tanouye, E.

1995 Merck's Osteoporosis Warnings Pave the Way for Its New Drug. Wall Street Journal, June 28: B1.

WDIO (Word Development Indicators On-Line)

2003 Health System statistics, Central African Republic.

2004 Health System and Population Statistics for Mali, Burkina Faso, Ghana, Central African Republic, and Zambia.

Woo, S.-B., J. W. Hellstein, and J. R. Kaimar

2006 Systematic Review: Bisphosphonates and Osteonecrosis of the Jaws. Annals of Internal Medicine 144(10):753–761.

CHAPTER TEN
DEADLY EMBRACE
Psychoactive Medication, Psychiatry, and the Pharmaceutical Industry

Michael Oldani

Over the last decade adolescents and young adults have increasingly killed both others and themselves as well as suffered "sudden death" while taking prescribed psychoactive medication. These cases range from the dramatic and sensational (e.g., Cho Seung Hui, the Korean student who killed 32 students and himself at Virginia Tech University) to many other less publicly visible examples. The deaths have polarized both the general public and the medical community into a "handgun-like" argument: Is it the medication or the (mentally ill) person who is harming himself or others? Are the selective serotonin reuptake inhibitor (SSRI) class of compounds or stimulants such as Adderall (mixed salts of a single entity amphetamine product), actually killer commodities? Or, are the deaths attributed to these compounds simply anomalies, coincidence, or human acts that a chemical compound could never induce (nor prevent)? One may start to think that changes in package insert labeling mandated by the FDA regarding SRRIs and the issue of suicidality have begun to limit the prescribing of this particular class of compounds, but that has not occurred. One may also conclude that when an entire country such as Canada pulls Adderall off the market due to unexplained deaths in patients, other countries would consider a similar policy, but this has not occurred either. In fact, the contrary is occurring. Psychotropic prescribing, in particular for children and adolescents in the United States, has reached unprecedented heights.

Moreover, as concerned scholars and medical clinicians raise cautionary flags regarding the deadly risks of psychoactive compounds, they continue to be prescribed across a range of disorders and patient types. In fact, an alarming trend is the eagerness of *parents* to embrace psychoactive drugs for managing complex psychosocial disorders in their children (Oldani 2006). This began in earnest in the 1990s with demand for Ritalin (methylphenidate) to treat ADHD and more recently with an *emerging* childhood disorder, such as "bipolar disorder." In the latter case there is great concern about the prescribing of psychopharmaceuticals that are considered powerful and what that may due to the developing brains of young children. Moreover, growth of Ritalin use over the last two decades provides an important example of how psychoactive medication continues to be used in all human life stages. According to a former director of the National Institute of Mental Health (NIMH), "the market" created a downward creep, which forced the NIMH to fund studies of the drug in these younger children, which subsequently created more "clinical" justification for stimulant prescribing in younger and younger children—a type of prescribing circularity (Oldani 2006). In general, eagerness to medicate can lead to the prescribing of psychotropics as "diagnostic tests" (Oldani 2006), which create symptom relief and eventually a diagnosed mental health disorder (and cultural label), such as "bipolar disorder," is placed upon the patient. In the meantime, young patients end up being prescribed powerful psychoactive medications, often for life, with little concern for short-term or long-term side effects (Healy 2004). And most recently, drugs like Strattera (atomoxetine), a nonstimulant treatment for ADHD, and Concerta, a long-acting form of methylphenidate, have been granted "adult" indications for the treatment of ADHD by the Food and Drug Administration, thus expanding the life cycle of a pharmaceutical (van der Geest et al. 1996) into virtually all human life stages—the SSRIs being another example.

There does exist, however, a growing concern from various scholars and clinicians regarding the overprescribing of these drugs and the associated side effects, including the death of mentally ill patients. In short, the killer status of these drugs is being debated and *played out* in the medical marketplace on an everyday basis. In this chapter, I address this issue by looking at how the "killer" status of these compounds remains *in limbo* and actually out of public/everyday discourse. I draw upon various primary and secondary sources to show how young persons are increasingly put at risk as prescriptions continue to increase and how the *acceptance of risk* is engineered through pharmaceutical industry practices. In particular, I draw upon the work of former pharmaceutical industry insiders as well as use both my autoethnographic experiences as a former pharmaceutical salesperson, or "drug rep" during the 1990s, and my current ethnographic research as a trained medical anthropologist. My work and the work of other scholars will outline how psychiatry continues to have a deep involvement with the pharmaceutical industry and a growing dependence on psychopharmacological cures when managing populations of mentally ill patients. These patients, who increasingly can be described as a type of "treatment naïve" population (Petryna 2003), will be discussed as well. In particular, the treatment-naïve family provides a lucrative, yet highly risky environment for prescribing psychoactive medication: a site to examine the potentially deadly embrace between doctors, consumers, and drugs.

A critical issue for any killer commodity and the protection of the general public continues to be *transparency*. The current growth of prescribing (and consumer desire for) psychoactive medication makes the issue of transparency all the more salient in the realm of pharmaceutical industry practices. This chapter shows conclusively how increasing the transparency regarding the relationship between psychiatric experts and the pharmaceutical industry will go far in understanding how potentially killer commodities can remain highly prescribed medications, used across all age groups in North America.

Modern Biopsychiatry: Caught between Killer Commodities and Killer Markets

In the 1990s pharmaceutical salespersons, or drug reps, in Wisconsin often described the selective serotonin reuptake inhibitor (SSRI) market, which through the late 1990s included Prozac (fluoxetine), Zoloft (sertraline), and Paxil (paroxetine), as *a killer market*. I know this firsthand because I sold and promoted Zoloft (sertraline) from 1992 to 1998 for Pfizer, Inc. (Elliot 2006, Oldani 2002, 2004, 2006). Drug reps used the term *killer* to refer to the market growth and dominance the SSRIs were experiencing as a class of medication for treating mental health disorders (i.e., these medications were *killing* the competition, namely older antidepressant compounds, such as the generic tricyclic antidepressants). *All* SSRIs that have been marketed in the United States (e.g., Prozac, Paxil, Zoloft, Celexa, and Lexapro) have eventually attained "blockbuster" status—one billion dollars or more in annual sales during their patent life. Lexapro (escitalopram oxalate) and Celexa (citalopram), both developed and marketed by Forest Pharmaceuticals, Inc., represent a unique molecular path to blockbuster sales. Celexa was aggressively marketed by Forest and quickly became the most prescribed SSRI in the late 1990s. However, its patent life was shortened in the United States and the company filed a new patent for citalopram's racemic isomer—escitalopram (the "mirror" image of citalopram)—thus easily creating the number-one prescribed SSRI by psychiatrists.

By 2006, introducing a SSRI to the U.S. market, or a close pharmacological cousin, such as an SNRI, almost guaranteed a blockbuster drug. (SNRI stands for serotonin and norepinephrine reuptake inhibitors, which are currently on the U.S. market in the form of Effexor (venlafaxine HCl) and Cymbalta (duloxetine HCl). These drugs are often referred to as the "next generation" of serotonergic agents used for depression and other mental health disorders.

As a drug rep in the 1990s, I could clearly see that the SSRIs' market dominance killed the (older generic) competition, even if they worked no better than older drugs and induced more suicide than the tricyclic antidepressants in clinical trials (Healy 2004:80–81). Nevertheless, by 2004 when Vioxx and Bextra were being pulled from the market by the FDA for killing patients, the same types of questions were being asked by the FDA concerning the SSRI-class compounds and increased risk for death, specifically suicide and suicidality. The FDA wanted to know if the SSRIs increased the risk of suicidality in young persons—children and adolescents. Suicidality refers to thoughts or actions that are focused on and can lead to self-harm. In the recent past manufacturers of SSRIs (i.e., GlaxoSmithKline, makers of Paxil) "sanitized" the language of suicidality by referring to it in clinical trials and scientific journals as "emotional lability" (Healy 2004:284–289). In many ways the question of suicidality has become an extremely difficult question to answer definitively for any psychotropic compound, in particular, for the SSRIs. Psychiatry rapidly accepted these new drugs because of their presumed safety. This growing acceptance allowed biopsychiatry to finally overtake the psychodynamic (i.e., Freudian) model of mental illness.

Tayna Luhrmann (2000) in her landmark work, *Of Two Minds*, ethnographically documented this growing chasm between biomedical and psychodynamic treatments of mental illness. Luhrmann discusses in detail how this split was fueled by the increasing reliance on the *Diagnostic and Statistical Manual of Depression* (DSM), in particular the post-Freudian DSM III-Revised (1980). Although she does not make a direct connection, it's quite apparent that the move toward biologically based psychiatry was also accelerated through advances in psychopharmacology. On a more concrete level, I observed this reliance over a period of two decades as I moved from an industry "insider" (Oldani 2002) to a critical medical anthropologist. A brief chronicle of the psychiatric acceptance of SSRI treatment helps illustrate the importance of looking at the "pharmaceuticalization" (Reynolds Whyte et al. 2002) of this medical specialty.

In 1990, I had less than a year's experience as a pharmaceutical salesperson when my district manager asked me to attend a lecture by a well-known, "academic" Wisconsin psychiatrist. It was unknown to this doctor at the time that he would become a future "champion" (in industry sales jargon) for the SSRI class of antidepressants. My sales manager wanted to hear "what he had to say," because most of the newer sales reps (myself included) had no experience in the mental health marketplace. (Older reps in the district had sold benzodiazepines and antipsychotic medications in the 1970s and 1980s.) I can remember the talk well because it was clear that this psychiatrist, Dr. T, was *skeptical* of the new SSRI class of "compounds," as he described them at the time, which only consisted of Prozac. He was speaking at a continuing medical education retreat in the north woods of Wisconsin that was well attended by the state's contingent of psychiatrists. He told the psychiatrists in the audience to "stick with the tried and true . . . the TCAs [tricyclic antidepressants]." My manager felt this made sense at the time because TCAs, according to him, were psychiatry's "bread and butter." These drugs, because they were "dangerous" (i.e., they could cause fatal heart arrhythmias when taken in large quantities), required an expert for dosage titration—the psychiatrist. At that time, primary care doctors were writing prescriptions for TCAs, but only in low doses and not for depression, but for sleep problems. Company X's market research in 1990 revealed that "depression" was still a taboo word in primary care. Patients who may have satisfied the DSM symptomatology for major depression were more comfortable discussing associated problems, such as sleep, backache, and other bodily sites of pain.

Dr. T's skepticism seems otherworldly when I compare it to his current practice almost 15 years later. By the time I left Pfizer in 1998, Dr. T and his partner, Dr. V, another esteemed Wisconsin psychiatrist, were actually beginning to speak for Pfizer (and Lilly, the maker of Prozac) on a routine basis. Their talks were on the educational side of the expert-speaker spectrum, meaning just having them present a topic (e.g., problems in the mental health treatment of women) through an industry grant, had quite a bit of currency—increased a drug rep's (and in turn their SSRI's) credibility with local doctors.

It was not until six years later (in 2004) while doing ethnographic work in Winnipeg, Manitoba, that I next heard Dr. T's name. I was at a grand rounds presentation and the speaker was David Healy (mentioned throughout this chapter). He was presenting his "Let Them Eat Prozac" lecture to the audience. (He wrote a book with the same title, published in 2004.) Aside from the bombastic title, he was presenting a well-researched cultural and pharmaceutical history of psychotropic prescribing and industry marketing campaigns over the past 50 years. He then began to discuss issues of suicidality with the SSRIs, namely how the industry had sanitized the language of suicide in published clinical trials and that "negative" trials showing increased risk were never published (Whittington et al. 2004). Healy then said something that he felt represented the *counterdiscourse*, or argument, to his analysis. In other words, he was showing the audience a statement from an "expert" used by Big Pharma to counter arguments such as his. Paraphrasing from my field notes: *The benefits of SSRI treatment far outweigh any of the possible risks of suicidality, which is an inherent symptom in many of the patients we treat.* The actual quote that Dr. Healy was referring to was from none other than Dr. T, who had become a de facto industry spokesperson! He was providing sound bites to counter all of the negative publicity starting to circulate around the entire class of SSRIs. Dr. T had traveled a 15-year road from skepticism to unquestioning support of SSRIs.

In 2005, I returned to live in Milwaukee and soon realized Dr. T (and Dr. V) had become true champions for SSRIs (Oldani 2006). I was informed by a current Pfizer representative/anthropological informant that the two psychiatrists are no longer affiliated with their previous academic center in Wisconsin. They had started up their own, independent psychiatric research center. And according to this drug rep, most of their money now comes from doing psychopharmacological studies. The phrase she used to describe their new brick-and-mortar operation was "Pfizer and Lilly built their clinic." The representative then told me they both speak for most of the major drug companies that are involved in the mental health-care marketplace and continue to speak for her.

Lastly, there was also another significant moment during the David Healy grand rounds talk mentioned above and this occurred during the question-and-answer session of his presentation. Many doctors in the audience seemed satisfied with his overall argument—that SSRIs appear to be riskier than previously thought and that they work no better than older agents. However, a local psychiatrist stood up and launched a tirade against the entire presentation. He called it "anecdotal" and "partial," based on "case studies." Then this psychiatrist, who was having a very visceral reaction (red, sweating, and voice raised), told Dr. Healy that "these drugs relieve suffering" and Healy was "wrong!" Dr. Healy stuck to his main points when responding, which was that regardless of the efficacy seen with these drugs, there are significant safety issues, particularly in vulnerable populations, such as children. I, on the other hand, could not take my eyes of the disgruntled psychiatrist, who listened to Healy's response while shaking his head no. This was a pivotal moment in my thinking regarding psychiatry and this specialty's reliance on SSRIs. The psychiatrist at grand rounds and Dr. T and Dr. V's shift in thinking went beyond clinical or medical science: psychiatrists *believed* in the *pharmacological efficacy* of these drugs to relieve patient suffering. Dr. T and Dr. V.'s belief is hard to gauge, but obviously their conviction reflects how they have benefited financially and professionally from their continued support of the biopsychiatric paradigm and psychopharmaceutical treatments.

Fortunately for medical consumers, states such as Minnesota and Vermont have begun to establish laws requiring more transparency regarding financial ties between doctors and the pharmaceutical industry (Meier 2007). A recent article in the *New York Times* (Harris and Roberts 2007) focused on psychiatrists and used these data to track the prescribing practices, expert speaker funding, and clinical trial administration of several doctors. The article highlighted the case of Dr. Faruk Abuzzahab, who over the last ten years has had his medical license suspended for seven months and restricted for two years. Yet, he continues to be funded by the pharmaceutical industry to oversee and conduct clinical trials and *to speak* to his colleagues about trial results (i.e., about how well the medication presumably works). According to the report, "he had helped study many of the most popular drugs in psychiatry, including [the SSRIs] Paxil, Prozac, Zoloft, and the atypical antipychotics Risperdal, Seroquel, and Zyprexa" (Harris and Roberts 2007:A1). The problem with Dr. Abuzzahab (and other "clinicians" noted in the article) is that their aggressive and unethical recruitment of study participants has put many patients at high risk for side effects and led to the death of many others.

Tragically, one patient of Dr. Abuzzahab, Susan Endersbe, who battled depression all of her life, checked herself into a Minnesota hospital in May 1994. After three weeks, she was feeling better on her prescribed medication and felt ready to leave. However, she was referred to Dr. Abuzzahab and she agreed to participate in a drug study he was being paid to conduct. (Her "suicidal tendencies" should have excluded her.) Dr. Abuzzahab stopped giving her the effective medication she had been taking and she was forced to wait nearly two weeks before receiving either an experimental drug or placebo. While waiting, the psychiatrist continued to record Susan's adverse effects as "0" (to keep her in the study), while nurses documented a steady decline. She even expressed reservations about going off "all of her medications" and began to speak repeatedly about killing herself—stating she planned to jump off a bridge (Harris and Roberts 2007:A20).

Dr. Abuzzahab, seemingly in denial, wrote in her chart that Susan was "medically improving" and allowed her at one point to visit her apartment alone (a violation of the study's protocol), even after she had spoken of suicide the night before. She left the hospital and two hours later jumped to her death off a local bridge. In another case the Minnesota Medical Board investigated why Dr. Abuzzahab abruptly discharged a suicidal patient (a Mr. Olson). He told the board "if a patient is determined to kill himself, he can't be prevented from doing it and hospitalization postpones the event." However, Mr. Olson mentioned to his sister (before he killed himself) that Dr. Abuzzahab told him by not agreeing to enroll in the study that "you're wasting my time and the hospital's" (Harris and Roberts 2007:A20).

These cases of preventable death highlight how the need for clinical trial results, fueled by a profit-driven medical-pharmaceutical complex, has allowed clinicians to compromise their ethics and patient care. The suicides reported in this article are deaths from psychoactive medication *by association*. The makers of psychoactive medication have the financial resources and the "structural force" (Applbaum 2004) to fund clinical trials worldwide and find willing doctors to run the studies (or hire outside companies who find the doctors). These clinicians are then responsible for finding willing (i.e., consenting) patients to participate in clinical trials. This report reveals that many patients would most likely be unwilling if not for their naïve trust in the experts charged with managing their psychiatric treatment. Outside of these tragic deaths, the most disturbing aspect of this report is the fact that many "psychiatric experts" with questionable medical ethics continue to speak (paid for by pharmaceutical companies) to community-based doctors about drug therapies *and* to conduct clinical trials. This generates more pharmaceutical prescriptions for powerful medications that are supported by clinical research that is increasingly being called into question regarding patient recruitment, study design, and end results. Returning to Dr. Abuzzahab, he continues to be paid by the pharmaceutical industry and is currently running a clinical trial for the Japanese company Takeda (for the sleep aid Rozerem). (He was conducting a trial for Eisai [for the Alzheimer's drug Aricept, marketed by Pfizer, Inc. in the United States] but was deemed "not qualified" after the *Times* inquiry.) And he continues to speak for and to run clinical trials for the U.S. company AstraZeneca.

On an everyday level "Big Pharma" continues to employ these "clinicians" for two reasons: they write a tremendous amount of psychoactive medication (i.e., generate prescriptions and sales at a local level) and they impact the prescribing habits of other doctors, such as fellow psychiatrists *and* both internal medicine doctors and family/general practitioners, where the bulk of all psychoactive medication is prescribed (Valenstein 1997). There exists a collective "unknowningness" (or a false confidence) by these doctors regarding how "expert" speakers form their opinions. Dr. Abuzzahab is paid to use his "expertise" to impact other doctors' prescribing habits regarding powerful psychoactive medication using the data from his own unethical and bogus clinical trials. According to industry norms, he actually has received a small amount of expert-speaker funding. Dr. Simon, mentioned in the same *New York Times* article, earned more than $350,000 from five drugmakers from 1998 to 2005 (Eli Lilly, the maker of Prozac and Zyprexa, paid more than $314,000 of this sum) (Harris and Roberts 2007:A20). This amount of money clearly reflects *the market* for his expertise—his talks must have had the desired effect of generating more prescriptions, or companies would not continue to pay him. And Dr. Simon clearly understands his clout—"I am respected by my peers" (Harris and Roberts 2007:A20). It has been my experience that experts making this sort of income are actually very clever salespersons for whatever product they happen to be presenting. Psychiatrists I recruited as expert speakers when I was a pharmaceutical representative in the 1990s often surprised me with their sales acumen; knowing how to plant questions in the audience in order to have a more effective and credible presentation; spinning negative questions about side effects into selling opportunities; and eventually *selling themselves* to corporate management (Oldani 2002).

These cases show that as psychiatry stakes its collective reputation on the psychopharmacological management of mental disorders—the outgrowth of a biopsychiatric paradigm—a clinical infrastructure has emerged that can lead to patient death. Risk exists for patients on several levels—questionable medical doctors (with dubious prescribing habits), unethical clinical trials, the dissemination of poorly run (and poorly understood) clinical trial results by so-called experts to local doctors, and of course the pharmacological effects of the medication itself. In particular, the SSRIs, which represent the cornerstone of the psychopharmacological turn in modern medicine (Healy 1997), are being reassessed as more risky for *life-threatening* side effects than previously believed. A growing literature indicates that some patient populations are at serious risk for suicidal behavior due to the "activation" of the serotonergic system (and also due to the abrupt withdrawal of medication) when prescribed an SSRI, in particular for children (Law 2006; Healy 2006). More important, there is evidence that shows the pharmaceutical industry has tried to withhold this information (or "sanitize" side effects) from doctors, the general public, and regulatory bodies, such as the FDA.

The "Treatment-Naïve" Consumer

Adriana Petryna has described certain vulnerable populations that become participants in clinical trials as "treatment naïve" (2003). These populations emerged during her investigation of another killer commodity, the antibiotic Trovan (trovafloxicin), which was eventually restricted by the FDA for causing sudden death in patients. Her work focused on how Trovan was studied in highly vulnerable African patients who had meningitis. A clinical trial was conducted in Nigeria, which compared Trovan-treated patients with Rocephin (ceftriaxone)-treated patients, but the Rocephin was administered to patients at suboptimal doses and several participants died. Pfizer, the maker of Trovan, has been sued by the families of these victims.

During my ethnographic work in Manitoba, I began to see another kind of "treatment-naïve" population—the average, middle-class family in search of psychotropic medication for their children. I became interested in how parents might be *shopping* for the right kind of prescription (specifically an SSRI or a stimulant medication), or *script* in pharmaceutical jargon, to help a child with either a behavioral and/or mood problem that was having a negative impact on family life or family dynamics. During this time the word *script* began to take on a dual meaning. Parents were shopping for a pharmaceutical pre-"script"-ion, which is part of medical and pharmaceutical jargon (i.e., doctors write scripts and pharmacists fill scripts). And, I eventually came to realize that parents were following a pharmaceutical industry–mediated *cultural script* (or narrative) that plotted out, scene by scene, the ways in which parents could secure a pharmaceutical prescription for a child. In short, I came to understand parents, children, and their families as *filling* (both) *scripts* (Oldani 2006, 2007).

As my fieldwork progressed, I began to collect larger narratives that showed how families were willing to place children on powerful medication, which an emerging critically based literature would describe as risky in terms of life-threatening side effects. Methodologically, I observed clinical encounters between families and doctors of various specialties (e.g., pediatricians, psychiatrists, family practitioners, etc.). I then *followed* the script home with the patient(s) where I conducted follow-up interviews regarding how "the medication was working"—a multisited approach (Marcus 1998). From the various cases I collected during fieldwork there emerged one household that presents an exemplary case of treatment naïveté. On the one hand, this case could be considered a *success story* of SSRI efficacy by the industry and many psychiatrists (i.e., there was symptom relief for the patient), and indeed it was deemed a success by the parents. On the other hand, this mainstream Canadian family's use of psychotropic medication highlights the risky business (i.e., the unspoken/unknown risks) of SSRI prescribing within a family. A condensed narrative of this family will illustrate this point further.

I met "Henry" and his parents, "Louise" and "Dan," during a clinical encounter with a Winnipeg pediatrician. Henry's parents were hoping to get a medication that "worked better" than Prozac, which their son had tried and eventually became lethargic while taking. The main parental concern was that Henry, a ten-year-old, was "doing fine at school but not at home." In fact he showed "superior ability" in school; teachers said he was "bound for success." But his behavior at home showed classic signs of sibling rivalry (with a younger brother), acting out, and sabotaging family events. His parents were at their "wit's end" and "walking on eggshells around him." He also had problems sleeping and would obsessively worry about current events. After talking to Henry, the pediatrician met with the parents and suggested a psychiatrist. The doctor then told them that he would respond well to medication. The dad wanted to know if the anxiety was connected to all this defiance. The dad didn't really believe in medicating his kids, partly, because Henry had been to this clinic before and tried Prozac and became "a bump on a log." Henry's mom was upset because she "didn't know how to help her son." The doctor listened and the parents eventually agreed with the referral, but they weren't completely satisfied with the visit—no prescription medication was offered.

Two months later I visited with this white, Canadian, middle-class family on a cold Winnipeg evening, and the entire family mood had changed. The parents were relaxed for the interview and seemed to be very happy, which was a complete turnaround emotionally from their tense frustration at the clinic months before. Henry had eventually seen a child psychiatrist and had been prescribed the SSRI Celexa for "worrying disease." I asked if Henry had changed and the response from Dad was "big time." I was told he was sleeping better, not staying up and worrying about things, and cooperating better with family members. Overall, the family was elated because they had dealt with Henry's anxious symptoms for five years and had finally restored what they described to me as "family harmony." When I asked Henry's father if he had changed his mind about medications (and psychiatry), he reluctantly nodded "yes." Although he added that some day he wanted to "take" Henry off of Celexa.

As my home interview progressed, I was struck by both the family's seemingly rapid acceptance of pharmaceutical treatment, and the parent's ability to overlook a key side effect of Celexa. If you recall, Prozac had made Henry act like "a bump on a log." During the interview, Henry came into the living room and politely interrupted our discussion a few times saying he was "feeling tired," which can be one of the side effects of Celexa as well. His parents told him he could go to bed after he finished his reading (i.e., homework) for school. His parents told me "he is sleeping better," that is, he wasn't lying in bed worrying about world events any longer. However, each time Henry interrupted us to complain about homework his parents had to prod him a little with encouraging words and then he left the room to complete his work. I found this interesting, and somewhat distressing, because according to Henry's clinical history, he was a *voracious reader.* In fact, his parents had indicated to his pediatrician that he "loved to read" and said that he would stay up all night reading both assigned and unassigned schoolbooks. It was noted in his chart that during the previous summer he had read over 63 books, to the astonishment of his teachers.

In my final assessment, I realized Henry's parents were not overly concerned with this change (or loss) in Henry's personality or scholastic ability because Celexa had helped to restore "family harmony." The family was functioning again, which had been the parents' desire at the outset—first failing with Prozac, then succeeding with Celexa.

As our interview continued, I asked the mom why she didn't have any problems trying these different psychoactive medications on her son. (Essentially using medication as their own familial "diagnostic test," until they found the right balance between efficacy and side effects.) Henry's mother told me that she felt all of his problems, his "worrying disease" in particular, was genetic and stressed to me that "there's anxiety in the family." She then looked at me and said, "I take Naprosyn [a pain medication] for PMS," known clinically as premenstrual disphoric disorder, or PMDD. (Henry's mother actually meant nefazadone [brand name Serzone], which she realized after getting up to find her prescription bottle; Naprosyn (naprozen) being an over-the-counter analgesic.) I looked at her husband with a curious glance, and he smiled. Henry's dad then reiterated to me that if he "can take his son off the medication some day he would," but for now it was quite evident this wasn't going to happen anytime soon. The final thing that I recorded that night was Henry's mother telling me what her son told her at his last visit to the doctor. He said: "Don't take me off this medicine." Her feeling was that Henry had realized his behavior was better *and* this change was pleasing his parents. In the short-term, the medication improved family affect.

Scripting Family Life, while Increasing Risk

As I drove home on the frigid streets of Winnipeg after my visit with Dan and Louise, I kept ruminating on the apparent happiness and harmony that this family was experiencing. I also kept thinking about a comment Louise made that there were "no side effects" with Celexa. The fact of the matter was that Henry's improvement could be tied specifically to a more mild side effect of Celexa—sleepiness. However, his parents saw this as part of the drug's efficacy and not as a side effect, as they did with Prozac. For whatever (biochemical) reason, Celexa made Henry sleepy at night, which is desired by most parents for their children, and not during the day like Prozac, which drove Henry's parents to discontinue that medication. I, too, was caught up (even seduced) in the family's psychopharmacological transformation. Later, when I began to analyze my field notes, I realized that this side effect of sleepiness had actually altered Henry's intellectual abilities as well. In my field notes I had recorded that Henry's teachers had said that he was "bound for success," while expressing shock that he was a problem at home. I recalled during my first observation with Henry and a pediatrician, that the doctor had noted how he read over 60 books for a summer reading program, which was well over the required number. His parents had also told the doctor he could stay up all night and read. Celexa, which his parents thought of as a "clean drug," had altered Henry's desire for reading (and doing his homework). During my follow-up interview with the family, Henry kept interrupting our discussion in order to tell his parents he wanted to go to bed, and he had to be prodded by his parents to find and finish his homework. This change in Henry's ability to read, which could be understood as an alteration of his personhood (i.e., Henry may be a gifted child), added a new dimension to this family's psychopharmacological transformation. Henry's desire to make his parents happy may cost him something valuable in the long term (Oldani 2006).

I continued to observe clinical encounters between parents and doctors after Henry's case and to document parental demand for SSRIs and psychotropic medication in general. I observed and/or was described such practices as: Mothers phoning a child psychiatrist for a script of Strattera, before it was on the Canadian market; a mother and daughter demanding from their family doctor that "we both need Celexa"; and, a father requesting a script for Strattera because it worked so well for *his son's* ADHD. These clinical experiences mirrored what was being reported by the U.S. popular press as well. For example, *Time* magazine had a brief article in 2001 about Ritalin acting as "mother's little helper." This article chronicled a case in which a mother and her son started Ritalin on the same day (Ripley 2001).

It wasn't until the summer of 2005, when I was perusing through an *In Style* magazine, that I was actually able to see how the pharmaceutical industry had come to script out (or emplot) what families ideally could become on SSRIs. An advertisement caught my eye and took me right back to Henry's family. I was introduced to "Dot," who is a recurring character in a series of Zoloft advertisements that script (or plot) the way a consumer can empower their way to an SSRI prescription. The inviting and playful plot of the Zoloft graphic advertisement has become the dominant narrative or pharmaceutical plot for generating psychoactive pharmaceutical prescriptions throughout North America.

The script lays out a series of exchanges and practices (i.e., each individual scene) that a mentally ill consumer and/or parent/guardian can follow in order to have both a patient's pharmaceutical script and the script of a happy family life (ful)filled. Moreover, this advertisement clearly shows how the industry has made "the family" a key site for generating prescriptions. Although "Kathy's story" is fictional, it is quite apparent when visiting the websites of large multinational drug companies that they are actively collecting and promoting patient "success stories" or testimonials to the life-changing aspects of a particular pharmaceutical product. "Kathy's story" appears to be one such outcome of collecting these "ethnomarketing" cases. In other words, the industry has done its own research on the everyday reality of how patients are involved in the prescription-writing process. This Zoloft advertisement represents only an imagined or ideal form of a pharmaceutical family, which is presented *as free of side effects*—similar to what Henry's parents experienced with Celexa.

Nevertheless, there remains a naïveté by consumers (and clinicians) regarding the more serious side effects of the SSRI class of medications. All one has to do is look directly below the Zoloft graphic advertisement *and read* the bold print to realize there are potentially serious side effects with Zoloft and/or any SSRI treatment, in particular for younger persons. It specifically states:

> Depression is a serious mental condition, which can lead to suicidal thoughts and behavior. A combined analysis of 9 antidepressants showed an increased risk from 2% to 4% in people under 18. This risk must be balanced with the medical need. Those starting medication should be watched closely for suicidal thoughts, worsening of depression, or unusual changes in behavior. In children and teens, Zoloft is only approved for use in those with obsessive-compulsive disorder.

This change in package-insert wording occurred after the FDA advisory meeting on SSRIs in 2004, which I mentioned at the outset of this chapter. It is important to note that advertisers do extensive research on advertisements, and I was informed by the president of an advertising firm that handles several major pharmaceutical accounts that all side-effect information in print/Internet advertising is positioned on the page to minimize impact. In his words, "the average person does not see it." He went on to explain that the "important" messages concerning drug efficacy (in this case to cure depression and improve family life) do make it into our mental consciousness/unconsciousness, which these firms ensure by extensive market research with doctors and consumers (Bioethics and Pharmaceuticals Workshop, University of Minnesota 2007).

During the summer of 2004, I addressed this issue of suicidality and SSRIs with a busy psychiatrist in Milwaukee, Wisconsin. She told me that she was "furious" about the whole issue. At first I thought she was referring to the way the industry withheld side-effect data concerning the SSRIs and suicidality. Instead, she was furious at the "media and liberals, like you! Who keep planting this idea that these drugs are dangerous." She told me that she routinely tells her patients who come in with questions about "killing themselves" while taking these meds to "stop surfing the Internet" and that "these drugs are safe! Period." This is a busy psychiatrist whom I have known since the mid-1990s, when she was a medical student and I was a drug rep. Our thinking about the SSRIs has diverged as she has become a "high prescriber" (Oldani 2002, 2004; Elliot 2006) of SSRIs, and I have become a medical anthropologist.

In fact, this ethnographic anecdote reflects a more general attitude I have encountered even at the highest bureaucratic level of mental health management. In the spring of 2005 the NIMH sent out calls for studies concerning the issue of SSRIs and suicidality in young persons, which reflected the growing literature pointing toward an increased risk. I informally submitted via e-mail a proposal for a study to follow families with children who were newly prescribed SSRIs for depression. I made the mistake of including the case of Henry in which I hypothesized parents, like his, were sometimes "too eager" to find pharmaceutical cures for problems (and behaviors) related to family dynamics. An NIMH clinician quickly read my proposal and returned it stating that I should "ask for money from the Scientologists"—an organization symbolic of antipsychiatry and in particular, against the use of psychoactive medication. This exchange with the NIMH reflected the intellectual, financial, and structural investment this organization has made through the use of SSRIs, and psychoactive medication in general, to treat a host of mental illnesses. To be fair, my grant was eventually "scored" (in 2006) and described as "timely and important," but not funded. Thus, there seems to be a growing concern within the NIMH regarding the issue of serious side effects and the SSRI class of medications and the risk of prescribing these drugs in younger populations. In fact, the NIMH has publicly solicited for more clinical research to examine the issue of selective serotonin reuptake inhibitors and suicidality (NIH 2005).

The Risky Business of Psychotropic Prescribing for Patients/Consumers

Interestingly, the issue of suicidality never came up with Henry's parents during our time together. In fact, Henry's parents were completely unaware that Celexa was indicated *only* for adults. I brought this up at one point during our interview, and they became slightly confused when I started discussing pediatric indications and the FDA and Health Canada. For their particular family situation this drug was *clean*, and I could tell they did not feel good about my probing questions regarding indications and serious side effects. Moreover, several months after my interview in November 2003, I learned that Serzone (nefazodone HCL), the non-SSRI antidepressant that Henry's mother was being prescribed "off label" (neither Health Canada or FDA approved) for "PMS" (i.e., PMDD—premenstrual dysphoric disorder), was being pulled off the Canadian market by its manufacturer, Bristol-Myers Squibb, along with one other generic formulation, Lin-nefazodone, manufactured by Linsson, Inc. Health Canada was overseeing the removal, which was based on 38 cases of liver-related adverse effects and one death in Canada since its introduction to the Canadian market in 1994. Health Canada was encouraging a "transition period" by doctors to switch patients to other medications as well as to ensure that the other six generic manufacturers of nefazodone follow a similar market removal system (Health Canada 2006). Serzone was pulled off the U.S. market by Bristol-Myers Squibb on June 14, 2004, for similar reasons, including "fatal liver damage," and, at that time, generic sales were being *continued.*

When I rethink this ethnographic case, I keep coming back to the fact many of Henry's problems were due to his lack of sleep. His worrying would keep him up at night, which led to behavioral (and mood) problems during the day. In the end Celexa, with all its inherent risk of suicidality, helped him sleep better at night. This seemed to improve his mood and behavior and subsequently his family relations. I keep asking myself, why wasn't Henry prescribed a sleep aid first? Maybe a mild tranquilizer to help him sleep—something that does not have the associated risk of suicidality in young persons. Yet, I also realized after reading David Healy's (2006) very keen historical analysis of SSRI marketing as well as analyzing my own clinical ethnographic observations and interviews, that this would be virtually impossible in today's medical marketplace to happen. The manufacturers of SSRIs have strategically positioned themselves (after securing the major depression marketplace) to dominate the anxiety market as well. And to quote Healy (2006:75) directly: "Clinical trials have become embodied in treatment algorithms and protocols drawn by experts—many of whom have affiliations with pharmaceutical companies—that rank pharmacotherapy as the leading option for the management of nervousness in children." This is now the therapeutic terrain of the SSRIs, which was previously the domain of tranquilizers such as Valium. Interestingly, Healy argues that clinically tranquilizers, such as the benzodiazepine class of compounds or even therapeutically used opioids, are less addictive (i.e., less dependence or possibility of withdrawal symptoms after discontinuation) than the SSRIs, which runs counter to current, mainstream medical common sense (Healy 2006:81; Medawar 1997; Medawar et al. 2003). The dominant pharmaceutical script for depression, anxiety, and other mental disorders today remains an SSRI prescription. Yet, these scripts carry many more risks, from the mundane to the severe, for the average consumer.

The risk of death and/or killing oneself or another remains the most controversial. For example, members of Chris Pittman's family, in a well-chronicled case in the media, claim that this 15-year-old boy murdered his paternal grandparents when he experienced "SSRI-induced mania" after he was prescribed Zoloft in 2001. Zoloft is only approved for use in children with OCD (obsessive compulsive disorder), but in this case it was prescribed for pediatric depression. Zoloft had been prescribed as a substitute for another antidepressant he had been taking at a psychiatric center. Soon after this change in medication, his grandparents took him back to their house to live, where the murders occurred. Chris Pittman lost his Zoloft defense and was eventually sentenced to 30 years in prison (Online Lawyers 2006).

There are of course other highly publicized cases such as the Pittman example that have tried to link SSRI-induced mania or anxiety to violence, murder, and suicides. The infamous Columbine High School murders in the United States would be another example. Eric Harris, one of the shooters that day who later killed himself, had been prescribed an SSRI. One expert on the SSRIs, Dr. Ann Blake, author of *Prozac: Panacea or Pandora?* has gone on record stating that "every single school shooting can be traced back to the use of these drugs" (Law 2006:112). Prozac went on trial for the first time in 1994, when 47-year-old Joseph Wesbecker, who was taking the medication, returned to his former place of work where he shot 20 people, killing eight, and then killed himself. Law (2006:110–112) argues convincingly that two events overshadowed this trial, greatly reducing the amount of public attention and scrutiny toward Prozac (and other newer SSRIs). First was the O. J. Simpson trial, which was happening at the same time. And second was the amount of positive attention Prozac was receiving because of Peter Kramer's book

Listening to Prozac. Nevertheless, Lilly, the maker of Prozac, won the case, after a "vigorous defense" and, according to journalists following the case, was exonerated in the court of public opinion. In other words, Prozac appeared very safe and effective in changing brain chemistry in only the right direction—improving mental health (Law 2006:110–112).

In 2001 the scientific/medical and legal community began to shift their opinions regarding the safety and widespread usage of SSRIs. First, a Wyoming judge ordered GlaxoSmithKline to pay $6.4 million in compensation to the surviving relatives of a 60-year-old man, Donald Schell. He had killed his wife, daughter, and granddaughter in 1998 while on Paxil. Similar to the Lilly case mentioned above, GlaxoSmithKline argued that it was the mental illness that killed these people and not the drug. However, in this case the SSRI manufacturer lost and immediately appealed (Law 2006:112). By 2000 there was a growing body of scientific and medical literature that indicated SSRIs were indeed causing an increase in "akathisia"—severe anxiety, which can lead to thoughts of suicide or violence. For example, a well-known experiment by David Healy (who is mentioned above) looked at how 20 *healthy volunteers* with no record of depression responded to SSRI treatment. Two of the participants became suicidal (Law: 2006). David Healy has also presented detailed case studies of mentally ill patients whose suicidal thoughts and acts ended abruptly after discontinuing treatment with Prozac (Healy 2004:40–48). By the early 2000s the issue of akathisia, suicidality, and the SSRIs had become a topic of critical importance. And subsequently, individuals who had experienced akathisia began to take action. SSRI-survivor communities emerged, such as the Prozac Support Group, which between 1999 and 2002 received 4,000 calls from fellow sufferers (Law 2006).

Clearly the question of the killer status of SSRIs has become divisive. Communities of supporters and detractors have emerged over the last 15 years, with the FDA (in the United States) finding itself squarely in the middle of the debate. The FDA is supposed to be a buffer between the public health of citizens and corporations. However, its objective eye, if you will, has been slowly eroded by pharmaceutical industry money and conflicts of interests between expert medical/scientific advisers and Big Pharma (Critser 2005). Nevertheless, the FDA was forced to review data concerning the SSRIs and suicidality in 2004 after the UK equivalent of the FDA had discovered that GlaxoSmithKline had indeed withheld (or suppressed) information on this possible side effect (Healy 2006). The FDA, after convening a special advisory panel regarding suicidality and children, responded by requiring the makers of SSRIs and SNRIS to change the labeling in their respective package inserts (PIs). The current universal SSRI package insert states:

> Suicidality in Children and Adolescents—Antidepressants increased the risk of suicidal thinking and behavior (suicidality) in short-term studies in children and adolescents with major depressive disorder (MDD) and other psychiatric disorders. . . . No suicides occurred in [clinical] trials. (Lilly, Inc. 2006)

The final sentence is a bit misleading because suicides have occurred for patients taking SSRIs, and these data were submitted to the FDA for licensing (Healy 2006:70, table 1). Healy's interpretation of the data suggests that in general SSRIs *do not* lower suicide rates for mentally ill patients. Regardless, it is now clear that the FDA has interpreted the data concerning SSRIs, children, and suicidality as a serious clinical and psychiatric matter. Prescribing SSRIs appears riskier in some populations than was previously understood to be the case. Interestingly, the onus on monitoring children and adolescents for "unusual changes in behavior" has been placed on families and caregivers, which in turn must be communicated with the prescriber. On page ten of the Prozac package insert under "WARNINGS" more specific instructions are given:

> Families and caregivers of pediatric patients being treated with antidepressants for major depressive disorder or other indications, both psychiatric and nonpsychiatric, should be alerted about the need to monitor patients for the emergence of agitation, irritability, unusual changes in behavior, and the other symptoms described above, as well as the emergence of suicidality, and to report such symptoms immediately to health care providers.

Although this labeling could be interpreted as damaging to the SSRI marketplace, these drugs remain on the market and are highly prescribed—a $19 billion global market (Law 2006:105). In short, the manufacturers of SSRIs have been successful in sustaining a killer market in part by admitting (at least to the FDA) that there does exist an increased risk of suicidality in some patients while getting the FDA to include families and caregivers in the pharmacotherapeutic process, to become more involved (and responsible) in monitoring their children. This does seem like an advantage to the industry if and when new legal cases emerge regarding the safety and killer status of these mediations. If parents (and doctors) fail to monitor these young patients closely, as instructed by the package insert, then who will be at fault in the eyes of the court?

Final Discussion—The Role of Experts

The multinational pharmaceutical industry constantly requires new (and expanded) markets for their products. They have enough resources at their disposal to change the mental health landscape of an entire nation-state. New indications also can lead to new markets. For example, pediatric indications have become a fast and easy way to extend the patent life (and general market life) of a drug. The math is simple, but the risks appear high as children become increasingly (over)medicated. Should families and parents be more aware of the risks? Of course. However, the current system in the United States remains flawed when multinational pharmaceutical corporations can keep products available on the market for pediatric use with virtually no restrictions for usage; when the management of risk has been inscribed via the package insert and become the responsibility of parents! In other words, doctors continue to write SSRI scripts for children because they legally can, which in turn has been greatly impacted by consumer demand and direct-to-consumer advertising.

Recently the use of amphetamines, such as Ritalin and Adderall, which are used to treat childhood disorders such as attention-deficit/hyperactivity disorder (ADHD), has been linked to sudden death in children. Canada was the first country to react to children dying on these medications. On February 9, 2005, Health Canada suspended the "market authorization" of Adderall XR, an extended release formulation of Adderall that is used to treat ADHD. Health Canada advised patients who were then being treated with Adderall XR to consult their physician immediately about the use of the drug and to select alternative treatments. Why? A thorough review of safety information provided by the manufacturer (Shire Biochem, Inc.) indicated that there were 20 international reports of sudden death in patients taking either Adderall or Adderall XR. These deaths were not associated with overdose, misuse, or abuse. There were 12 reports of stroke, two in children. Overall, 14 deaths occurred in children and six in adults. The United States eventually reacted through the FDA by having another black box warning added to the package insert of amphetamines (including methylphenidate) used to treat ADHD.

The *Washington Post* reported on February 15, 2005, that because of the Health Canada decision, the FDA had reviewed the safety data of Adderall and Adderall XR and concluded that the drug should not be given to patients/children with "structural cardiac abnormalities," such as heart murmurs. However, neither form of the drug was being removed from the U.S. market (Ritalin and related compounds have since added a warning to their package inserts regarding possible cardio-toxicity). Dr. Joseph Biederman, chief of pediatric psychopharmacology at Massachusetts General Hospital, was quoted as saying you need to put a "denominator" of 30 million patient (prescriptions written) under these 20 deaths. The FDA said this number of deaths was not uncommon for the number of scripts written. The *Post* did report that some physicians were considering switching. "You always have to be extra careful with kids." Neither form has been studied in children under the age of six (*Washington Post* 2005). Dr. Biederman was following a common outline (or script) for risk management within the U.S. health marketplace: Find an expert or a pharmaceutical industry champion of a disease/disorder and its prescription drug treatment, and if there is a crisis, have him or her reassure the medical community and consumers about the drug's safety *and* efficacy. In this script, it comes down to *a numbers game* (i.e., more simple math).

It is important to highlight that Dr. Biederman is involved in another type of numbers game. He runs one of the largest child and adult ADHD treatment and research centers in the country. His clinic has received grant support from Shire Laboratories, Inc., Eli Lilly & Co., Pfizer Pharmaceuticals, Cephalon Pharmaceuticals, Janssen Pharmaceuticals, Neurosearch Pharmaceuticals, Stanley Medical Institute, Lilly Foundation, Prechter Foundation, NIMH, NICHD, and NIDA. He has served on the speaker's bureau for Eli Lilly & Co., Pfizer Pharmaceuticals, Novartis Pharmaceuticals, Wyeth Ayerst, Shire Laboratories Inc., McNeil Pharmaceuticals, and Cephalon Pharmaceuticals. Dr. Biederman is on the advisory board for Shire Laboratories, Inc., Eli Lilly & Co., CellTech, Novartis Pharmaceuticals, Janssen Pharmaceuticals, Johnson and Johnson, Pfizer Pharmaceuticals,

Cephalon Pharmaceuticals, New River Pharmaceuticals, and Sanofi-Synthe (ADHDhome 2008). Needless to say, an expert such as Dr. Biederman, as well as other clinical experts involved with the pharmaceutical-industrial complex, has a vested interest in not making a hasty decision regarding the side effects of psychoactive drug treatment. Needless to say, Health Canada, under pressure from various groups in the United States, allowed for the return of Adderall to the Canadian market in August 2005 (FDA 2005).

On February 15, 2005, I accessed the Adderall website (www.adderallxr.com) of Shire Pharmaceuticals and there was no mention of the Health Canada decision. The Internet site was consistent with other prescription drug sites and provided links to product information, safety, education, and so forth, along with a now-common image on many pharmaceutical product websites. In this version, there was a happy pair of males, a father and son, smiling and hugging and/or wrestling (perhaps both were being prescribed Adderall XR, which is indicated for children and adults). This was a grim reminder that as debates continue, the pharmaceutical industry continues to *promote*, *prescribe*, and *profit* from this increasingly risky reality.

Obviously, no pharmaceutical product remains risk free. Answering the many questions and problems related to the "killer status" of SSRIs (and other psychoactive medications) remains a difficult task and requires constant vigilance by concerned investigators. As outlined above, *causation* (some may say blame) concerning the killer status and potentially deadly risk(s) of prescribing psychoactive mediation lies with pharmaceutical industry-supported *experts*. In many ways the killer status of psychoactive medication will be determined by how the scientific and medical data are interpreted by clinical experts and whether or not they are influenced consciously (or unconsciously) by the industry. It is also important to note that increased scrutiny by scholars interested in "critical pharmaceutical studies" (Oldani 2006) has created more transparency regarding how the pharmaceutical industry conducts business.

David Healy is one such example—an expert who has placed the critical mirror back on to the pharmaceutical industry and his own profession of psychiatry. However, the cultural currency and impact of an expert such as Healy remains low when compared with the pharmaceutical industry experts who continuously help determine the everyday and commonsense approach doctors and medical consumers take with powerful psychotropic medication and the treatment of mental health disorders. Healy (2007) has stated publicly that we are on the brink of "pharmageddon," when the house of cards of psychotropic prescribing will crumble. In a more optimistic vein, some experts have decided to navigate and embrace a dual role of pharmaceutical industry expert *and* consumer advocate.

When GlaxoSmithKline settled a lawsuit with the State of New York over the SSRI Paxil (regarding the fact the company had failed to publicize all pediatric trials of Paxil, including ones which showed an increase in suicidality), the company took the unusual step of posting on a website the results of *all* clinical trials for Paxil and other drugs (Meier 2007). Dr. Nissen and a colleague at the Cleveland Clinic quickly analyzed the data for another GSK drug—the billion-dollar blockbuster diabetes drug Avandia (rosiglitazone). What they found in the newly transparent data was that patients prescribed Avandia were at "significant increase in the risk of myocardial infarction" (Nissen and Wolski 2007). This information created a drop in Avandia prescribing and a drop in sales of roughly 30 percent in the first half of 2007 for a drug that generated $3.2 billion in sales in 2006. Obviously, pharmaceutical industry transparency can have a significant impact on the lives of medical consumers. Dr. Nissen continues to be a controversial figure because of his public health advocacy as drug industry "watchdog" and his ties to the pharmaceutical industry; namely taking money from companies to conduct clinical trials. He continues to call himself "an insider and outsider at the same time" who wants "to fix the FDA," and he has had a significant impact on dangerous pharmaceuticals (Saul 2007:1). He has helped to keep both Bristol Myers Squibb's experimental diabetes drug, Pargluva, and Merck's son of Vioxx, Arcoxia, off the market as well as being part of the push to remove Vioxx from the market.

Nevertheless, what remains disconcerting is the number of *mainstream* experts who continue to fall on the side of powerful pharmaceutical interests, fostering consumer confidence and a dangerous *treatment naïveté* regarding the dangers and risks of prescribing psychotropic medication. These experts as well as Big Pharma have worked to keep the killer status of psychopharmaceuticals in limbo while the industry maximizes profitable drugs. It's increasingly clear to many scholars and advocates that a definite correlation exists between the use of psychotropic medication, in particular the SSRI antidepressants, and violence, ranging from killing oneself and others to "bizarre behavior." The International Coalition for Drug Awareness keeps a current list of cases related to antidepressantinduced violence. As of the writing of this chapter, the coalition has documented over 1,300 cases, many of which ended tragically in multiple deaths (International Coalition for Drug Awareness 2007). The correlation between these medications and violent outcomes appears very clear. However, the question of actual *causation* remains in limbo—still a matter of expert research, discussion, and opinion. Thus, as prescribing doctors and millions of consumers embrace these commodities for mental health treatment, the battle for clarity and transparency regarding the killer status of these drugs continues on.

References

ADHDhome

2008 CME Information/Disclosure of Conflicts of Interest. Electronic document, www.adhdhome.org/cme_information.html#interest.

American Psychiatric Association

1980 Diagnostic and Statistical Manual of Mental Disorders, 3rd ed. Washington, DC: American Psychiatric Association.

Applbaum, K.

2004 How to Organize a Psychiatric Congress. Anthropology Quarterly 77:303–310.

Bioethics and Pharmaceuticals Workshop

2007 Interdisciplinary Symposia, Center for Bioethics, University of Minnesota, organizer: Carl Elliot, April 12–14.

Critser, Greg

2005 Generation Rx: How Prescription Drugs Are Altering American Lives Minds, and Bodies. New York: Houghton Mifflin.

Elliot, Carl

2006 The Drug Pushers. Atlantic Monthly, April: 2–13.

FDA (Food and Drug Administration)

2005 Electronic document, www.fda.gov/cder/drug/infopage/adderall.

Harris, Gardiner, and Janet Roberts

2007 After Sanctions, Doctors Get Drug Company Pay, New York Times. Electronic document, http://www.nytimes.com/2007/06/03/health/03docs.html.

Health Canada

2006 Electronic document, www.hc-sc.gc.ca/english/protection/warnings/2003/200383.htm, accessed January 10, 2005.

Healy, David
1997 The Anti-Depressant Era. Cambridge, MA: Harvard University Press.
2002 The Creation of Psychopharmacology. Cambridge, MA: Harvard University Press.
2004 Let Them Eat Prozac: The Unhealthy Relationship between the Pharmaceutical Industry and Depression. New York: New York University Press.
2006 The New Medical Oikumene. *In* Global Pharmaceuticals: Ethics, Markets, Practices. A. Petryna, A. Lakoff, and A. Kleinman, eds. Pp. 61–84. Durham: Duke University Press.
2007 Paper presented at Psychopharmacology in a Globalizing World: The Social Lives of Psychiatric Medication. Advanced Study Institute Workshop, McGill University. June 12–15.

International Coalition for Drug Awareness
2007 Electronic document, www.drugawareness.org/home.html, accessed July 21, 2007.

Law, Jacky
2006 Big Pharma: Exposing the Global Healthcare Agenda. New York: Carroll and Graf.

Lilly, Inc.
2006 Electronic document, www.prozac.com, accessed August 1, 2007.

Luhrmann, Tayna
2000 Of Two Minds: The Growing Disorder in American Psychiatry. New York: Knopf.

Marcus, George
1998 Ethnography through Thick and Thin. Princeton, NJ: Princeton University Press, pp. 79–104.

Medawar, Charles
1997 The Antidepressant Web. International Journal of Risk and Safety in Medicine 10:75–126.

Medawar, Charles, Andrew Herxheimer, Andrew Bell, and Shelly Jofre
2003 Paroxetine, Panorama and User Reporting of ADRS. Consumer Intelligence Matters in Clinical Practice and Post-Marketing Drug Surveillance. International Journal of Risk and Safety in Medicine 15:161–169.

Meier, Barry
2007 For Drug Makers, a Downside to Full Disclosure. New York Times, May 23. Electronic document, http://www.nytimes.com/2007/05/23/business/23drug.html, accessed June 30, 2007.

NIH (National Institutes of Health)
2005 Antidepressant Treatment and Suicidality (RO1; expired: 2005). National Institutes of Health. Electronic document, www.grants.nih.gov/grants/guide/rfa-files/RFA-MH-06-001.html.

Nissen, S., and K. Wolski

2007 Effect of Rosiglitazone on the Risk of Myocardial Infarction and Death from Cardiovascular Causes. New England Journal of Medicine 356(24):2457–2471.

Oldani, Michael J.

2002 Tales from the "Script": An Insider/Outsider View of Pharmaceutical Sales Practices. Kroeber Anthropological Society Papers 87:147–176.

2004 Thick Prescriptions: Toward an Interpretation of Pharmaceutical Sales. Medical Anthropology Quarterly 18(3):325–356.

2006 Filling Scripts: A Multisited Ethnography of Pharmaceutical Sales Practices, Psychiatric Prescribing, and Phamily Life in North America. Dissertation. Department of Anthropology, Princeton University.

2007 Can Doctors Take Back the Script? Understanding the Total System of Prescription Generation. Atrium: The Report of the Northwestern Medical Humanities and Bioethics Program, Fall.

Online Lawyers

2006 Electronic document, www.onlinelawyersource.com/news/zoloft-case .html, accessed July 31, 2006.

Petryna, Adriana

2003 Ethical Variability: Drug Development and Globalizing Clinical Trials. American Ethnologist 32(2):183–197.

Reynolds Whyte, S., S. van der Geest, and A. Hardon

2002 Social Lives of Medicines. Cambridge: Cambridge University Press.

Ripley, Amanda

2001 Ritalin: Mother's Little Helper. Time, February 12: 73.

Saul, S.

2007 Drug Safety Critic Hurls Darts from the Inside. New York Times. Electronic document, www.nytimes.com/2007/07/22/business/22nissen.html?ei=5070&en=212 ae981dd1a40c&ex=11856816000&emc=eta1&pagewanted=print.

Van der Geest, S., Susan Reynolds Whyte, and Anita Hardon

1996 The Anthropology of Pharmaceuticals: A Biographical Approach. Annual Review of Anthropology 25:153–178.

Valenstein, Elliot

1997 Blaming the Brain: The Truth about Drugs and Mental Health. Toronto: Free Press.

Washington Post

2005 Adderall: A Stroke of Bad News. Electronic document, www .washingtonpost.com/wp-dyn/articles/a24764-2005Feb14.html.

Whittington, C. J., T. Kendall, P. Fonagy, D. Cottrell, A. Cotgrove, and E. Boddington

2004 Selective Serotonin Reuptake Inhibitors in Childhood Depression: Systematic Review of Published Versus Unpublished Data. Lancet 363:1341–1345.

CHAPTER ELEVEN

A GUINEA PIG'S WAGE

Risk and Commoditization in Pharmaceutical Research in America

Roberto Abadie

> You are not thinking that these things [experimental drugs] are going to give you cancer five years from now, or that you might have a high level of radiation in your body
>
> —Grandpa Guinea Pig, January 5, 2005

On June 16, 2001, the *New York Times* reported the death of a healthy 24-year-old female who volunteered for an asthma study at Johns Hopkins University. The story revealed that a few days into the trial she felt very sick. She was discharged and sent home. Within some hours she checked into the emergency room at a local hospital and fell into a coma. She remained in this state until her death a month later. She had received $375 for participating in seven to nine sessions as an outpatient in the clinical drug study.

This tragic death touched me deeply, since I had also volunteered as a paid healthy human subject for phase I trials. During the last months of 1998 while I was pursuing my MA in Quebec City, I volunteered on a couple of occasions as an inpatient for Anapharm, a major CRO (contract research organization) performing phase I trials for local and international pharmaceutical companies which had their headquarters a few blocks away from my campus at Université Laval in Saint-Foy. The research facility was a functional, flat, uninviting five-story building, no doubt a fine expression of the Soviet-style architecture of the 1960s and 1970s that also shaped the university campus. Anapharm's staff was organized along a very clear division of labor: women were in charge of technical work while males performed the research and managerial tasks. Among the volunteers was a mix of unemployed, mentally disabled, artists, and university students. The research floor was crowded; dozens of double bunk beds were aligned in facing rows. A yellow light went on at night after the regular lights went off. Cash was handed to us in envelopes the last day of the trial, on our way out.

The first drug I tested was a new version of a drug to combat heartburn and gastritis that was already on the market. For a five-day, inpatient study I received $550 Canadian dollars. The second trial was a new drug to increase appetite in terminal patients with HIV or cancer. This experimental drug did not increase my appetite, but the trial definitely contributed to an increase of my diminished bank account savings by $800. I am sure, in retrospect, that the "financial compensation for my time and travel expenses," as the pharmaceutical industry regularly frames volunteers' participation in the trials, did not compensate for the risks I faced, the pain of endless blood extractions, and the boredom of spending hours doing nothing but watching TV.

The death of a paid subject at Johns Hopkins—a very dramatic death, but by no means a unique one—poses new questions in relation to commoditization in trials research, risks, and the ethical regulations protecting human subjects' participation that have not been addressed thus far. For example, does monetary compensation distort volunteers' perception of risks? What is the effect of market recruitment on the ethical regulations protecting human subjects in the experimental phases of drug trials research?

Focusing on ethnographic research of "first in man" phase I trials in a northern American city,[1] this chapter attempts to provide answers to these questions while offering some public policy recommendations intended to limit the risk paid subjects face in clinical trials drug research. Fieldwork was conducted between July 2003 and January 2005 among a group of self-defined professional "guinea pigs" volunteering as paid subjects for phase I clinical trials.[2]

Commoditization of the body in clinical trials research has increased significantly with the emergence of market-recruited patients, which replaced "captive" populations in the 1980s due to concerns that prisoners could not give proper informed consent because of institutional constraints. As a result, the industry had to find a new, suitable population to test the safety of a drug, creating in the process a new occupational category: the professional guinea pig.

The prospect of "easy, quick money" was enough to motivate mainly poor, unemployed, working-class individuals to become trials subjects and enter into the "economy of the flesh." The participation of paid research subjects in clinical trials research is only one of the examples of body commoditization in biomedical research.

Recent technological advances in transplantation techniques, artificial reproduction, and drug development have resulted in the increasing commoditization of the body (Scheper-Hughes and Wacquant 2003; Sharp 2000; Erickson and Cheney, this volume). Currently, there is a local and international market for major organs like the heart, kidney, and liver; body tissue; reproductive material such as sperm and eggs; plasma; and even hair.

In fact, this process of body commoditization is not new in American history where corpses have been sold to dissectionists, anatomists, and surgeons. Other forms of commoditization include the enslavement of human beings and the current use of reproductively rich products or tissues reaped from the dead (Sharp 2006). In keeping with these developments, there has been a growing scholarly interest in the commoditization of the body in medicine (Sharp 2000; Scheper-Hughes 2000; Nelkin and Andrews 2001; Moore 1999; and Marshall 1992). According to Sharp, organ transfer—like many new biotechnologies—elicits a powerful social anxiety in the public, which in turn leads to the industry's denial of body commoditization. She notes, "body commoditization—especially within the highly celebrated arena of organ transplantation—quickly erodes an already shaky public investment in medical trust. In response to such deep concerns, the transplant industry has generated an array of powerful euphemistic devices that obscure the commoditization of cadaveric donors and its parts" (Sharp 2006:17). According to Sharp, the reference to the commoditization of the body is avoided by using the rhetoric of the "gift" through which organ transfer is equated with "donating life" and organs with "precious resources" to be "harvested." For Sharp, these semantic choices make it possible to avoid references to the trauma, suffering, and death involved in removing organs from the donors. As a result, the language of the gift economy mystifies key aspects of organ transfer.

As with organ transplantation, pharmaceutical corporations appear to avoid references to commoditization of the body in their clinical trials, presumably in an attempt to maintain public trust. In clinical trials research, one can observe a discursive practice similar to that observed by Sharp in relation to organ transfer. This practice contributes to the industry's denial of the commoditization of volunteers' bodies. Subjects are labeled by the industry with the oxymoron of "paid volunteer," as it is claimed that they are being compensated not for their labor but for their "time and travel expenses."

It is not only organ transplantation that has the capacity to elicit anxiety in American society. A similar anxiety can be detected in clinical trials research. Clinical trials research based on market-recruited subjects provides the basis for drug development and patenting that has made the pharmaceutical industry one of the largest and most profitable sectors of the American economy. However, the commoditization of the body in clinical trials, as in other domains in biomedicine, elicits a profound distrust among the public about potential abuses from corporations seeking financial gain to the detriment of the well-being of research subjects or the larger drug-consuming public.

For example, a popular novel by John Le Carré, *The Constant Gardener*, and the movie based on the book both present abuses by a pharmaceutical company conducting clinical trials among poor, disenfranchised African residents; both elicited numerous questions about the ethics of clinical trials in third world countries. These artistic productions expressed criticism of the pharmaceutical industry and also of Western governments and agencies for exploiting the poor for commercial and national gain and exposed the ethical abuses involved in clinical research in developing countries. While clinical trials in developed countries do not usually elicit the same degree of attention or anxiety, recently a very serious episode during a trial sponsored by Parexel in England brought up public concerns that the pharmaceutical industry might abuse volunteers in its search for profits.[3] The recent market withdrawal of and subsequent lawsuits over Vioxx, a pain medication, due to evidence that Merck, its producer, manipulated evidence of increased risk of heart attack, elicited concerns among drug consumers and the general public.

My findings suggest that the commoditization process shapes volunteers' perceptions and responses to risk. More important, the reliance of the pharmaceutical industry on a group of professional research subjects might pose unforeseen risks, such as synergistic drug interactions and long-term effects. While some of the potential risks are relatively well known and clearly established as ADR (adverse drug reactions) or secondary effects, the experimental nature of phase I clinical trials might expose subjects to risks neither volunteers nor the industry might be aware of. Compared to coal miners, asbestos workers, or other types of workers exposed to industrial pollution, professional trial subjects are exposed to risks which are much less understood and documented. This is partially explained by the relatively recent professionalization of trial subjects dating from the mid-1970s, and by the dispersion of professional guinea pigs, who are always moving from one trial to another, obscuring the collective recognition of adverse effects. In addition, the pharmaceutical industry does not keep detailed records of subjects' participation in trials and might be unaware of this problem. Besides, it might have little or no interest in such a follow-up, which could jeopardize the current development of clinical trials research based on the professionalization of research subjects.

Another area of concern is that by exposing a particular socioeconomic group of volunteers to such risks, commoditization in phase I trials research distorts major ethical principles and guidelines regulating the protection of human subjects participating in research as contained in the Belmont Report. The shift from a captive population to a market-recruited population unfairly targets a particular socioeconomic group of individuals, creating thereby a new type of captive and vulnerable population. Paradoxically, this is the situation the Belmont Report intended to eliminate when it was formulated.

The Experimental Nature of Phase I Clinical Trials and the Use of Randomized Clinical Trial Designs

Phase I clinical trials employ healthy human volunteers to test new drugs under development by the pharmaceutical industry, not for therapeutic efficacy, but for drug safety. Phase I trials are designed to identify any danger associated with using the drug or compound under study and is the first time a chemical compound is tested in human beings after having been tested in laboratories and then in animals. After a drug is proven safe in phase I, then it goes through phase II and III trials, which involve larger groups of volunteers. While phase II also continues to test the drug for safety, this phase and the next one are intended to test for therapeutic benefits. If the drug proves to be safe and therapeutically useful, it then receives FDA approval and goes on the market.

Phase I trials are conducted either at pharmaceutical industry research sites, at contracted sites in university settings, or at sites held by independent contractors called contract research organizations (CROs). At this stage, the professional knowledge involved in drug development is mostly supplied by biostatisticians and experts in toxicology. In contrast to later phases in drug research, no specialized knowledge about a particular disease or medical condition is required.

Phase I clinical trials are designed as controlled experiments that follow an experimental design. The trials are devised to obtain information about how the human body responds to a particular substance, what the levels of toxicity are, and how the drug is absorbed and eliminated. As previously mentioned, this phase is not designed to test therapeutic effects on the volunteers.

According to Center Watch, an information services company monitoring clinical research, there were more than 80,000 clinical trials being conducted in 2002 in the United States alone. Impressive as this number is, it represents only a fraction of the total number of trials being conducted globally. Abroad, especially in third world countries, companies are not required to use the same standards of human subject protection as in the United States. Since 1980, looking to speed up the drug approval process and in the context of an increasing concentration and internationalization of clinical trials drug research, pharmaceutical industries have shipped many clinical trials abroad, mainly to developing countries, where ethical regulations are more relaxed, nonexistent, or unenforced and where trials can find a large population of willing, poor, disenfranchised subjects, who enter the trials induced by the prospects of getting access to health care, drugs, medical supervision, and financial rewards (Petryna 2006:193).

Human subjects engage in the phase I trials not to seek a therapeutic benefit or for altruistic motives but rather for financial gain (Weinstein 2001). Clinical trials for phase I drugs in the area where I conducted my research typically offer between $200 and $400 per day to volunteers. Compensation for engagement in a trial might range between $1,200 for three or four days in less intensive trials to $5,000 for volunteering for three or four weeks in more extended ones; on occasion a trial might need even more time to be completed, with even higher payment going to volunteers. Volunteers might have occasional jobs on the side, often in the service economy as cooks, painters, office cleaners, and construction workers, among others. However, for many participants clinical trials become their full-time job; full-time volunteers might enroll in five to eight trials a year, deriving a total estimated income of $15,000 to $20,000 in exceptionally good years. Experienced research subjects that I met during my fieldwork had participated in 40, 50, and even more phase I trials over the course of a few years.

Risk and Commoditization of the Body in Phase I Trials

As Mary Douglas reminds us, risks are individually perceived but socially constructed. Risk in the context of clinical trials research is understood by disciplines such as medicine, epidemiology, and pharmacology as a quantitative, bounded, and discrete phenomenon that can be objectively measured and dealt with. From this technoscientific perspective, risks can be expressed statistically, providing the basis for neutral decisions about causation, safety, and dosage. However, social scientists have shown that assessing risk in clinical trials research is a contingent social process.

Focusing on the way scientists detect adverse drug reactions at the trials and in postmarketing phases, Corrigan (2002) argues that scientific knowledge and practices are shaped by epistemological, political, and institutional arrangements to produce the scientists' risk assessments. According to this author, although scientists present their findings as "ready made" (that is, as finished and stable), risks assessments are fluid and dependent upon a kind of knowledge that is always in the making. As I will show in this chapter, Corrigan's argument can also be extended to the scientific assessment of long-term risks and synergistic interactions among paid "guinea pigs" enrolled in trials research. Far from being settled, the issue is obscured by the shifting nature of toxicological knowledge coupled with administrative and financial interests.

In turn, Abraham (1994) argues that adverse drug reactions are not neutrally assessed as scientists claim. Instead, Abraham shows how the scientific assessment of some drug trials is influenced by pharmaceutical companies' financial interests, which play a significant role by ignoring, dismissing, or obfuscating unfavorable results—a pattern reported in several other chapters in this book. Abraham points to the political and economic elements shaping governmental regulation of new drugs both in the United States and the UK. He argues that neoliberal policies weakened the regulatory powers of the state in both countries, leaving the pharmaceutical companies in a better position to influence regulations. The author suggests that this outcome compromises public safety and calls for active public control and citizens' participation to ensure stricter drug regulation procedures.

The Construction of Risk among Paid Subjects

Risk perception among professional guinea pigs is shaped by their clinical trial experiences and interactions with other volunteers, as well as by their need for drug trial income. In this sense, risk perception is thus closely related to the socialization into being or becoming a professional guinea pig.

Paid subjects share narratives about which kind of trials are risky and which ones are not, and also how to deal with these situations. Local knowledge shapes the social construction of risk and the strategies volunteers choose to implement to cope with the risks they perceive. A quick reference to frequently told guinea pig jokes involving risk provides clues into the socially constructed character of risk in this population.

Humorous tales describing bizarre experiments or risky situations form a critical part of guinea pig folklore. For example, some jokes depict an operation to remove and reattach the pinky toe for $5,000, or to remove the heart and "put it back in" for $10,000. These jokes were first introduced by the head researchers at a local university hospital, and quickly picked up by professional guinea pigs. The popularity of the jokes reflects not only paid subjects' awareness of the commoditization of their own bodies but also their anxieties around the risks they might face as paid subjects.

Volunteers not only share jokes about risks, but more important, they also consult each other about potential risks they might face in a prospective trial, especially if the drug is not a marketed drug, and thus has not been tested yet in humans. In addition, volunteers might search the Internet and sometimes ask individuals with medical training if they have doubts about the drug being tested.

The required signing of the informed consent form at the beginning of the trial provides the most relevant institutional opportunity to discuss risks volunteers might encounter. This document details the design, procedures, potential risks, and benefits of the study and is perceived by volunteers to be the main source of information about the trial. The informed consent form is the most important source of information for volunteers about the trial for phase I. While ethics regulations establish the avoidance of technical or professional jargon in the disclosure of information contained in the form, this requirement is not followed in phase I trials. Instead of using plain language to disclose risks and benefits, the informed consent form utilizes a language that obscures the risks involved in participation. Euphemistic terms along with hypertechnical language are used to avoid references to risks, suffering, and death.

One professional subject who has been doing clinical trials for more than ten years explains his anxiety over this point:

> This is an example for a study I did once. They were reading down the Informed Consent and they were going like, this is a Phase 1 study. First time in man, we did it with animals already and she is saying that the dose, 20 times over the normal rate, would produce an antiepileptic reaction in 60% of the animals. And I was like: "what is an antiepileptic reaction?" she paused, "well, it is when your heart stops beating and your lung stops breathing," then I said: "that means that you are dead?" and she replied: "as long as it doesn't start again, yes." That's good to know. (White mouse 2004)

The informed consent process, the screening, and the lengthy inpatient trials offer opportunities for close interaction among volunteers. The latter especially provides less experienced members an opportunity to expand their understanding of the way trials are organized, which risks they might face, and how to deal with them.

The social construction of risk among professional guinea pigs is based on two different but complementary classifications. On the one hand, risk is constructed along a temporal dimension that differentiates between short-term risks and long-term risks. On the other hand, risk is placed in a hierarchy from low risk, to medium risk, to high risk. Paid subjects' concerns are located in the present and are related to the trial they are currently volunteering for and the consideration only of its short-term effects. A volunteer who has done more than 40 trials over a five-year period elaborates on the perception of risks as related to the conditions of a given trial:

> Nobody thinks a lot about Long Term Risks. It is like getting a job in a restaurant; the neighborhood with a lot of crime, a far away train, whatever. You are thinking about a short-term problem, you are not thinking about what is going to bother you five years from now. You are thinking how am I gonna get to this job and how I am getting my weekly paycheck for this job. And with a trial it's the same thing. You are not thinking that these things are going to give you cancer five years from now, or that you might have a high level of radiation in your body. (Grandpa Guinea Pig 2005)

Trial subjects are not thinking that they might become ill years after the trial. Instead, they are worried about short-term considerations, such as acceptance into the trial, and then they focus on the schedule in order to receive the financial compensation for doing so.

While influenced by scientific constructions of risk, professional guinea pigs' understandings of risk are shaped as well by the experience and knowledge gained through their participation as paid subjects. Low-risk studies are considered to be those that involve drugs that are already in the market and present few or no side effects, even at the high doses administered during the trial. A new brand of Tylenol, or a similar pain medication, would be placed in this category and would constitute the most popular trial choice among professional guinea pigs.

Paid subjects perceive most clinical trials as presenting a moderate risk level. This evaluation is based on two elements. First, they view a trial as "a carefully controlled situation," an assessment that is based on the scientific design of the trial and the ethical regulations about the use of human subjects which, in their view, helps limit risk levels. The second element shaping the volunteers' perception of a moderate risk level in trials is their conviction that serious adverse effects or dangerous situations are exceptional in their trial experiences as paid guinea pigs.

While the majority of the trials are placed in the medium risk category by volunteers, some trials are perceived as presenting a high risk. New experimental drugs, and in particular, those that change the immunological system, or psychiatric drugs that alter the chemical structure of the brain are considered to be high risk. Experimental studies involving genetic drug testing and sleep deprivation studies are also a source of major concern. Volunteers rank experimental drugs as riskier than marketed drugs. Their assumption is that a marketed drug has already been tested in healthy volunteers in phase I, but also in later phases, and by a much larger population after it has reached the market. In contrast, an experimental drug, or "first in man," as it is called by volunteers, does not offer this safeguard.

Experimental drugs are believed to present a higher risk than nonexperimental drugs, but this assessment is relative and rests upon such factors as their chemical composition and established side effects. It is in this sense then that research subjects perceive an experimental drug that acts as a blood thinner or a bone strengthener as less risky than experimental psychiatric or HIV drugs—which are believed to be very toxic, based on the side effects listed in the informed consent forms. While some volunteers' views that experimental drugs present a higher risk than experimental drugs are also shared by scientists, the way volunteers understand and deal with the risks they face is heavily influenced by local knowledge about their bodies and biological processes.

Professional guinea pigs provide a series of "horror" stories depicting volunteers' experiences in trials. In such stories, psychiatric drugs stand at the top of their risk hierarchy, eliciting a very strong negative response. Drug trials involving psychological drugs that change the chemistry of the brain stand at the top of their risk hierarchy:

> Psychiatric trials are for a couple of reasons very different from trials of non-psychotropic drugs because they involve your mind. You are renting your mind and your body at the same time instead of just your body. It is a completely different economic deal. Secondly, in the psychotropic drug trials, people are writing diseases into existence. You cannot fake fast heartbeat into existence; you cannot make people believe that the heart is beating faster. I put a stethoscope into your chest and check your fucking heartbeat, that's simple. They cannot invent your blood pressure but they can invent your depression, they can invent your mood. And they can change the interpretation of what you say according to what the drug market wants. The marketing department writes the label of the

> drug, not the fucking doctors, the scientists. It is the marketing department. And they also write the disclaimers, fight the lawsuits. Blame the disease, not the drug. Like, he is getting into middle age, a lot of time on its hands and is getting a little raunchy goes into the psychiatrist for a little talk, gets put on Prozac and two weeks later he slaughters the whole family with a rifle and blows his own brain out. Tell me it is not the fucking Prozac! That is what I think, fuck you, fuck you. And it happens over and over again and the lawsuits get buried by companies that put a lot of money to quiet people down. (Grandpa Guinea Pig 2005)

This volunteer's strong opinion about clinical trials involving psychotropic drugs echoes professional guinea pigs concerns with these trials, and offers a powerful contrast to the usual, more neutral, way in which they talk about risks they face in clinical trials. Following a long-established Western tradition, the mind is perceived as separate from the body, a locus of reason and rationality, giving the mind a privileged position vis–à-vis other body organs.

Research subjects believe that risk can be known, and then, managed. While this perspective on risk is based on their particular trial experiences and understandings, it also helps volunteers to sustain their confidence and to keep volunteering. Local knowledge influences not only the way risk is constructed in this group, but also the ways in which they attempt to manage the risks they face.

Classification, and in particular the structuring of risk hierarchies, is a way in which volunteers deal with risk anxiety and attempt to manage risks. In addition, the strategies professional guinea pigs implement thus can be summarized as avoidance of trials they place at the top of their risk hierarchy, quitting the trial if risks were not foreseen but appear to be present during the trial, and cleansing practices intended to "wash out" harmful trial substances.

If a trial is perceived as being very high risk, volunteers might avoid the trial altogether, if possible. The prospect of obtaining the financial compensation along with their dependency upon trial income, however, might lead volunteers to participate in trials they wouldn't be inclined to join based on their perception of risk. The majority of experienced guinea pigs report having participated in at least one trial they labeled "too risky" because they were enticed by the promise of substantial financial gain. At the same time, experienced volunteers say that they have at least once turned down a trial because they felt it presented risks that were not acceptable.

A more extreme variation of this strategy of risk management is to abandon the trial. This is a very rare measure, and few professional guinea pigs use it as a last resort. However infrequent, sometimes the drug has secondary effects, which are harder to endure than the volunteers had anticipated. If the volunteer manages to show that these effects are the direct result of the trial, then he or she might be able to leave the trial, sometimes receiving payment for the full amount, sometimes a prorated portion of the trial completed. While there is no penalty involved in leaving the trial in such circumstances (except loss of payment), making the case is not easy, and failure to do so can be financially costly for participants. In addition, some volunteers fear that leaving a study before completion might compromise their chances to be accepted in future studies.

Finally, some professional guinea pigs believe that certain substances help them to "clean the blood" and to detoxify the body from the chemicals they absorbed during the trial. The assumption behind these practices is that the chemical substances are only contained in the blood and urine. If a few days after the drug intake is completed, drug remains cannot be found in blood and urine tests, then research subjects assume that there is none in their bodies. This assumption is shared by most professional guinea pigs, which in turn helps explain the fact that they do not continue to pay a lot of attention to their "cleansing" practices other than drinking water, a standard procedure suggested usually by the nurses or doctors conducting the trials.

Volunteers resort to other methods on special occasions, for example, after a very long and demanding trial, when they fear that the drug administered had a particular toxicity or if they are planning to do another trial soon after finishing one. Unsweetened cranberry juice is a standard "cleansing" staple among trial volunteers and is believed to help absorb, metabolize, and eliminate toxic trial substances. The practice of drinking water to "flush out" toxic remains or consuming cranberry juice is inspired by recommendations received at trial sites, usually in the form of a handout given by staff.

In addition, trial subjects resort to the use of herbs like goldenseal or marigold flowers as a way of "keeping the blood fresh and clean." Goldenseal, according to the zine *Guinea Pig Zero*, is "said to have a dramatic cleansing power, and is recommended by herbalists for removing the toxins related to alcohol, coffee, nicotine and other substances from blood."

A small group of volunteers in the anarchist community sometimes attempt to implement diets in which they only eat apples for some days, or yogurt, based on the belief that this will help "clean" their bodies. The use of herbs and organic methods of cleansing is preferred in the anarchist community. Although anarchist volunteers usually eat meat in the trials, mainly due to their lack of choice (researchers require them to follow a standard diet that proscribes vegetarian staples), they live in communities that practice vegetarianism and value organic diets and healing practices. Professional subjects who are not affiliated with an anarchist group commonly prefer a chemical approach, using blood supplements that contain iron, which helps rebuild the blood supply.

Despite their efforts to manage risk, the market recruitment of paid volunteers for phase I research places subjects at risks they are unable or unwilling to recognize. As a regular participant in trials put it: "you become addicted to the trials, to the easy money." The need to secure an income leads some volunteers to underestimate long-term risks.

Enticed by financial rewards, many volunteers remain in trials for many years, thereby potentially exposing themselves to synergistic drug interactions and long-term effects. The social organization of the clinical trials and the guinea pigs' lifestyle makes it difficult for them to become aware of these interactions and effects that might surface sometimes many years after a trial is completed. While volunteers maintain close interaction during the trials, which might last from a few days up to a few weeks, once the trial is over they usually do not remain in contact. Some leave for other cities looking for new trial opportunities. Even the more stable community of professional anarchist guinea pigs is highly mobile and in constant flux.

This fact contrasts with the stability of other categories of workers performing toxic or dangerous trades, such as coal miners, or those exposed to asbestos or other industrial pollutants. It was only over extended periods of sharing experiences that these workers developed an awareness of risk in contrast to that offered by the industry. Additionally, other categories of workers in dangerous trades commonly participate in organizations, such as unions, that can help to spot and act on risks. In the case of professional guinea pigs their mobility, lack of organization, and their relative anonymity conspire against this possibility. The fluidity and instability of the guinea-pig workplace resembles that of migrant agricultural workers who face similar problems associated with toxic substances.

The lack of a centralized register of human subjects volunteering for phase I trials might also obscure the existence of the problem for the pharmaceutical industry and regulatory agencies like the FDA. Aggravating the problem is the fact that while individual research sites keep lists of volunteers for recruiting purposes they do not record their history of clinical trial participation, making it impossible to know how many trials, how often, and to which substances volunteers were exposed.

In addition, conspiring against the recognition of the need to study long-term risk is the fact that the pharmaceutical industry has no incentive to invest in such research and that the FDA has not given consideration to the fact the there is a segment of the workforce that depends on serial involvement in pharmaceutical clinical trials and could be subject to synergistic effects.

The Effects of Body Commoditization in Phase I Trials on the Ethical Principles Regulating the Participation of Human Subjects in Research

Body commoditization in phase I trials subverts basic ethical principles and guidelines regulating the participation of human subjects in research. In particular, commoditization challenges the Belmont Report, which was formulated in the mid-1970s to protect human subjects and sets the foundation of the architecture of the informed-consent process and current ethics regulations protecting the participation of research volunteers.

In 1979 the Belmont Report summarized the basic ethical principles identified by the National Commission for the Protection of Human Subjects of Biomedical and Behavioral Research. The document begins with a brief introduction of ethical principles and guidelines for research involving human subjects, followed by a section setting the boundaries between practice and research. This section outlines the main ethical principles that have become established in human subject research: respect, beneficence, justice, and avoidance of malfeasance. The final section outlines the application of these principles in relation to informed consent, the assessment of risk and benefit, and the selection of subjects.

As we see from my study, the existence of market-recruited subjects in phase I clinical trials raises questions with regard to the principle of justice. According to the Belmont Report, an injustice in research occurs when "some benefit to which a person is entitled is denied without good reason or when some burden is imposed unduly" (1979:5). The case used to exemplify this principle in the report is the Tuskegee syphilis study in which poor rural black men were denied existing treatment in order not to interrupt the research project. It is a good example, since the withdrawal of existing therapy illustrates both the denial of a benefit to which patients are entitled and also the imposition of an undue burden on study participants. The document argues that the selection of research subjects needs to be scrutinized in order to determine whether some classes (e.g., welfare patients, particular racial and ethnic minorities, or persons confined to institutions) are being systematically selected simply because of their easy availability, their compromised position, or their manipulability, rather than for reasons directly related to the problem being studied (Belmont Report 1979:6). The section of the report that illustrates the application of the principle of justice to the selection of subjects provides further evidence of the articulation of the principle with the practice. According to the text, the principle of justice while applied to the selection of subjects needs to accommodate two levels: the social and the individual. Individual justice requires that researchers exhibit fairness in the selection of subjects. Social justice establishes the need to distinguish between "classes of subjects that ought, and ought not, to participate in any particular kind of research, based on the ability of members of that class to bear the burdens and on the appropriateness of placing further burdens on already burdened persons" (Belmont Report 1979:9). The document further notes that "some populations, especially institutionalized ones, are already burdened in many ways by their infirmities and environments. When research is proposed that involves risks and does not include a therapeutic component, other less burdened classes of persons should be called upon first to accept these risks of research" (Belmont Report 1979:9).

This is a revelatory statement concerning the philosophy behind the formulation of this document. The Belmont Report, imbued with a progressive ideology of human rights and the protection of vulnerable groups, seeks to protect vulnerable groups from possible abuses in research. Drawing from past abuses where institutionalized populations of orphaned children, the mentally ill, and prisoners had been exploited, the document intends to set standards to prevent this from happening again, particularly when there is no therapeutic gain involved. While the document makes no mention of phase I trials, it is possible that this situation was in the authors' minds, since a number of abuses had been reported in prisoner populations volunteering for such trials, and this population was regarded in the document as unable to give proper, "free" informed consent. The question remains, which would be a less-burdened class of persons who should be called upon first to accept these risks of research? There is no direct reference to the question of market-recruited populations. However, the authors caution against the effects of economic disadvantage on the unfair recruitment of vulnerable research subjects. As the document states, "one special instance of injustice results from the involvement of vulnerable subjects. Certain groups, such as racial minorities, the economically disadvantaged, the very sick, and the institutionalized may continually be sought as research subjects, owing to their ready availability in settings where research is conducted. Given their dependent status and their frequently compromised capacity for free consent, they should be protected against the danger of being involved in research solely for administrative convenience, or because they are easy to manipulate as a result of their illness or socioeconomic condition" (Belmont Report 1979:10).

It seems that current market recruitment for phase I trials research constitutes a challenge to the standards set by the Belmont Report. Many paid subjects for nontherapeutic trials are poor and constitute clearly the "economically disadvantaged" the report was concerned about. Not all volunteers are poor, however. While few if any are rich, this research has shown that for some volunteers being a professional guinea pig is an occupation. It is clear, however, that the transition from an institutionalized to a market-recruited population has produced a segment of that working class composed of professional subjects that depend upon continuous participation in clinical trials research, which in turn relies on their continuous participation to operate correctly. In this sense, the shift toward a paid research subject has produced a new group of "captive" volunteers, subjected to the risks and hazards of clinical trials science, capital investment, and socioeconomics. It is hard to anticipate the detrimental effects of this change on the new emergent population of professional guinea pigs. As mentioned, the social organization of phase I trials in America conspires against the recognition of possible synergistic interaction among drugs or of long-term consequences of being a regular clinical trial subject.

Continuous trial participation might expose volunteers to long-term effects and synergistic drug interactions, which can burden their lives. Recognition of this fact by the pharmaceutical industry, governmental regulatory agencies, and local IRBs would challenge the current organization of phase I clinical trials research and might explain why the problem has not yet been addressed.

Some Public Policy Recommendations

Risk is embedded in the structure of clinical trials involving human subjects. Producing knowledge about new potential drugs and drug regimes involves dealing with unknown or unforeseen outcomes. As in the past, it is the vulnerable, the desperate, or the poor who bear the burden in trials research at home and abroad. Market recruitment is perceived as a legitimate mechanism of risk allocation, where individuals freely consent to place their bodies at risk in exchange for financial rewards. However, the reliance on such recruitment mechanisms should not validate the current social organization of trials, especially the risk level subjects are exposed to today. While I believe trials research involving healthy volunteers is needed, I do not suggest that all risks can be eliminated. What we as a society can do is at least make clear the level of risk we are willing to accept. Placing individuals at risk for the benefit of the common good is a social decision. Thus, we can decide who will suffer the risk burden, establish conditions to minimize risk exposure, and maximize benefits for trial participants and the society as a whole. The following suggestions point to a more equitable distribution of risk in the management of trials in accordance with the Belmont Report's aim to protect vulnerable socioeconomic groups from the "undue burden" involved in research:

1. To restrict the number of trials, diminishing thereby drug exposure and potential adverse effects. Since this would change some aspects of the market-based organization of trials research, it could encounter stiff resistance from the pharmaceutical industry. However, from the point of view of larger social

interests, there is no harm involved in this measure. Most trials are conducted on "me too drugs," that is, versions of drugs that are already on the market. This increases the industry's profits, allowing them to extend patent protection and capture or expand market share, while exposing volunteers to risk with no scientific advancement.

2. To carry out scientific, impartial studies of possible drug interactions in the short term, but also over extended periods of time, attempting to prevent long-term toxicity and synergistic effects.

3. The need to keep detailed records documenting the participation of paid volunteers in trials research. Of particular relevance is information about the identity of volunteers, as well as how often, where, and in which trials they participate.

4. To recognize volunteers' participation as labor. We should recognize that paid subjects place their bodies at the service of scientific research and are not just contributing their "time and effort" (even if theirs is, as they themselves note, a "weird" type of work). Acceptance of this point should improve their contractual relationship, affording labor protections guaranteed to other workers in risky environments.

The current corporatization of the FDA tends more toward facilitating a good business climate than to public intervention and is not adequate to the implementation of any of these recommendations. In addition, these recommendations also challenge the industry's and governmental agencies' denial of commoditization in phase I trials research. Thus, implementing these recommendations might require a concerted effort on the part of civil society to reassess issues of commoditization, risk, and ethics in trials research.

Notes

1. To avoid legal complications and to protect informants, I have decided not to name names, therefore no direct reference to institutions or places is made and made-up pseudonyms are employed when referencing individuals.

2. This research was conducted with the generous assistance of grants from the Wenner-Gren Foundation for Anthropological Research and the Horowitz Foundation for Social Policy.

3. Lawrence K. Altman, "US to Investigate Death in an Asthma Study." *New York Times*, March 16, 2006.

References

Abraham, John
1994 Science, Politics and the Pharmaceutical Industry. London: UCL Press.

Angell, Marcia
2004 The Truth about the Drug Companies: How They Deceive Us and What to Do about It. New York: Random House.

Barber, Bernard
1973 Research on Human Subjects; Problems of Social Control in Medical Experimentation. New York: Russell Sage Foundation.
1980 Informed Consent in Medical Therapy and Research. New Brunswick, NJ: Rutgers University Press.

Baer, Hans
1992 The Politics of Public Health. Medical Anthropology 6(2):176–178.
2003 Biomedicine and Alternative Healing Systems in America: Issues of Class, Race, Ethnicity and Gender. Madison: University of Wisconsin Press.

Belmont Report
1979 Ethical Principles and Guidelines for the Protection of Human Subjects of Research. The National Commission for the Protection of Human Subjects of Biomedical and Behavioral Research. April 18.

Corrigan, Oonagh P.
2002 A Risky Business: The Detection of Adverse Drug Reaction in Clinical Trials and Post Marketing Exercises. Social Science and Medicine 55(3):497–507.

Das, Veena
1999 Public Good, Ethics, and Everyday Life. Beyond the Boundaries of Bioethics. Bioethics and Beyond. Daedalus 128(Fall):99–134.

Douglas, Mary, and Aaron Wildavsky
1981 Risk and Culture. Berkeley: University of California Press.

Farmer, Paul
1992 AIDS and Accusation: Haiti and the Geography of Blame. Berkeley: University of California Press.

2001 Infections and Inequalities. The Modern Plagues. Berkeley: University of California Press.
2002 Pathologies of Power: Health, Human Rights, and the New War on the Poor. Berkeley: University of California Press.

Fisher, Michael
1998 Emergent Forms of Life: Anthropologies of Late or Post-Modernities. Annual Review of Anthropology 28:455–478.

Fox, Renee
1974 Experiment Perilous. Physicians and Patients Facing the Unknown. Philadelphia: University of Pennsylvania Press.
1961 Physicians on the Drug Industry Side of the Prescription Blank: Their Dual Commitment to Medical Science and Business. Journal of Business and Human Behaviour 3(2):3–16.
1990 The Evolution of American Bioethics: A Sociological Perspective. *In* Social Science Perspectives on Medical Ethics. George Weisz, ed. Pp. 201–220. Philadelphia: University of Pennsylvania Press.

Gray, Bradford H.
1975 Human Subjects in Medical Experimentation. New York: Wiley.

Harrington, Anne
1997 The Placebo Effect: An Interdisciplinary Exploration. Cambridge, MA: Harvard University Press.

Helms, Bob
1996–2000 Guinea Pig Zero: A Journal for Human Research Subjects. Philadelphia: Bob Helms Publisher.

Higby, George J., and Elaine C. Stroud, eds.
1990 Pill Peddlers: Essays on the History of the Pharmaceutical Industry. Madison: American Institute for the History of Pharmacy.

Hogshire, Jim
1992 Sell Yourself to Science. Port Townsend, WA: Loompanics.

Hornblum, Allen M.
1998 Acres of Skin: Human Experimentation at Holmesburg Prison. New York: Routledge.

Jones, James H.
1981 Bad Blood. The Tuskegee Syphilis Experiment. New York: Free Press.

Katz, Jay
1972 Experimentation with Human Beings. New York: Russell Sage Foundation.
1984 The Silent World of Doctor and Patient. New York: Free Press.

Lederer, Susan
1992 Orphans as Guinea Pigs: American Children and Medical Experimenters, 1890–1930. *In* In the Name of the Child: Health

and Welfare, 1880–1940. Roger Cooter, ed. New York: Routledge.
1995 Subjected to Science: Human Experimentation in America before the Second World War. Baltimore, MD: Johns Hopkins University Press.

Liebenau, Jonathan
1986 Medical Science and Medical Industry: The Formation of the American Pharmaceutical Industry. Baltimore, MD: Johns Hopkins University Press.

Lindenbaum, Shirley, and Margaret Lock, eds.
1996 Knowledge, Power and Practice: The Anthropology of Medicine and Everyday Life. Berkeley: University of California Press.

Lock, Margaret, Allan Young, and Alberto Cambrosio, eds.
1999 Living and Working with the New Medical Technologies. Cambridge, UK: Cambridge University Press.

Mahoney, Tom
1959 The Merchants of Life: An Account of the American Pharmaceutical Industry. New York: Harper.

Marks, Harry
1997 The Progress of Experiment: Science and Therapeutic Reform in the United States, 1900–90. Cambridge, UK: Cambridge University Press.

Marshall, Patricia
1992 Anthropology and Bioethics. Medical Anthropology Quarterly 6(1):49–73.

Marshall, Patricia, and Barbara Koening
2004 Accounting for Culture in a Globalized Ethics. Journal of Law, Medicine, and Ethics 32(2):252–266.

McNeil, Paul M.
1992 The Ethics and Politics of Human Experimentation. Hong Kong: Cambridge University Press.

Meyer, Peter B.
1974 Drug Experiments on Prisoners. Lexington, MA: Lexington Books.

Moerman, Daniel
2000 Cultural Variations in the Placebo Effect: Ulcers, Anxiety and Blood Pressure. Medical Anthropology Quarterly 14(1):51–72.

Moore, Lisa
1999 On the Construction of Male Differences: Marketing Variations in Technosemen. Men & Masculinities 1(4): 339–359.

Moreno, Jonathan
2000 Undue Risk: Secret State Experiments on Humans. New York: W. H. Freeman.
Nelkin, Dorothy, and Lori Andrews
2001 Body Bazaar: The Market for Human Tissue in the Bioetechnology Age. New York: Crown.
Pappworth, Maurice H.
1967 Human Guinea Pigs: Experimentation on Man. Boston: Beacon Press.
Parascandola, John
1985 Industrial Research Comes of Age. Pharmacy in History 27 (Fall):12–21.
1998 The Development of American Pharmacology: John Abel and the Shaping of a Discipline. Baltimore, MD: Johns Hopkins University Press.
Petryna, Adriana
2006 Globalizing Human Subjects Research. *In* Global Pharmaceuticals: Ethics, Markets, Practices. Adriana Petryna, Andrew Lakoff, and Arthur Kleinman, eds. Durham, NC: Duke University Press.
Rajan, Kaushink S.
2004 Subjects of Speculation: Emergent life Sciences and Market Logics in the United States and India. American Anthropologist 107(1):19–30.
Reynolds Whyte, Sjaak Van der Geest, and Anita Hardon
2000 Social Lives of Medicines. Cambridge: Cambridge University Press.
Rosner, David, and Gerald Markowitz
1988 Deadly Dust: Silicosis and the Politics of Occupational Disease in Twentieth-Century America. Princeton, NJ: Princeton University Press.
2000 Deceit and Denial: The Deadly Politics of Industrial Production. Berkeley: University of California Press.
Scheper-Hughes, Nancy
2000 The Global Traffic in Organs. Current Anthropology 41(2):191–224.
Scheper-Hughes, Nancy, and Loïc Wacquant, eds.
2003 Commodifying Bodies. London: Sage.
Sharp, Leslie
2000 The Commodification of the Body and Its Parts. Annual Review of Anthropology 29:287–328.

2006 Strange Harvest: Organ Transplants, Denatured Bodies, and the Transformation of the Self. Berkeley: University of California Press.

Silverman, Milton, and Philip R. Lee
1974 Pills, Profits and Politics. Berkeley: University of California Press.

Susser, Ida
1982 Norman Street: Poverty and Politics in an Urban Neighborhood. New York: Oxford University Press.
1996 The Construction of Poverty and Homelessness in US Cities. Annual Review of Anthropology 25:411–435.

Temin, Peter
1980 Taking Your Medicine: Drug Regulation in the United States. Cambridge, MA: Harvard University Press.

Van der Geest, Sjaak, Susan Reynolds Whyte, and Anita Hardon
1996 The Anthropology of Pharmaceuticals: A Biographical Approach. Annual Review of Anthropology 25:153–178.

Vuckovic, Nancy, and Mark Nichter
1997 Changing Patterns of Pharmaceutical Practice in the United States. Social Science Medicine 44:1285–1302.

Weinstein, Matthew
2001 A Public Culture for Guinea Pigs: U.S. Human Research Subjects after the Tuskegee Study. Science as Culture 10:195–223.

CHAPTER TWELVE

CORROSION IN THE SYSTEM

The Community Health By-Products of Pharmaceutical Production in Northern Puerto Rico

Alexa S. Dietrich

> Now we also hold ourselves accountable for how we produce those medicines.
>
> Focusing on the economic, social, and environmental impacts of our businesses and operations.
>
> We must operate our business in a manner that protects human health, the environment, our employees and the communities in which we operate.
>
> —Representative quotes from pharmaceutical companies' literature

As the sun was disappearing and the crowd began to gather for the first night of the annual patron saint festival of Nocorá[1] *I was as excited as everyone else. But while the locals clustered in groups around the wooden racing horse machines, bought* bacalaitos *(codfish fritters) and beer, and waited for the live music to start, I had finally arranged an introduction to "the biggest environmentalist in Nocorá." Don Lirio listened attentively while I described my interests and then hastened to invite me to the next meeting of the* Comité para Defender el Ambiente Nocoreño (*Committee to Defend the Environment of Nocorá,* CDAN), *digging in his pockets for a piece of paper on which to draw a map to their headquarters. "We can tell you much about the pharmaceuticals," he assured me, meaning the drug companies, "and also about the particular environmental problems of our barrio, about* la planta. *We have struggled for more than 20 years." He paused. "If you have a camera, you should bring it," he said. "We'll show you many things . . . and then you can make up your own mind what you think."*

I returned with my friend Benicia to our folding chairs, and I noticed she was grinning. "It will be good for you to talk to Lirio and his group," she said. "I don't agree with his politics at all, he's independentista,[2] *you know, but he is very, very dedicated. You'll learn a lot."*

She suddenly grabbed my arm and instead of sitting down, she pulled me in another direction, waving at another man I did not know. "I want to say hello to Francisco, too, and I'll introduce you. We're colleagues, but he used to work in Environmental Health. If anyone knows about la contaminación, *he does."*

Francisco also nodded with vague interest in my project, and when I said, "I want to learn about the impact of the pharmaceuticals on the lives of Nocoreños," he slowly drew his fingers across his neck, saying nothing, and making a tight grimace. I glanced over to Benicia, and she unhelpfully widened her eyes, but made no attempt to break up our conversation. I leaned closer to Francisco. "Do you mean that these are questions I shouldn't be asking?" I asked in a low voice, hoping I didn't sound nervous.

*He grinned and shook his head. "It's that I can tell you in one sentence how they impact our lives." He paused, and leaned toward me until our faces were quite close. "*El impacto es . . . nos matan.*" The impact is . . . they're killing us. His tone was calm, quite simply matter-of-fact. "Oh, not today, not tomorrow, but little by little . . . it will kill us all."*

According to the Pharmaceutical Industry Association of Puerto Rico (PIAPR), the pharmaceutical industry "represents over 26% of the work force generated in the manufacturing sector" on the island (approximately 30,000 jobs), generating an additional 96,000 jobs in related or supporting industries. It is the source of 25 percent of the island's $72.4 billion GDP and accounted for 64 percent of all island exports in 2004 (Pharmaceutical Industry Association of Puerto Rico 2005). While average wages in the drug sector are among the highest on the island, and the jobs at all levels of skill very much in demand, wages remain lower than the average for the same pharmaceutical jobs on the mainland. There can be no question of the importance of the industry in the overall Puerto Rican economy; in north coast Nocorá, however, even with the highest drug factory to resident ratio in the world, the 2000 Census still reports that the unemployment rate is 24 percent, compared to the rest of the island at 19 percent. Instead of providing local jobs, the pharmaceuticals pay local taxes, which in turn fund half the municipal budget of Nocorá, the highest per capita on the island. Unfortunately, the drug industry has also supplied the air and water of Nocorá with a level of pollution that remains notorious throughout the island.

Medical anthropologists (see particularly Whyte et al. 2002; van der Geest and Whyte 1991), as well as practitioners of critical medical anthropology (CMA) (see Nichter 1996; Petryna et al. 2006; see also Oldani and Singer and Baer this volume; Singer 2007) have undertaken a number of excellent analyses of the nature and impact of legal drug products, their roles in the market and in social life, and intellectual property issues (to name a few areas). However, there has thus far been little work bridging the critical medical anthropology of pharmaceutical products with the political ecology of health. This chapter is primarily concerned with a community-health case study of Nocorá, thereby adding further perspective to the key CMA questions raised by the killer commodity framework with respect to drug *production*: namely, What is the extent of damage caused by (the creation of) these products? How is the damage caused, and how can further damage be avoided through new public health and/or environmental policies?

In this example, by-products, rather than traditionally defined commodities, are the focus: that which is produced as a side effect of the making of those "useful" things that "can be turned to commercial or other advantage" (Webster's Dictionary online 2006). In the process of pharmaceutical production there are various by-products, many of which are washed away in wastewater following the process of chemical synthesis, or in the flushing of solvents used to clean manufacturing equipment during routine maintenance. Between 1988 and 2004 (the period for which public data are available) the local pharmaceutical manufacturing facilities released into the Nocorá Regional Wastewater Treatment Plant (NWTP) over 47 million pounds of toxic chemicals (as reported to the Federal Toxic Releases Inventory [TRI]). Ammonia, chloroform, dichloromethane, methanol, nitrate compounds, formaldehyde, and toluene are a few of the monitored chemicals that contributed to the treatment plant's influent stream. Since 1983, and into the present, residents of Barrio Tipan, in which the NWTP is located, have struggled against the resulting pollution in their environment and its health and quality-of-life consequences.

As Singer noted in his 1998 rapprochement with a proposed "new biocultural synthesis" in anthropology, conventional medical anthropology, in making the much-touted distinction between "illness" and "disease" (i.e., between reported health problems and clinically diagnosed health problems), has detrimentally contributed to the idea that health problems recognized by authorized clinical (or in this case public health) sources are "culture-free [and] politically neutral" (p. 107). This distinction is replicated time and again in epidemiological encounters with environmentally damaged communities, in which the standard tools of public health often fail to quantify the social, psychological, and indeed physical suffering of residents of polluted areas (see e.g., Brown 1992). In some cases these failures are the consequence of the limits of methodological approaches for measuring environmental exposures, especially past exposures: in the most well-known example, cancer clusters, the U.S. Centers for Disease Control and Prevention states clearly that even after a cluster is confirmed, "follow-up investigations can be done, but can take years to complete and the results are generally inconclusive (e.g., usually, no cause is found)" (National Center for Environmental Health 2005). In cases like that of Barrio Tipan in Nocorá, however, the power structure of the local community, and the influence of corporations within local government, may play a more direct role in whether or not a community's health complaints receive a fair evaluation from the public health establishment.

By examining the interplay of community-based activists with the pharmaceutical industry and local government, this chapter shows how the community health interests of Tipan have been pushed aside in favor of a broader narrative of economic progress both for the municipality of Nocorá and for its patron industry. In the category of "community health interests" I include negative physical health outcomes likely related to the pollution (based on community-gathered data, as well as data from my fieldwork). But what is most obviously being killed is their overall quality of life and psychological (and communal) sense of well-being as much as their physical persons in some easily measurable, epidemiologic sense.

I also suggest that given the level of political-economic, as well as social, power wielded by the pharmaceutical corporations in Nocorá, they have no need to ally themselves with government and against people. They could quite easily use their influence to materially improve the lives of their residential "neighbors," and yet choose actively not to do so. Their unwillingness to truly think outside the traditional patron-client model of corporate-community relationships proves them not to be transformative corporate citizens, as their public relations materials would like to broadcast (and as exemplified by the quotes on this chapter's first page), but rather a business-as-usual public health nuisance.

The project on which this chapter is based involved a total of 18 months of fieldwork in Puerto Rico (16 consecutive), framed around the basic questions, *Are the four multinational pharmaceutical companies with facilities in Nocorá an integrated part of the local community, as they claim to be? If so, how do they participate in that community, and how are they viewed by local residents?* And finally, *Can we truly speak of corporations as local citizens, as is becoming common parlance in their public relations?* While the theoretical and applied legal question of how corporations came to be considered *persons* under U.S. law is beyond the scope of this chapter (see, e.g., Hartmann 2002), corporate personhood and citizenship are important considerations for thinking about how corporate entities behave in the social sphere, and how they treat other entities within that sphere. In this chapter it is important to pay attention to the points at which the pharmaceutical companies claim membership in the Nocorá community, when they wish to be exempted from responsibilities, and when and how their acts of self-interest are justified.

The sampling strategy for the study was generally purposive, with the goal of gaining a broadly representative sample of the Nocorá community within three general sectors: 1) residents and their interest groups; 2) government workers and elected leaders; and 3) for-profit and not-for-profit corporate entities. I did several door-to-door samples in Barrio Tipan to access residents who were not actively involved in grassroots activities, as well as spent time with activist residents. I also sampled the rest of the municipality in locations where people used services that were sponsored by the companies, and may therefore have had positive associations with them (such as the library and cultural center—these were convenience samples, supplemented by general participant observation activities). This group included residents of some areas that have been exposed in the past 35 years to as much air pollution (in TRI-reported poundage) as the NWTP has received water pollutants, but where there has never been significant grassroots environmental activism. I surveyed a majority of health-care workers from the local health center, as well as a large portion of the elementary school teachers and principals in the Nocorá school district, in which the companies generally claim to practice much of their corporate citizenship/philanthropy. I also interviewed and observed the activities of corporate and nonprofit representatives who worked in the field of community relations and the environment, and in corporate social responsibility.

In addition to in-depth interviews and surveys (which yielded many qualitative comments and observations in the course of being administered), I conducted substantial participant observation in a wide variety of community-based activities, government and organization meetings, and of course in the everyday social contexts that are the bread and butter of traditional anthropological fieldwork. I argue that a deeper-than-surface investigation of the community of Nocorá gives ample cause for concern about past and current attitudes and trends in corporate-community power relations (see also Nash and Kirsch 1988), as well as future developments in the growing field of "corporate social responsibility" (CSR). As I have discussed elsewhere, the pharmaceuticals have shown themselves quite adept at mastering the emerging rhetoric of CSR (Dietrich 2006), but both words and actions must be examined, and in conjunction with one another, in order to assess whether a corporation truly acts in socially responsible ways.

This chapter gives a brief history of how the pharmaceutical factories arrived in Nocorá, and will contextualize the inception of the Nocorá Regional Wastewater Treatment Plant and its relationship to its industrial sponsors. Then, further describing the problems arising from its poor operations and its highly toxic influent, the chapter will draw on both ethnographic and community-gathered data to argue that 1) residents of Barrio Tipan (in which the NWTP is located) indeed have suffered as a consequence of the toxic wastes processed in their vicinity; 2) that the pharmaceutical companies that produced these wastes and the governmental bodies responsible for protecting local residents actively allowed this suffering to continue for decades; and 3) that had the pharmaceutical companies acted in the "good citizen/neighbor" spirit which they publicly espouse, the problems in Barrio Tipan would have long ago been resolved.

At the beginning of my study of Nocorá, I discovered that there had been two previous studies of the town, both of which took place when the local industry was still the production of sugarcane. The initial project, part of the classic People of Puerto Rico study (Steward et al. 1956), focused on the cultural influences of the local mode of production—a government-owned sugar plantation. Padilla Seda's 1948 observations concluded that though the public corporation had indeed the "social objective of distributing work and dividing profits" (Padilla Seda 1956:265), the end result was rather, in the words of a prominent official of the Land Authority, that it did "not distribute wealth, but poverty" (p. 312). Padilla Seda notes that there remained many cultural holdovers from the days of the haciendas, particularly the political and economic attitudes of dependence, and a personal quality to relationships of power more typical of patron-client relationships than political participation in electoral politics or union activities. Shadows of these relationships, and of their overall community impact, linger on in local residents' relations with their new patrons, the pharmaceutical companies and the alcalde, or mayor, of Nocorá, whose municipal government is in active partnership with the corporations.

Barrio Tipan, coincidentally the subsite of both previous studies of Nocorá (see also Seda Bonilla 1964), had its beginnings as an informal settlement of sugarcane workers near the beach. It was formalized in the 1950s by the allotment of land parcels and government-subsidized building projects in which neighbors provided the labor to build one another's houses. To the east of the original Tipan settlement, on the other side of an area of mangroves and closer to the water lies Tipanito, a more recent settlement of "urbanized" *parcelas*, meaning chiefly that the neighborhoods are planned, with paved streets and set housing lots. Tipan, Tipanito, and the Tipanito extension, to the south, comprise, as of the 2000 Census, 359 housing units. Tipan (in general referring to the whole area) is now the site of the only grassroots environmental movement in Nocorá, in part, perhaps, because unlike other equally polluted areas closer to the factories, Tipan is generally ignored in the planning of "community activities" sponsored by the pharmaceutical companies.

The closing of the Nocorá sugar operations created a serious economic vacuum for those laborers of Nocorá who did not choose labor migration to the United States. As in other parts of the island, including neighboring municipalities, the leaders of Nocorá sought to attract industries of higher technologies so that their residents could find better-paying work. Initially these industries included canning and food processing, to complement the Land Authority's new local agricultural endeavor, pineapple cultivation. While petrochemical companies were drawn to the southern coast, the large quantities of high-quality groundwater located in aquifers along the northern coast served to lure a number of chemical companies to Nocorá. The available water was in need of little treatment prior to industrial use, and the companies were permitted by the commonwealth to drill their own wells, and extract tens of millions of gallons, daily, cost free.

Once established, the drug companies (the names of which, at least in their present incarnations, would be immediately recognizable to most readers) had to plan for the disposal of their copious liquid waste. Typical of waste-management practices at the time, one popular solution was for industries to reinject liquid wastes into wells drilled especially for that purpose, or into water wells that had been sucked dry by the industry.

Injection of waste was one solution; discharging it into the Bajas River was another; disposing of it in sinkholes which are natural to the region (García 1982), or depositing it in local landfills (Agencia EFE 1998) were still others. Many informants in the community, particularly the fishermen, vividly describe not only the change in coastal water quality during this era, but also the marked drop in aquatic life. It became apparent in the mid-1970s that another solution was necessary, in part because the contamination from the practices described had unexpectedly breached the very aquifer so necessary to the industries. In addition, the need for waste disposal was expected to rise significantly, as the municipal government in conjunction with Fomento (the Commonwealth Development Agency), was planning to build even more chemical factories in the same area (García 1977; Goitía n.d.).

There was at this time a local wastewater treatment facility for the municipality, only capable of handling domestic wastewater and rain runoff. There is some evidence that new factories being built were nevertheless being given permission to hook up waste pipes to the original plant (García 1975). In a compromise that recognized the inadequacies of a new primary treatment plant to process industrial waste, the industries of Bajas and Nocorá agreed to sponsor the construction of a secondary treatment facility (Goitía n.d.). The new plant was financed substantially by a cooperative group of the local pharmaceuticals, which formed a nonprofit corporation (the Nocorá Consortium) to administer the funding for the building and continued maintenance of the treatment plant. At a capacity of 8.3 MGD (million gallons daily), approximately 70 percent of the NWTP influent comes from the industries located further inland.

A Solution and Its Problems

The planning for the new treatment plant did not go unnoticed by environmental activists (López Acevedo 1976; Partido Socialista Puertorriqueño 1977). However, as with many environmental mobilizations in Puerto Rico, many people interpreted the concern as "*cosa de independentistas*"—more agitations by those who favored independence for the island. One longtime socialist activist lamented to me: "They never listen, just because we're socialists. But this wasn't about socialism." His sentiment was echoed in barrio Solita of the Cacique municipality, where a primarily domestic treatment plant is located, and where residents are now active in community planning and social justice movements. "Activists came through here when PRASA was going to build our plant with flyers, knocking on doors—and everyone said, 'Oh, they're just agitating.' But now we're sorry we didn't listen."

Ricardo Solano, a chemist who was one of the founding members of the activist group CDAN, remembers the establishment of the NWTP a little differently than the official version, in which a secondary treatment protocol was deemed sufficient. "The government promised us a tertiary-level treatment plant," he told me with quiet vehemence. "We had community presentations, we asked questions. They promised us a sophisticated plant, capable of treating whatever the industries sent down the pipeline. And they never delivered it."

The plant was planned in two stages, and the primary treatment facility became operational in August 1977, receiving permission from the EPA to accept domestic waste, industrial waste from the food processing factories, and some "weak wastes" from one of the pharmaceutical factories. Following treatment, the wastewater from the plant passed through a pipe to an ocean outfall pipe 815 meters (about 1/2 a mile) offshore (Goitía n.d.). The building of the outfall pipe was the source of one of the earliest controversies involving the plant.

"It was supposed to be a mile and a half," Reynaldo San Pareil, former president of CDAN, told me. "The fishermen will tell you. They know that pipe isn't what they said it would be. It's from them that we've learned about many of the effects of the plant, things they see because they're on the water." The fishermen of Nocorá were particularly adamant about two things: 1) the building of the outfall pipe had not gone as planned, and therefore they were extremely skeptical as to where the treated waters from the plant were ending up, and 2) since the establishment of the pharmaceuticals and their so-called waste treatment solution, the fish and other local sea life had gone from a one-time overabundance to nearly zero.

About the building of the pipe I heard the same story many times, the core of which was as follows: In the preliminary plans (which Ricardo Solano and others describe as those which were proposed to the community in initial public presentations and which convinced the community that they would suffer no harm as a consequence of the plant) the outfall pipe was designed to extend approximately 1.5 miles out to sea to ensure an adequate "mixing zone" for the treated waste. The mixing zone for wastewater has the theoretical benefit of further diluting the waste with high concentrations of water (in this case the Atlantic Ocean) so as to reduce the waste-to-water ratio to near negligible levels. However, during the construction of the pipe, the ocean was so fierce that one construction boat was lost, and the completion of the original design distance was deemed impossible. The project was amended, presumably with the approval of the commonwealth's Environmental Quality Board (EQB), and the final distance is now cited at half a mile (Goitía n.d.). For some this was simply evidence that the Puerto Rico Aqueduct and Sewer Authority (PRASA), with the rubber stamp of the EQB, always amended its projects for its own convenience regardless of environmental or structural consequences. This became a recurring theme in my discussions with the Tipan community.

For others it appeared more sinister. One man who had gotten work driving some of the consulting engineers on the project around town professed deep doubts about the true nature of the mixing zone. "They claimed the pipe was done. Then they put something, a red dye of some kind, into the system, to see where it came out. When it didn't arrive, they said that meant it was mixing really well, that it was good. Me, I think they have no idea where the pipe ends."

The secondary treatment phase of the plant was inaugurated in 1981, and within two years there was already evidence of severe problems—and evidence of the difficulty of getting those problems recognized. In a memo to the EPA Caribbean field office in June 1983, an EPA engineer reported his communications with the earliest incarnation of the group CDAN, and his subsequent inspection of the NWTP (Campos Bistani 1983). The primary complaint emerging from the community was a phrase that would become ubiquitous in Nocorá for the next 20-plus years, and that would recur repeatedly in my fieldwork: bad odors (*malos olores*).

It should be noted that this simple phrase has a way of sounding at times silly, at times quaint. A bad odor, in common parlance, is something that causes social discomfort more than physical. A bad odor is, in the words of the EPA memo, a "nuisance." It is presumed to be not a big deal, certainly not something for an entire community to coalesce around. It does not sound, to a layperson, like the reasonable basis for a lawsuit, or for a public health study.

As noted in general in the wastewater treatment literature, however, the monitoring of both odors and corrosion is a constant and serious concern for treatment systems, and the two are in fact often correlated (Witherspoon et al. 2004). For the town of Nocorá the subject of *malos olores* (also called *olores objetables*, or objectionable odors) is likewise a very serious one, whether the odors come from the NWTP or directly from the factories. Due to the technical challenges involved in measuring environmental exposures and linking them directly to disease, I will not argue that the disposal of pharmaceutical waste is killing the neighbors of Tipan in a strict epidemiological sense. Rather, the point I wish to demonstrate is that 20 years of pollution and inaction on the part of the polluters have robbed Tipanecos of "*what matters most: life and the potential it holds when we are feeling our best*," to borrow a phrase from the public relations materials of a local pharmaceutical company (emphasis added).

In the case of many industrial pollution examples, it is typical for past (and sometimes current) polluters to claim previous ignorance of the potential for harm of their products or by-products, and to earnestly display present-day environmental accomplishments. One environmental expert I interviewed even made this argument on behalf of the Nocorá pharmaceuticals, assuring me that "abuse in general [in industry] was out of ignorance." However, the "we didn't know" claim in the case of the Nocorá Consortium and the NWTP does not, as one might say, hold water, given PRASA's well-known, abysmally poor maintenance track record (see

Estado Libre Asociado de Puerto Rico 2004), corroborated by the earliest reports from regulatory inspectors of the Nocorá treatment plant.

The 12-page report to the EPA field office (Campos Bistani 1983) is an impressive compendium of operational problems at the NWTP in Tipan, including inoperable machinery due to disrepair and/or severe corrosion, uncalibrated and/or nonfunctioning monitoring instruments, and significant inconsistencies in monitoring records. The inspector noted, "there is no way the plant can be run effectively if the instrumentation deficiencies are not corrected."

One of the two primary settling tanks was completely out of operation and looked "corroded in most of its metal parts and is [sic] in very poor condition." He further observed that one of the two aerated grit chambers for the initial removal of sand and other solids appeared "not to have been in operation for weeks" (Campos Bistani 1983).

The inspector also found what he considered to be evidence of several violations of the National Pollutant Discharge Elimination System (NPDES) permit, including the effluent limitation, monitoring requirements, and special discharge conditions. According to the permit, only the seven original pharmaceutical partners were identified by PRASA as "major contributing industries authorized to discharge" at the plant. However, PRASA had failed to identify to the enforcement agencies nine other industrial users of the NWTP. He noted that the color of the effluent passing through to the ocean outfall was sufficiently black to alter the color of the receiving water, in spite of the mixing zone. He also noted it had a "very offensive smell."

A significant finding of this 1983 inspection was that it appeared that the design of the plant and the way in which it was used had diverged substantially, and there was little or no consideration by those who had planned the plant of what would be the result of an increasing industrial usage, apart from an increased quantity of liquid. According to the inspection, the plant was receiving far below its raw capacity volume of influent, and yet failing utterly to treat the wastes contained within that influent. For the residents of Barrio Tipan the consequences of these outrageous operating conditions were frequent clouds of noxious fumes emanating from a number of locations at the plant, which floated into their homes causing respiratory problems, nausea, severe eye irritation, and often severe lack of sleep.

Within several months of this inspection the community had experienced no substantial relief from their situation, causing the *Comité para Defender el Ambiente Nocoreño* to once again contact the EPA, this time at the regional level in New York. In October 1983 CDAN received a highly unsatisfactory response from that office. Admittedly, accession to CDAN's request that the facility be closed until the problems could be resolved was an unlikely outcome, and the EPA was justified in pointing out that without the plant the industries in the area would have nowhere to dispose of waste and would have to stop production (Schafer 1983). In what was to become a familiar refrain from EPA officials, the EPA administrator suggested that such changes would cause layoffs of local employees, an outcome she presumed no one wanted.

As representative of CDAN, Ricardo Solano had received both this October letter and the field inspection memo of a few months earlier. A comparison of both documents is instructive to understanding the pattern of contradiction which would characterize the community-government-industry interactions for the next 20 years. Both documents address the question of possible violations of the NPDES permit. As mentioned previously, the field inspection memo (Campos Bistani 1983) described several suspected violations, relating, among other areas, to the quality of the effluent discharge. In contrast, the regional administrator's letter states:

> The Environmental Protection Agency (EPA) has been closely monitoring the [Nocorá] facility with respect to compliance with its National Pollutant Discharge Elimination System (NPDES) permit. According to monthly sampling reports that are submitted to the EPA, the facility is consistently in compliance with its effluent limitations. Furthermore, a sampling survey conducted by EPA in April, 1983 also indicated compliance with effluent limitations for a wide range of parameters. (Schafer 1983)

Given the discrepancy between the lack of operational functioning found by the inspector in June 1983, and the confidence expressed by the regional office with regard to self-reported compliance only a few months later, it is not surprising that the residents of Barrio Tipan were soon trying to gather their own evidence.

Sitting at Don Reynaldo's kitchen table, I am flipping through photographs and come across one I recognize. "Look, it's Don Gabriel," I say, holding up the picture. "He's so young." This is a relative statement, since the Don Gabriel I know, a fisherman and active member of CDAN, has a head of pure white hair. The one staring out of the photograph, holding up a manhole cover so the camera can see the inside of the sewer, is far less wrinkled and has hair of iron gray. I flip through and see groups of men standing over a sewer pipe, pictures taken in Tipan and in downtown Nocorá. An election poster marks the year as 1984.

"That was before my time," Don Reynaldo says, looking carefully. "But the one of Gabriel I think is meant to show the damage in the pipe. When the sewers are built they have metal ladders into them, you know, at the manholes. When the residents opened them up, they found the ladders had been eaten away, corroded completely."

The next time I see him I ask Don Gabriel about the manholes, and he laughs. "Didn't you hear about the manholes? Sometimes, whatever they were putting in the pipe, it would mix all up, and smell terrible. The air coming out of the manholes would make you choke. But even worse, sometimes the manhole covers would explode! Pow, clear into the air!"

The September 2003 report, "EPA's National Pretreatment Program, 1973–2003: Thirty Years of Protecting the Environment," gives credence to these fantastical-sounding reports of explosions and other disaster-quality events from the Tipan activists, citing the following areas as arguments in favor of a rigorous pretreatment program:

- *Protecting the physical integrity of the sewer system.* Volatile organic compounds discharged to sewers may accumulate in the head space of sewer lines, increasing the potential for explosions that may cause significant damage. Discharge limitations and management practices required by the pretreatment program reduce the likelihood of such catastrophes.

- *Preventing the buildup of poisonous gases.* Discharges of toxic organics can generate poisonous gases, through various kinds of mixing and chemical reactions. Appropriate pretreatment discharge limits prevent this gas build up. (US-EPA Office of Water 2003)

This same report lauds the achievements of the EPA's pretreatment program for industrial discharges into publicly owned treatment works (POTWs, such as the Tipan treatment plant), noting as an example a major dropoff in the transfer of toxic organic chemicals to POTWs nationwide beginning in 1988. These nationwide numbers overall fell rapidly between 1988 and 1990, reaching a low-level plateau in 1994.

However, it was not until 1990 that the EPA first published an "Effluent Guidelines Plan (55 FR 80), in which schedules were established for developing new and revised effluent guidelines for several industry categories," including the pharmaceuticals (Federal Register 1998). Charging that this plan did not sufficiently meet the requirements of the Clean Water Act, a lawsuit was quickly filed by public interest groups, and in 1992 a consent decree required that the EPA begin developing a special rule for the pharmaceutical industry. This process, which began in 1992, required that a rule be proposed by 1995, to go into effect in 1998, and to require full compliance by 2001.[3]

Examining the Toxic Registry Inventory (TRI) summaries for the year 2003, and comparing them to the years 1988 to 2002, the effect of the pretreatment rule on the release of toxins, particularly toxic organics, is impressive. As mentioned earlier, between 1988 and 2002, those pharmaceutical industries permitted to send wastewater into the Nocorá WTP released over 47 million pounds of TRI-monitored chemicals. The most recent data indicate that they are now mainly releasing the less toxic pollutants for which reporting is required, and in much lesser quantities. From the time the plant opened (1981) through 1987 there are no public data.

When asked about the pretreatment rule, one pharmaceutical environmental manager extolled the virtues, quite rightly, of their on-site pretreatment system, which according to an environmental engineer who oversaw the project, is absolutely state-of-the-art. Praise of their technological achievements aside, however, the manager did express some personal-corporate resentment of the pretreatment regulations:

> Each company paid a percentage to build the [regional] plant, and still pays, by percentage, for its maintenance. This percentage gives each company rights to put a certain amount of BOD into the system. But now with the pretreatment required, we're putting almost zero BOD

> into the system. So pretreatment regulations have really taken away property rights that we bought and paid for. . . . That's another way of looking at it.

While this argument might hold sway in an unregulated market system, the manager seemed unaware of a basic legal principle: property rights of corporations, as legally created entities, are only those which are granted by law. However, as entities with no natural lifespan, it is perhaps not surprising that the corporate view of law is more negotiable and flexible than it might otherwise be. Corporations, like their polluting by-products, may very well outlive the laws that regulate them. (See e.g., Hartmann 2002 for a discussion of corporations and the law.)

With the stakes of a class-action lawsuit like the one Tipanecos filed in 2000 running high, it is understandable that few managers volunteered their views on the case, or even on their relationship to Barrio Tipan in general. However, as in the quote above, their statements clearly show that their attitudes toward pollution are not proactive, but are more concerned with getting what they paid for. Another environmental manager, who also had community-relations experience because of local pollution issues, generously praised his own company's preemptive stance on chemical leaks. "I have always been proud to work for a company like SuperMed," he said. "Leaks happen," he continued with a shrug, explaining that it was always better to use aboveground pipes for toxic wastes, because then leaks cannot cause as much damage. He presented this view as general knowledge among environmental engineers. If this was indeed the case, and underground pipes, like those delivering the industrial influent to the NWTP, are more potentially hazardous, one might ask why they should not receive regular monitoring, an approach which might, for example, reveal excessive corrosion before it had consumed the iron ladders in their entirety. But as informants consistently reported on this question, the companies had always taken pains to assert that once the wastes entered the "shared" portion of the pipe, they were no longer individually liable for the pipe maintenance, in part because it became impossible to identify which industrial source was "at fault." Again, a concern with costs, in this case, paying for something that might not be their problem, was paramount.

On the one occasion when a pharmaceutical representative did divulge his perspective on the Tipan legal case to me, it was equally revealing:

> There is a group, down by the beach, that has a lawsuit . . . and they really might win, might get some money. But they're not really suffering. They didn't know they had problems until some big lawyers from San Juan, and those environmentalists told them they were suffering. And now, they could really get some money for that.

Emergent Health Concerns

From the beginning of the NWTP's operations residents of Tipan reported health problems associated with the odors (Campos Bistani 1983). The symptoms they describe are primarily respiratory, as well as burning of the eyes and nasal passages. They also frequently report symptoms that are more difficult to define in strict clinical terms, but which are nevertheless indicative of disturbed health, particularly if they are chronic; for example, the frequently occurring odors of both domestic waste and chemicals were reported by residents to cause nausea so acute that they could not eat. The sudden arrival of strong odors was credited with profoundly disturbing the sleep patterns of residents, preventing them from falling asleep as well as waking them in the middle of the night.

For residents of Barrio Tipan, antiquated notions of miasmic sickness, contamination produced by foul odors emanating from noxious waters, is no mere public health fairy tale. When Don Reynaldo arrived in Tipan in 1995, he coordinated some of his neighbors to write daily reports of the experience of *la peste*. "We call it *la peste*, because it is more than just a bad smell," Don Reynaldo explains. "You see, the word *peste*, it's like *pestilencia*, it gives the idea of sickness." Recognizing that reports from members of CDAN could perhaps be dismissed as "troublemaking" or "the usual suspects," he recruited three women from the neighborhood to do reports. "I had Beatriz [his wife] recruit women from her church, because they lived here, but also because of their religious dedication, no one would be able to accuse them of lying for me." He collected daily notes on their experience of *la peste* for several years in the mid-to-late 1990s, and sent copies, with his own reports, at weekly intervals, to pharmaceutical managers, PRASA officials, and managers of the NWTP, and at one point, to the union representative of the local PRASA workers. Excerpts from these reports eloquently describe both the chronicity and the intensity of the impact the emanations from the treatment plant had on barrio life:

> Friday: 5:00 a.m. It began. Very strong the kind of stink that leaves the eyes watery and burning. What is it going to take to make it stop? We are never going to be free! It began at 10:00 p.m. again!
>
> Sunday: 8:20 a.m., later 5:00 p.m.–11:59 p.m. Today was horrible, an incredibly strong odor of gas, I have had a headache for 3 days, and the odor of gas is affecting me very much.
>
> Monday: This morning very early at 5:30 a.m. the stink flooded my bedroom. Not only do we have to sleep with it, but now like an "alarm clock" it wakes us up! Who can eat breakfast like this!

Similarly compelling are the expressions of relief, gratitude, and even encouragement to the plant operators when the reporters have nothing to report: "Monday: Didn't feel the stink today! Not even at night. It's the way it should be."

In his cover letters to the reports Don Reynaldo often expressed not only the frustration and ill health of his community, but also a sense that if only their experience could be compassionately understood, then those who had the knowledge, the resources, and the power to either change the influent of the NWTP, or correctly maintain and operate the plant, would do so. In mid-1996 Don Reynaldo informed those receiving the reports that they would now be sent in English (San Pereil 1996), in hopes that this would facilitate understanding for any North Americans who were in management positions in both PRASA and the pharmaceuticals. As most Puerto Ricans in high positions are also likely to be able to at least read English, the reports remained accessible to them. On New Year's Eve of that year Don Reynaldo wrote:

> Last day of the year and the problems of the odors have not been solved. This is destroying our health, it is impossible for us to enjoy our life, because the odors come into our houses making us unhappy, making us sick, and not able to rest because of the gases that come from the Plant.

> What is causing all these problems? . . . This not only makes us sick, but it also contaminates our surroundings, and who knows, problems in other areas. We hope that *deep in your hearts* you really want to do your best to help solve this problem. Something you have promised *so many times* that you will do.

Though Don Reynaldo continued to express his courteous, if desperate-sounding, hope that between the companies and PRASA a solution would be reached, through some combination of better maintenance and supervision of the NWTP, CDAN had begun considering other options, and they began sending information to an environmental lawyer. However, nearly another four years would pass before CDAN and Don Reynaldo would take the drastic step of naming not only PRASA, but the corporate pharmaceutical members of the Nocorá Consortium, in a lawsuit filed in February 2000. Shortly thereafter, residents began to notice a significant improvement, though there are still periodic problems. CDAN members believe, and the ethnographic evidence supports the idea, that without the threat of a court order for oversight, the Consortium and PRASA will have no incentives to keep the plant under control.

The lawsuit did not endear CDAN to the pharmaceuticals—nor to their elected officials. The position of the Nocorá municipal government as it was expressed to me is that organized communities are a positive force in the life of the municipality. Speaking of CDAN and the community activism in Tipan, a high-ranking official familiar with environmental issues told me that "the plant has improved because it was *obligated* to by the community. The municipality, too, has supported the community's efforts, we've given them money to help their organization, brought in experts to work on the problems." Without prompting he brought up the lawsuit himself, claiming that it had been an important part of the improvement process, providing a certain kind of pressure, because "bad publicity doesn't interest the industries."

The municipal administration has, however, also played a role in trying to destabilize CDAN's legal efforts. One of the "helping" actions promised was to arrange an epidemiological study that would establish whether the gaseous emissions from the treatment plant, particularly hydrogen sulfide and volatile organic compounds, were causing the widely reported respiratory ailments in the neighborhood. The study, on behalf of

Tipanecos, was to be organized through the mayor's office by means of the regional health department. When it was arranged, the group's outside environmental advisers asked for a copy of the questionnaire in advance. It turned out to be a basic survey, "to show that health problems were from smoking, hygiene, etc., with *no attempt to measure air quality*," the environmental consultants stated. Follow-up interviews in the Environmental Health Division confirmed the intent of the study. Said one health worker: "When I found out they were going to use the survey to blame the community, I refused to work on it." When questioned, a supervisor familiar with the project gave me a confused look, saying, "a simple sanitary survey was what was requested of us"; a survey that would not have answered whether an association existed between the NWTP gases and respiratory disease. The point person for the mayor in dealing with such arrangements, the environmental director, had a master's degree in public health—it can only be assumed he would have known the difference between various epidemiological study designs.

The officially sanctioned sanitary survey was halted by Don Reynaldo and CDAN, but as part of the process of planning their lawsuit, the group had also made an effort to collect its own data, a classic example of what Phil Brown has called "popular epidemiology" (Brown 1992). In 2000 the U.S. Census identified 359 households as comprising the urbanized areas of Tipan; in 1997 CDAN was able to collect health data from 353 households in that area.

As an epidemiologist, I would not present table 12.1 as definitive proof that asthma or other respiratory ailments are endemic to Barrio Tipan, or that their root cause is to be found at the NWTP. However, given the available data (which sometimes list health issues as present in the household without identifying individual sufferers), the statistics below do suggest a generalized burden of suffering across households. The

Table 12.1. Households Reporting One or More Members with Respiratory Complaints

Condition	*Percent*
Asthma alone (does not include undiagnosed chronic difficulty breathing)	37.7
Nonasthma chronic respiratory infections (including chronic cold)	46.7
Total asthma and/or other chronic respiratory infection	84.4

numbers also indicate a substantial burden of care and/or chronic symptom management that is distributed widely in Tipan—a measure of community health seldom addressed by traditional epidemiologic methods. Furthermore, when viewed in light of two recent studies of asthma in Puerto Rico, the above figures represent a problem that was worth seriously investigating. A study of island Puerto Rican homes (Montealegre et al. 2004) suggests that traditional indoor exposures (e.g., mold and dust) are less relevant to asthma locally, in good part because the homes are so well ventilated, as is the case in Tipan. Another recent study (Pérez-Perdomo et al. 2003) using Behavioral Risk Factor Surveillance Survey (BRFSS) data concluded that asthma prevalence among island-dwelling Puerto Ricans did not differ among age groups, people smoking at least 100 cigarettes in an entire lifetime, or physical activity, some of the "usual suspects" of asthma.

Together these two studies suggest that Barrio Tipan's data on asthma and chronic respiratory problems did indeed deserve the attention of a specially tailored study, taking into account not solely the usual individual behavioral variables, but external air quality as well (such as might freely blow into well-ventilated houses from nearby sources). Admittedly, the Department of Health does not always have the resources to conduct complex studies that focus on small groups of people. However, scarce resources were not the basis of the failure to accurately quantify Tipan's health. In an effort to avoid the bad publicity that "doesn't interest the industries," the municipal government requested a study that would collect only enough information to effectively blame the residents (by means of their behaviors) for any pattern of disease, effectively exonerating their local corporate citizens.

While the mayor would likely have either supported or been neutral about a suit naming only PRASA as a defendant, he has been much colder to Barrio Tipan since they threatened the pharmaceuticals, the backbone of Nocorá's economy, and an integral part of the mayor's vision for its future growth and development. In spite of the widespread acknowledgment, including by municipal insiders, that the suit was an essential catalyst to recent improvements which have been made, Barrio Tipan has become increasingly isolated and actively removed from participation in the sociopolitical life of Nocorá. Major development projects are soon to be carried out in Tipan, and the community is not being kept well informed about the emerging plans, including major land rezoning and other changes. The mayor's vision of Tipan's future will certainly affect present and future residents, particularly those low-income families for whom housing is being built on the other side of the fence from the treatment plant.

Given the persistent complaints of residents; their proactive involvement in a variety of problem-solving efforts, both independent (prying up manhole covers) and cooperative (decades-old industry-government-resident committees); and the acknowledgment of a problem by representatives of PRASA, local government, and the pharmaceutical companies, it is hard to understand how the *malos olores* problem could remain unresolved. Given the abysmally poor track record of PRASA's environmental compliance (see Estado Libre Asociado de Puerto Rico 2004; Huertas 2004), "*los grandes*" (as Tipanecos sometimes refer to those with more power than they have, in this case the mayor, the pharmaceuticals, the Environmental Quality Board of Puerto Rico, and the EPA) should have been alert from the beginning to the need for more effective monitoring and oversight of the plant. However, other documents suggest that the industry was most concerned with meeting the demands of technical compliance without sacrificing their competitive edge in production.

A 1994 memo from an industry environmental compliance specialist, once a high-ranking member of the Environmental Quality Board (EQB), makes this perspective clear (PRASA Memo 1994). The purpose of the memo, outlining a request for an exception to the present permit of the NWTP, emphasizes the costs of requiring the plant to meet treatment specifications as its effluent exited the plant and entered the outfall pipe (the usual place to measure compliance and where, it should be recalled, the 1983 inspection noted a foul-smelling black effluent, which the inspector believed had discolored the ocean water in spite of the mixing zone).[4]

In the case of the Nocorá WTP it was never just the destination of the treated waters that gave cause for concern, but the quality of influent into the plant, as well as the gases released during the treatment process. The better the treatment, the fewer locations in the process to release gases, as well as the higher the quality of the water being put into the ocean, where local fishermen sought their livelihoods. However, when the first organized threat of legal action was raised in the mid-1990s, the pharmaceuticals made it clear that they preferred that water quality not be measured at either the influent site or the effluent site, *but at the mixing zone itself* (PRASA Memo 1994). This strategy clearly demonstrates that the only concern of the companies was with technical legal compliance with Clean Water Act regulations, and that any escaping pollutants occurring before that point (and their consequences) were unimportant.

If we consider the proposal to measure at the mixing zone to indicate indifference to the realities of both air and water pollution from the NWTP, the following quote from the same memo shows that minimizing costs is the main concern of the companies:

> Since it is in the interest of the Commonwealth of Puerto Rico to maintain and promote the selection of Puerto Rico as a suitable home for the pharmaceutical industry, the maximum operational flexibility of the [N]WTP should be made available. (PRASA Memo 1994)

Other documentation from about a year later also indicates that although the consortium was involved in trying to make improvements to the NWTP to minimize the odors reaching Tipan, its mandate was to "execute the best alternative at the least cost" (Roberts 1995). It is also important to note in the block quote above the thinly veiled threat that the pharmaceutical industry *as a whole* would likely abandon Puerto Rico if the proposal was not accepted. The threat of not just one factory abandoning the island, but an entire industry upon which the island's economy relies, if not entirely, then substantially, was not an idle one, even in 1994. By 1997, the pharmaceutical preparations industry had secured its place as the largest manufacturing employer in Puerto Rico (Southern Technology Council/Southern Growth Policies Board 2000).

While the industrial nature of the influent has been largely resolved by the pretreatment regulations, the problems of hydrogen sulfide production and corrosion within the system remain constant for all treatment facilities. The literature on this issue agrees that only high-quality maintenance will prevent such odor- and pollution-related difficulties, a task at which PRASA has never excelled, even under the best of circumstances. The pharmaceuticals, as private partners with government in the business of the Nocorá treatment plant, have an ethical, if perhaps not a legal, obligation to the Tipan community. It requires that they effectively move beyond their traditional adversarial stance as the NWTP's penny-pinching banker, and demand higher-quality return for their investment in the plant. A recent audit by the island's Office of the Comptroller reports that though improvements have been made, PRASA (including the plant at Nocorá) still has serious management and maintenance problems with their water treatment plants (Estado Libre Asociado de Puerto Rico 2004). Perhaps such difficulties can be expected generally in a large public system such as PRASA—but if, as the mayor assured me, they are immediately responsive to urgent needs of the Nocorá plant, then surely Tipanecos should be able to expect better-than-average maintenance:

> They pay 80% of the operational costs of the plant, continuously. Whatever type of repair that needs to be made that is urgent, they come with their own people, in association with PRASA . . . wherever the necessary part is, in the world, by airplane or whatever, they bring it here . . . not for the protection or the health of the *pueblo*, you understand, but because it affects their production. But as a consequence, we have benefited, because the majority of Nocorá is now connected to a sewer system [author's note: though most of Tipan is not] . . . which has allowed the people to improve their health overall.

It would seem that the mayor, though he is an active partner of the local industry, is more pragmatic than complimentary in his view about the motives of the pharmaceuticals; it may well be that their supposed commitment (which much of the evidence would contradict) is merely one of mutually rewarding self-interest. However, if the pharmaceuticals have a real commitment to more than just compliance, as they would like the public to believe, they should certainly be treating the complaints of residents with the respect, and the action, they deserve.

Conclusion

In our conversations around his kitchen table, Don Reynaldo sometimes speaks with a thoughtful regret about suing the pharmaceuticals; at times he has said that he didn't want to name them, as well as PRASA, but he had no choice. "They always treated me politely, you know," he tells me one afternoon, a grave look on his face, "the one from SuperMed, particularly, he was always very gen-

tleman-like with me. I remember him telling me, 'Don Reynaldo, I think I see a light, it's a very small light, but I think there is a light at the end of the tunnel.' He always seemed like he wanted to help."

I ask Don Reynaldo when it was that the environmental engineer from SuperMed (whom I later interviewed) claimed to see this "light at the end of the tunnel." He guesses it was around 1998 or 1999, before the lawsuit, because they never talked after the suit was filed. I observe to Don Reynaldo that it is interesting that the pharmaceutical rep had predicted an end to the wastewater problems just around the time that the pretreatment regulation was handed down. I wonder aloud if the tiny light was 2001, when the industry was scheduled to require full compliance. He is quiet a moment, and then he says, "It could be. It could very well be."

The pharmaceutical representatives I worked with represented a range of attitudes toward the average citizens of the community of Nocorá. One from AlphaPharm in particular gave a much more convincing demonstration of his commitment to his job in "community affairs" than I would say was typical. Nevertheless, even this realistic, and I believe sincere, industry manager was ultimately unwilling, or perhaps unable, to concede the obvious advantages his company has when dealing with residents' complaints: money, connections, organization, and arguably a better public image than many local environmentalists. He said:

> If someone in the neighborhood has a problem, they should come to me. Like the woman who called because she thought our construction had caused the flooding on her street. She called, and I investigated. What I don't like is when outsiders come in and get involved. I don't think that's right.

Even when the pharmaceutical managers have a more humane outlook, they share a sense of entitlement to political and legal access, which they would readily deny residents seeking justice. They are quick to label nonresident environmentalists or other advocates "outsiders," though few, if any, of the managers themselves live in Nocorá.

Sound arguments exist against underinformed and reactive NIMBY (not in my backyard) activism (see especially Freeze 2000). The case of Tipan, the wastewater treatment plant, and the Nocorá pharmaceutical industry is not such a case. Rather, it exemplifies the attempts of a small community, unified by over 20 years of embodied physical experience and organized struggle, to have their right to well-being acknowledged and respected—to be free of the effects of poisonous by-products. Efforts to isolate and minimize the history of pollution in Tipan, using the narrative of economic progress for the rest of Nocorá and Puerto Rico as a supposedly self-evident trade-off, are not acceptable, particularly given the good citizenship and social responsibility claims made by these same companies and by locally elected political leaders. They must be held to a higher standard, one they espouse themselves.

In order to fully take into account the multilayered nature of the modern community of Nocorá, which residents, government officials, and companies alike will acknowledge includes a corporative element, I have included the perspectives of corporate representatives in my data gathering and analysis, rather than relying solely on a strict dependency, or axiomatically "anticorporate" angle. While I have sought to critique the naturalized structures, roles, and other power dynamics that contribute to health (or in this case its lack), I began the research from the perspective that the corporations and their representatives, too, had a story to tell; I designed the project with the intention, to a certain degree, to take the pharmaceutical corporations at their word with regard to their community-social behaviors. What I often found was that in seeking to explain their own perspectives, and defending typically self-protective corporate stances, pharmaceutical managers inadvertently revealed the hypocrisy of the practice of so-called corporate citizenship. Instead, with the assistance of government agencies and elected officials, the pharmaceutical companies of Nocorá have created an environment in which "what matters most: life and the potential it holds when we are feeling our best," is in practice treated if not with contempt, then as definitively less important than minimizing the costs of production for the world's most profitable industry (Public Citizen 2002).

Nevertheless, corporations, as we know, are made up of individuals whose behavior is influenced both by their position in the corporation as well as by other factors. Paying attention to the voices of the human players representing corporations fulfills critical medical anthropology's "approach in which symbols and meanings are neither obscured nor unduly empowered" (Singer 1998). An overly deterministic analysis of corporate managers as simply cogs in the machinery of capitalism diminishes their individual agency and responsibility as participants in damaging processes, as well as the potential for them to initiate positive change. It is these same managers, as the on-the-ground negotiators of corporate social responsibility, who have the potential to make the opening quotes of this chapter become something more of a reality, and pollution less of a quality-of-life killer.

Notes

1. Following the convention of previous studies of this town (Padilla Seda 1956; Seda Bonilla 1964), I use the fictitious names Nocorá (the municipality) and Tipan (the seaside barrio which is now home to the *Comité para Defender el Ambiente Nocoreño* and the regional wastewater treatment plant). All names of people, barrios, corporations, and groups are likewise fictitious, and some are presented here as composites. I follow this convention for two reasons: 1) to maintain the integrity of the previous studies, and 2) because many people spoke with me on the condition of confidentiality. It is not my intention to point a finger at any one person or corporation, but rather to emphasize the negative impact of *joint ventures* and *shared indifference*.

2. It is common practice in Puerto Rico to diminish the importance of something by associating it with the independence movement. This tactic can be successful for several reasons: 1) as a U.S. possession the historic relationship between nationalism and socialism in Puerto Rico has resulted in persecution of nationalists to the present day, and 2) many Puerto Ricans are skeptical of the economic viability of independence, and therefore of the judgment of *independentistas*. Environmentalism (as contrary to "progress") is frequently associated with them.

3. Notice and comment rule making, such as happens with agencies like the EPA, is time-consuming and requires significant external input, and the agency has to respond to all comments. It can easily take five to ten years.

4. This principle of the mixing zone (Alaska Division of Water Quality Standards 2005) is typically used as an economical way of achieving water quality for treated wastewaters that do not meet drinking water quality, being emitted into natural bodies of water.

References

Agencia EFE
1998 A pagar por la limpieza. *In* El Nuevo Día. Pp. 38. San Juan.

Alaska Division of Water Quality Standards
2005 2003–2005 Triennial Review: Mixing Zones Fact Sheet. Electronic document, www.state.ak.us/dec/water/wqsar/trireview/trireview.htm, accessed March 16, 2006.
Brown, Phil
1992 Popular Epidemiology and Toxic Waste Contamination: Lay and Professional Ways of Knowing. Journal of Health and Social Behavior 33(3):267–281.
Campos Bistani, Luis F.
1983 [Nocorá] Wastewater Treatment Plant. Memo to EPA Caribbean Field Office.
Dietrich, Alexa S.
2006 Downstream and Pushed Aside: Intra-community Competition for Health and Quality-of-Life in Puerto Rico. Paper presented at the Annual Meetings of the Society for Applied Anthropology/Society for Medical Anthropology. Vancouver, BC.
Estado Libre Asociado de Puerto Rico
2004 Informe de Auditoria CP-05-13 (Autoridad de Acueductos y Alcantarillados de Puerto Rico (PRASA)): Oficina del Controlar.
Federal Register
1998 Pharmaceutical Manufacturing Category Effluent Limitations Guidelines, Pretreatment Standards, and New Source Performance Standards; Final Rule, vol. 63, no. 182, 40 CFR parts 136 and 439.
Freeze, R. Allan
2000 The Environmental Pendulum: A Quest for the Truth about Toxic Chemicals, Human Health, and Environmental Protection. Berkeley: University of California Press.
García, Neftalí
1975 Informe Sobre Industria Químico-Farmacéutica y Plantas de Tratamiento: Archives SCTInc. Folder 1975: #7.
1977 Ni Una Química Ni Una Farmacéutica Mas Para el Área de [Bajas-Nocorá]: Misión Industrial y Servicios Legales.
1982 Acerca de la Contaminación de los Pozos de Agua Potable en [Cacique y Nocorá] con Tetraclouro de Carbono: Archives of SCT-Inc. Folder: 1982, #5.
Goitía, José R.
N.d. [Nocorá's] Regional Wastewater Treatment Plant: Puerto Rico Aqueduct and Sewer Authority.
Hartmann, Thom
2002 Unequal Protection: The Rise of Corporate Dominance and the Theft of Human Rights. Emmaus, PA: Rodale Books.

Huertas, Evelyn
2004 Impact and Environmental Risk of Discharges from Wastewater Treatment Plants of the Puerto Rico Aqueduct and Sewer Authority. MS thesis, Metropolitan University, Environmental Affairs Graduate School.

López Acevedo, Bernardo
1976 Desperdicios venenosos para la costa norte. *In* Claridad, 15 de mayo. Pp. 3. San Juan, PR.

Montealegre, F., B. Fernández, A. Delgado, L. Fernández, A. Román, D. Chardón, J. Rodríguez-Santana, V. Medina, D. Zavala, and M. Bayona
2004 Exposure Levels of Asthmatic Children to Allergens, Endotoxins, and Serine Proteases in a Tropical Environment. Journal of Asthma 41(4):485–496.

Nash, June, and Max Kirsch
1988 The Discourse of Medical Science in the Construction of Consensus between Corporation and Community. Medical Anthropology Quarterly 2(2):158–171.

National Center for Environmental Health
2005 About Cancer Clusters. Electronic document, www.cdc.gov/NCEH/clusters/about_clusters.htm, accessed June 18, 2006.

Nichter, Mark
1996 Pharmaceuticals, the Commodification of Health, and the Health Care-Medicine Use Transition. *In* Anthropology and International Health: Asian Case Studies, 2nd ed. M. Nichter and M. Nichter, eds. Amsterdam: Gordon and Breach.

Padilla Seda, Elena
1956 Nocorá: An Agrarian Reform Sugar Community in Puerto Rico. *In* The People of Puerto Rico: A Study in Social Anthropology. Julian H. Steward et al., eds. Pp. 265–313. Urbana: University of Illinois Press.

Partido Socialista Puertorriqueño
1977 Boletin Especial: Unete al Piquete del Partido Socialista Puertorriqueña—¡Salvemos Nuestras Playas y Nuestra Pesca! ¡Alto a la Contaminación!

Pérez-Perdomo, R., C. Pérez-Cardona, O. Disdier-Flores, and Y. Cintrón
2003 Prevalence and Correlates of Asthma in the Puerto Rican Population: Behavioral Risk Factor Surveillance System, 2000. Journal of Asthma 40(5):465–474.

Petryna, Adriana, Andrew Lakoff, and Arthur Kleinman, eds.
2006 Global Pharmaceuticals: Ethics, Markets, Practices. Durham, NC: Duke University Press.

Pharmaceutical Industry Association of Puerto Rico
2005 Homepage of the Pharmaceutical Industry Association of Puerto Rico. www.piapr.com, accessed March 2005.

PRASA Memo
1994 Status: Water Quality Certificate for the [N]WTP. Memo to: PRASA and Advisory Council Members. December 7, 1994.

Public Citizen
2002 Pharmaceuticals Rank as Most Profitable Industry, Again: "Druggernaut" Tops All Three Measures of Profits *In* New Fortune 500 Report. Electronic document, www.citizen.org/documents/fortune 500_2002erport.PDF.

Roberts, Blanca O.
1995 Women's Executive Leadership Program—30-Day Developmental Assignment: Summary of Activities while at the [Nocorá] City Hall—Environmental Directorate. Memo to the mayor of Nocorá. March 8, 1995.

San Pereil, Reynaldo [pseudonym]
1996 To [Managers of PRASA and Pharmaceutical Representatives to the Comite de Olores]: "El proposito de esta es para informarles que de ahora en adelante van a recibir tres reportes en ingles y uno en español."

Schafer, Jacqueline E.
1983 Letter to CDAN from EPA regional administrator. N.d. (received October 17, 1983).

Seda Bonilla, Edwin
1964 Interacción social y personalidad en una comunidad de Puerto Rico. San Juan, PR: Ediciones Juan Ponce de Leon.

Singer, Merrill
1998 The Development of Critical Medical Anthropology: Implications for Biological Anthropology. *In* Building a New Biocultural Synthesis: Political Economic Perspectives on Human Biology. A. Goodman and T. L. Leatherman, eds. Ann Arbor: University of Michigan Press.
2007 Drugging the Poor: Legal and Illegal Drugs and Social Inequality. Long Grove, IL: Waveland.

Southern Technology Council/Southern Growth Policies Board
2000 Invented Here: Toward an Innovation Driven Economy. Electronic document, www.southern.org/pubs/ih2000/pr.pdf.

Steward, Julian H., and others
1956 The People of Puerto Rico: A Study in Social Anthropology. Urbana: University of Illinois Press.

US-EPA Office of Water
2003 EPA's National Pretreatment Program, 1973–2003: Thirty Years of Protecting the Environment (EPA 833–F–03–001).

Van der Geest, Sjaak, and Susan Reynolds Whyte, eds.
1991 The Context of Medicines in Developing Countries: Studies in Pharmaceutical Anthropology. Amsterdam: Het Spinhuis.

Webster's Dictionary
2006 www.merriam-webster.com

Whyte, Susan Reynolds, Sjaak van der Geest, and Anita Hardon, eds.
2002 The Social Lives of Medicines. Cambridge, UK: Cambridge University Press.

Witherspoon, J., E. Allen, and C. Quigley
2004 Modelling to Assist in Wastewater Collection System Odour and Corrosion Potential Evaluations. Water Science Technology 50(4):177–183.

CHAPTER THIRTEEN

INVERTING THE KILLER COMMODITY MODEL

Withholding Medicines from the Poor

Michael Westerhaus and Arachu Castro

In August 2004, Apio Jane, a 26-year-old woman, grimaced in pain as she lay on an examination table in the acquired immunodeficiency syndrome (AIDS) clinic at St. Mary's Hospital Lacor in northern Uganda, an area stricken with a double affliction of poverty and war. Weighing just 32 kilograms, her ribs and cheekbones conspicuously protruded forward; her physician could stretch her hand across the width of the woman's abdomen. This woman was dying of AIDS. The woman's mother, also in the room, complained that she was tired—tired of the incessant hospital visits, tired of endless clinic lines, tired of bringing her daughter to the clinic when there was nothing the doctors could offer her. All of this transpired despite the fact that antiretroviral therapy (ART), which consists of a combination of life-saving AIDS medications, has been available since 1996—at least for some. Jane's story is one shared by many who are in urgent need of ART—2000 patients in Lacor hospital's catchment area, 4.7 million in sub-Saharan Africa, and 6.5 million throughout the world (World Health Organization 2005a:19). As pernicious as commodities can often be, the absence of needed commodities can be just as or even more deadly, and some of the reasons certain commodities are beyond the reach of those who need them may be the same as the reasons why killer commodities continue to be put on the market.

Much of this book focuses upon the grave harm done to public health by dangerous commercial products in today's capitalist world.

Yet the inverse also holds true—withholding certain products, such as medicines, can cause extraordinary morbidity and mortality, a painful fact to which the poor of the world can quite readily attest. Since the introduction of ART in 1996, mortality due to AIDS has dropped precipitously for those with access to the medicines (Hammer et al. 1997; Sterne et al. 2005). Although public health and medical practitioners continue to assemble a stultifying set of reasons—including lack of infrastructure, corrupt governments, poor adherence, and stigma—about why ART won't work in developing countries, this treatment approach has been shown to be equally effective in resource-poor and resource-rich settings (Castro and Farmer 2005; Severe et al. 2005; Weidle et al. 2002; Harries et al. 2001; Farmer et al. 2001; Müller et al. 1998). In the case of ART, it is the intentional absence of a life-saving commodity, rather than commodity presence, which is onerous. In other words, in this instance commodity absence kills people living with human immunodeficiency virus (HIV)/AIDS, a pattern that has been seen with other intentional commodity absences as well, such as medications for multidrug-resistant tuberculosis (MDR-TB) (Farmer 2003:179–195; Mukherjee et al. 2004).

The absence of ART is not an uncommon dilemma, particularly for the poor who simultaneously inherit both a high risk of HIV infection and a high likelihood of minimal access to ART. Given this morally untenable reality today, it is imperative to ask what forces determine the absence of ART across the world. In response to this question, health activists often readily ascribe blame to transnational corporations (TNCs). While certainly shouldering their burden of guilt, TNCs can't be singled out as solely responsible for the dismal access to ART in the world today. Generally, the global distribution of medicines and health care is the product of numerous forces and relationships—development and health strategies set forth by the United Nations (UN) and World Health Organization (WHO), global trade and investment policies engineered by the World Trade Organization (WTO), capitalism and free market ideology, gender inequality and socioeconomic disparities, and government and corporate interests and corruption, among others (Millen and Holtz 2000:221–222). In the same vein, political, economic, corporate, and social forces can either erect or demolish avenues for ART distribution (Westerhaus and Castro 2006).

In high-income settings such as the United States and European Union (EU) countries, patients, health-care professionals, government agencies, and pharmaceutical companies all engage in an economic tug-of-war to determine which medications are available, who receives those medications, and how much these medications cost. In low-income settings, however, the voices of the poor, who bear a disproportionate burden of global disease, are often silenced in conversations that determine drug distribution. Rather, it is representatives of multinational pharmaceutical companies, trade ministers of high- and low-income countries, WHO officials, and humanitarian organizations that do all the public talking and acting. Not surprisingly, all this work—which is often much heavier on the talking and lighter on the acting—has left far too many individuals infected with HIV without access to adequate health care and medications. The current lack of access to ART is an example of commodity absence at a monumentally devastating level.

In this chapter, we aim to scrutinize a specific determinant of the current global distribution of ART—intellectual property (IP) law and international trade agreements, and in this, this chapter reveals the important intersections of unhealthy health policy (Castro and Singer 2004) and the killer effects of commodity absence. As globalization further entrenches international links and relationships, the issue of intellectual property and its protection throughout the world has increasingly taken center stage. Momentum for the global expansion of intellectual property law, propelled primarily by the United States and EU countries which most multinational pharmaceutical companies call home, has materialized through WTO negotiations and intensified U.S. pursuit of "free" trade agreements with low- and middle-income countries. While we recognize that multiple factors influence access to ART, including poor drug quality, inadequate public health infrastructure, understaffed clinics and hospitals, lack of political commitment, and underfinancing of HIV treatment programs, we argue that patent law and the strengthening of this law in current U.S. trade agreements also poses a significant threat to access to medicines and demands attention in any analysis of global access to ART.

A number of underlying questions inform our exploration of this topic. Should matters of health constitute a state of exception from patent law? Do trade agreements with strengthened patent law disavow efforts to combat global disease, especially the AIDS pandemic? What potential benefits do bilateral, regional, and multilateral trade agreements have for resource-poor settings? Is it accurate to conceive of these trade agreements as "free"? Can the intellectual property components of trade agreements be designed in a manner that is mutually beneficial for the poor and for drug innovation? Ultimately, how can the human right to health be preserved in all the fanfare over intellectual property law and access to ART? These questions guide our analysis and are questions to which the poor deserve urgent, honest answers.

A Brief History of Intellectual Property Law

Recognizing the necessity of analyses that are "historically deep" (Farmer 2003:159), we believe that understanding today's story of the relationship between impeded access to ART and patents requires engagement with the gradual development of intellectual property (IP) law. The history of IP law provides an insightful reflection of the shifting economic priorities and relationships in the world. As Christopher May and Susan Sell, political scientists with extensive experience studying this subject, argue, "the history of intellectual property has been a *political economic* history; intellectual property has been the policy background among contending economic interests, politically driven governments, and contrasting philosophical traditions" (May and Sell 2006:204). Indeed, even a brief overview of IP history reveals that IP law has been closely tied to both power and wealth.

The origins of intellectual property in Europe have been traced to 15th-century Venetian authorities when, under pressure from craft guilds who desired to protect their profits, it enacted its patent statute in 1474, which created "for the first time a legal and institutional form of intellectual property rights [that] established the ownership of knowledge and was explicitly utilized to promote innovation" (May and Sell 2006:58–65). With time, the formalization of patent law spread across Europe—and eventually to the United States: in 1624, Britain, aiming to boost commerce, passed the Statute of Monopolies, which established a systematic method of processing invention patents; France and the United States established firm intellectual property law through legislation in 1791 and

1790, respectively (U.S. Patent and Trademark Office 2005; May and Sell 2006:104). This history reveals the formation of a progressively entangled relationship between the expansions in industry and individual profit interests and the development of IP law, a historical process which failed to incorporate the interests of the poor and disenfranchised.

As these sentiments spread geographically and interstate economic relationships strengthened, the need for international agreements on intellectual property became necessary. In 1873, United States and German inventors refused to participate in the World Exposition held in Vienna for fear that their ideas would not be adequately protected against theft, thus stirring cross-border discussions about the protection of intellectual property (May and Sell 2006:118–119). As a result, modern international patent law arose with the 1883 Paris Convention for the Protection of Industrial Property, which established a set of internationally agreed-upon rules, including that patents must be enforced for all products and must be filed in each country where protection is sought within the span of one year from the primary patent filing date. This agreement also gave states the permission to issue compulsory licenses, which are lawful circumventions of patents in which a third party is given permission to produce products without the patent holder's consent. In the Paris Convention, compulsory licenses were allowed primarily on the grounds that the patent holder was failing to make the product available to the public over a reasonable period of time (World Intellectual Property Organization 1883). On July 7, 1884, the Paris Convention was ratified by ten countries—Belgium, Brazil, Italy, Netherlands, France, Switzerland, Tunisia, United Kingdom, Portugal, and Spain—and the enforcement of patents at an international level, including those for pharmaceutical products, was born (World Intellectual Property Organization 2006).

Since that time, countries have, at varying paces and with variable amounts of external pressure, come to recognize the Paris Convention as favorable for their national interests. For example, the United States joined in 1887, Denmark in 1894, Germany and Mexico in 1903, Ireland in 1925, South Africa in 1947, and Haiti in 1958. By 1965, 70 countries had signed on to the Paris Convention (World Intellectual Property Organization 2006). As the number of member countries steadily increased, the need for an expanded regulatory body became evident. Thus, in 1967, the World Intellectual Property Organization (WIPO) was established to regulate the production, distribution, and use of knowledge.

Following the establishment of WIPO, the number of Paris Convention signatories continued to expand—75 in 1970, 87 in 1980, 97 in 1990, and 160 in 2000. Many developing countries joined between 1986 and 1994 or shortly thereafter because that period marked the delineation of the Trade-Related Aspects of Intellectual Property Rights (TRIPS) agreement, which required consent with and enforcement of many provisions in the Paris Convention in order for these countries to access expanded opportunities for foreign investment and trade. Today, the Paris Convention has 169 signatories, the most recent assenting members being Saudi Arabia, Pakistan, Namibia, and Andorra in 2004 and Comoros in 2005 (World Intellectual Property Organization 2006). Other than a few minor revisions, the basic precepts of the Paris Convention continue to form a global foundation for patent law.

Theoretically, the patenting of pharmaceutical products, or substances manufactured and sold for the explicit treatment of disease as conceptualized through a biomedical lens, was consensually agreed upon in the Paris Convention, as it states in article 1 that "industrial property shall be understood in the broadest sense and shall apply not only to industry and commerce proper, but likewise to agricultural and extractive industries and to all manufactured or natural products" (World Intellectual Property Organization 1883). However, in reality pharmaceutical patents have had a varied history across different geographic locales. In Europe, most countries originally distinguished between patents for pharmaceutical processes and products. For example, France banned the patenting of pharmaceutical products in 1844 and only completely lifted this ban in 1978; patents for pharmaceutical processes were allowed much earlier. Germany and Switzerland followed similar courses and only made pharmaceutical product patents available in 1967 and 1977, respectively, whereas pharmaceutical process patents were available in 1877 in Germany and 1907 in Switzerland. Spain only began applying its law for product patents in 1992 (Boldrin and Levine 2005:3–4). For most of these countries, pharmaceutical product patents were long seen as detrimental to public health and contrary to the common good.

In contrast to European countries, the United States, reflecting its long history of leading efforts to strengthen IP law, has allowed for both pharmaceutical process and product patents since the inception of its domestic patent law. This subject, however, has not been without controversy. Revealing the contentiousness of the debate even in the 19th century, physician F. E. Stewart warned of the hazards of pharmaceutical patenting, including increased drug costs for patients and the propensity of patents to turn medications into commodities as opposed to public goods available for the benefit of all (Stewart 1897:816B).

Despite such debates, the United States has consistently surged forward in expanding protection for IP. For example, the Drug Price Competition and Patent Term Restoration Act of 1984 (Hatch-Waxman Act) increased the length of patent protection to offset the regulatory requirements that slow market introduction of novel medicines (Angell 2004:178–180). The United States has and continues to export and strongly push for these sorts of expansionary, corporate-friendly IP rules to be adopted by all countries.

Intellectual Property Law Related to Public Health: TRIPS and Beyond

The early debates surrounding pharmaceutical patenting and IP law were mere microcosms of the intensified disputes about the role, value, and ethics of pharmaceutical patenting that would eventually unfold in the late 20th century as a result of the arrival of two seemingly distinct entities—AIDS and further internationalization of trade agreements and of rules governing intellectual property. Around the same time that the first recognized AIDS cases appeared in the early 1980s, there was mounting pressure for global standardization of strengthened intellectual property law and policing in order to parallel an expansion of international economic trade flows. Between 1986 and 1994, countries participating in the Uruguay round of trade negotiations developed the TRIPS agreement, a treaty which in part aimed to implement and enforce strengthened patent law throughout the world. These negotiations also gave birth to the WTO, which came into existence on January 1, 1995. Exactly a year later, the WIPO and the WTO entered into a cooperative agreement to share information and monitor the enforcement of TRIPS. As of 2005, the WTO had 149 member states, over two-thirds of which are low- and middle-income countries (World Trade Organization 2005).

The TRIPS agreement and the establishment of the WTO have profound implications for pharmaceutical patenting and global access to medicines. Originally, the TRIPS agreement required the standardization of intellectual property law for pharmaceutical patents among all member states by 2005 (World Trade Organization 1994:348). Essentially, the agreement prohibits the production, exportation, and importation of a generic drug for which a patent exists, hence making this really an issue of not just commodity absence but also commodity blockage. However, similar to the Paris Convention, the TRIPS agreement makes provisions for compulsory licensing, which could theoretically allow for breaking a pharmaceutical patent under the appropriate circumstances. Regarding the permitted circumstances for a compulsory license, the TRIPS agreement states:

> Such use may only be permitted if, prior to such use, the proposed user has made efforts to obtain authorization from the right holder on reasonable commercial terms and conditions and that such efforts have not been successful within a reasonable period of time. This requirement may be waived by a Member in the case of a national emergency or other circumstances of extreme urgency or in cases of public non-commercial use. (World Trade Organization 1994:333)

Vague and ill defined, this wording failed to explicitly define the circumstances under which compulsory licenses could be used, making its interpretation a point of considerable concern. What constituted a national emergency? Who would determine the legality of a compulsory license? Do health crises fall under the rubric of a national emergency? Does the AIDS pandemic qualify in severity and urgency as a national emergency?

Moreover, the TRIPS agreement stated that compulsory licenses were to be used "predominantly for the supply of the domestic market of the Member authorizing such use" (World Trade Organization 1994:333). This provision meant that countries would be required to have in-country manufacturing capacities for pharmaceuticals if they desired a compulsory license for generic drug production in the event of a health emergency. As most resource-poor countries lack the resources or infrastructure to produce medications, this stipulation meant that many countries, especially those most in need of ART, were not in a position to take advantage of the compulsory licensing provision unless allowed to parallel import—that is, import from a country that has purchased or produced medications within the legal boundaries of patent law and subsequently offers these medications for international resale. The TRIPS agreement explicitly says nothing about the legality of parallel importation (World Trade Organization 1994:323).

As these rules of a new world order governing patent law emerged, enormous concern was generated that the TRIPS agreement would compromise the protection of public health in low- and middle-income countries. Public health activists and academics argued that the TRIPS agreement would raise drug prices throughout the world and further curtail already limited access to medicines in low- and middle-income countries. Nongovernmental organizations (NGOs), such as Médecins Sans Frontières (MSF), Health Action International, and the Consumer Project on Technology, advocated that the WTO needed to explicitly establish that compulsory licenses could be used for essential medicines to protect public health ('t Hoen 2003:46). These issues took center stage at the 1999 WTO Ministerial Conference in Seattle. President Bill Clinton did announce a shift in U.S. policy regarding intellectual property law and access to medicines that would be more poor-friendly. But the talks eventually collapsed under the weight of intense antiglobalization protests in part directed against patent law rules in the TRIPS agreement. Of note, President Clinton did follow through on his promise by issuing a May 2000 Executive Order, which supported the use of compulsory licenses to increase access to HIV/AIDS medications in sub-Saharan Africa ('t Hoen 2003:47).

Prompted by these pointed calls for justice in international trade, WTO delegates gathered in Doha, Qatar, in 2001 and attempted to better define the boundaries of compulsory licensing. The delegates concluded the meeting by issuing a strong statement favoring the use of compulsory licensing in public health emergencies (World Trade Organization 2001). This statement, now referred to as the Doha Declaration, affirmed the priority of public health over patent status by stating:

> We agree that the TRIPS Agreement does not and should not prevent members from taking measures to protect public health. Accordingly,

> while reiterating our commitment to the TRIPS Agreement, we affirm that the Agreement can and should be interpreted and implemented in a manner supportive of WTO members' right to protect public health and, in particular, to promote access to medicines for all. Each member has the right to determine what constitutes a national emergency or other circumstances of extreme urgency, it being understood that public health crises, including those relating to HIV/AIDS, tuberculosis, malaria and other epidemics, can represent a national emergency or other circumstances of extreme urgency. (World Trade Organization 2001)

The Doha Declaration also stated that the least-developed countries (of 50 countries defined as such by the United Nations, 32 are WTO members) were not obliged to implement patent law for pharmaceuticals until January 1, 2016. Finally, the Doha Declaration acknowledged the shortsightedness of the TRIPS agreement rule mandating that countries could only break patents in public health emergencies in order to produce generic drugs "predominantly for the supply of the domestic market." Paragraph 6 of the Doha Declaration, thus its future reference as the "paragraph 6 problem," ordered the TRIPS council to develop a plan to resolve this conundrum by the end of 2002 (World Trade Organization 2001).

However, reaching consensus on the "paragraph 6 problem" was yet another task mired in a morass of contention, the lines of division falling between high-income countries and low- and middle-income countries. Not by chance, these same fault lines divided countries that had multinational pharmaceutical companies based in them from those that did not. The United States led an effort to restrict paragraph 6 of the Doha Declaration to certain diseases, namely, AIDS, malaria, tuberculosis, and other infectious diseases creating epidemics. Further, the United States worked to limit the number of countries that could benefit from the importation of generic medications (Loff 2002:1951). On August 30, 2003, the TRIPS council finally issued a decision that would serve as a temporary waiver to the TRIPS agreement restrictions. This waiver created a system in which a country with pharmaceutical manufacturing capacities could legally export generic medications to a country without manufacturing capacities. Both countries would need to declare a compulsory license and notify the WTO of these intentions (World Trade Organization 2003a). To curb fears that this system would undermine the patent system, Carlos Pérez del Castillo, the council's chairperson, concomitantly released a statement that strongly restricted use of this system to public health crises (World Trade Organization 2003b). This waiver would remain in place until a permanent amendment to the TRIPS agreement could be formulated.

Efforts to agree upon a permanent amendment to TRIPS were fraught with further discord. The United States and other developed countries argued for ratification of the temporary waiver, including the chairperson's statement, as a permanent amendment. On the other hand, developing countries, led by the African Group, argued that the temporary waiver included too many procedural obstacles that would still hinder access to essential medications for countries without domestic production capacity (Khor 2005). Further, MSF pointed out that no country had actually used the temporary amendment and argued that it would be unwise to make permanent something that had not been tested (Médecins Sans Frontières 2005a).

Despite these concerns, WTO members agreed in early December 2005, just prior to the WTO Ministerial Conference in Hong Kong, to make the temporary waiver permanent if at least two-thirds of the 148 WTO members ratified the amendment by December 1, 2007 (Cage 2005). The United States and the Pharmaceutical Research and Manufacturers of America (PhRMA) touted the amendment as "part of the wider national and international action, including many activities taken by PhRMA companies, to address the gravity of the public health problems afflicting many developing and least-developed countries" (Pharmaceutical Research and Manufacturers of America 2005).

Yet, do these acts of self-proclaimed generosity by the pharmaceutical industry and powerful governments such as the United States translate into tangible advances in access to essential medicines in low- and middle-income countries? Have all these shifts in intellectual property law benefited poor countries through increased technology transfer and innovation as PhRMA and the United States so readily assert? The case of access to ART is particularly poignant in answering these questions and casts considerable doubt on the veracity of claims that strengthened IP law will suit the poor. Sadly, the inverse is more likely true—that strengthened patent law threatens to further displace the hopes of HIV-positive patients living in poverty who desire health.

Access to Antiretrovirals and Patent Law

Currently, 40.3 million people in the world live with HIV. In 2005, 3.1 million people in the world died of AIDS; of these, about 570,000 were children (UNAIDS 2005). Given these circumstances, it is evident that addressing the issue of ART distribution requires urgency. Therefore, between December 2003 and 2005, the WHO led an effort to rapidly scale up HIV treatment throughout the world. This endeavor, known as the 3 by 5 Initiative, aimed to have three million people on ARV treatment by the end of 2005. During the initiative, the number of patients receiving ART in low- and middle-income countries increased from 400,000 to 1.3 million. Although short of the December 2005 goal, the initiative achieved significant progress in mobilizing the expansion of ARV treatment. The WHO estimates that between 250,000 and 350,000 premature deaths were averted due to the scale up in ART. Despite these successes, numerous challenges remain in efforts to continue improving access to ART. Some of the reasons cited by the WHO to explain the failure to reach the 3 by 5 Initiative's targets include poorly harmonized partnerships; constraints on the procurement and supply of drugs, diagnostics, and other commodities; strained human resources capacity and other critical weaknesses in health systems (e.g., lack of functional health centers for drug distribution and inadequate number of trained community health workers), and difficulties in ensuring equitable access (World Health Organization 2006b).

In addition to these challenges, a critical gaze must be fixed upon the interrelationship between intellectual property law and access to ART. Most types of antiretrovirals, of which 12 are included in the most recent WHO list of essential medicines, can be produced by generic manufacturers in India, where it is estimated that 5.1 million adults and children are living with HIV (World Health Organization 2005b:7–8; AMFAR 2004; UNAIDS 2004). Built upon substantial economic and infrastructural capabilities for drug production, Indian generic companies, such as Cipla and Ranbaxy, have become the major suppliers of low-cost ART regimens throughout the developing world: MSF estimates that 50 percent of these medications are produced in India (Médecins Sans Frontières 2005b). However, this supply of inexpensive generic antiretrovirals may soon end following India's enforcement of TRIPS-compliant patent law since January 1, 2005, as a consequence of stipulations laid out in the 1996 TRIPS Agreement. In March 2005, the Indian government passed amendments that boost intellectual property law and could hinder the future production of medications for health emergencies such as AIDS (McNeil 2005; New York Times 2005).

These developments generated concern that access to affordable ART, especially for second- and third-line antiretrovirals, may be severely constrained under India's enforcement of TRIPS. In a December 17, 2004, letter to the Indian minister of health, Jim Y. Kim, then director of the Department of HIV/AIDS at the WHO, cautioned India against implementing new patent laws that hinder public health efforts both within and outside of India (Kim 2004). Indian activists declared that "the Government is adopting a simplistic, conformist approach of hurriedly 'aligning' our Patent Law to the coercive version of TRIPS" and asserted that "the need of the hour is to follow a more creative and independent approach, while still remaining within the broad contours of TRIPS" (Joint Action Committee Against Amendment of the Indian Patents Act 2004).

The changes in India are emblematic of a general shift toward strengthened intellectual property law that raises considerable concern about whether the interests of the poor and public health really matter in WTO and patent-law decisions. After a period of extensive study by a committee of IP experts, the WHO identified global changes in IP law as a threat to the gains made in improving access to ART (World Health Organization 2006a). This work hints that, despite all the wrangling over the specific provisions of the TRIPS agreement and the self-proclaimed interest by multinational pharmaceutical companies and the U.S. government to promote global health, little has changed to suggest that WTO rules are actually promoting the betterment of global public health. In fact, compulsory licenses and other mechanisms offered for public health protection by the TRIPS agreement and the Doha Declaration have been rarely utilized (World Health Organization 2004; Oliveira et al. 2004). The exact procedures for issuing a compulsory license for ARV production remain unclear and largely untested. Significant international pressure also exists against declaring compulsory licenses, as seen when Brazil recently threatened to issue compulsory licenses for the ART medications efavirenz, lopinavir/ritonavir, and tenofovir (Adelman 2005; Kaiser Daily HIV/AIDS Report 2005a). For these reasons in part, only four countries—Malaysia, Indonesia, Zambia, and Mozambique—have thus far issued compulsory licenses for ARV production, all of them in 2004 (Consumer Project on Technology 2005; World Health Organization 2004).

Further, as stated earlier, no country has yet made use of the provisions instilled in the temporary, now permanent, waiver granted to solve the "paragraph 6 problem." Why might this be so? Certainly not because low- and middle-income countries don't have public health emergencies. Southern Africa is currently witnessing a decimation of its population by AIDS, while malaria kills around one million people, predominantly children, per year. Some might at this point recite the antiquated mantra that low- and middle-income governments are too corrupt and power seeking to actually care about the health of their populations. How then can we explain the health successes of countries such as Brazil, Cuba, and Thailand? Perhaps it is, as suggested by the African Group during the paragraph 6 discussions, that WTO rules are far too cumbersome and impractical for poor countries to navigate. Viewed in this light, the humanitarian motives pled by pharmaceutical companies and economically powerful governments are nothing more than empty lip service to counter growing calls for social justice in global health and in this are on par with similar lip service paid to "safety first" in the case of so many killer pharmaceutical commodities.

Pharmaceutical companies also argue that patents are central to the preservation of innovation. Yet, there is little evidence that current intellectual property law creates incentives for the development of new drugs. An analysis of a small sample of pharmaceutical inventive activity before and after compulsory licensing showed no uniform decline in scientific innovation, challenging the assumption that patent protection is necessary to foster the development of new drugs (Chien 2003). Furthermore, current patent protections do not necessarily create financial incentives for the development of desperately needed drugs, such as a malaria vaccine, in poor countries: between 1975 and 1997, only 13 out of 1,223 newly developed drugs were targeted toward diseases which disproportionately affect poor countries and account for a large bulk of global disease (Pécoul et al. 1999).

In support of the research-based pharmaceutical companies, some argue that patent laws have historically played very little role in inhibiting access to essential medicines in the developing world—instead asserting that poverty and poor health infrastructure are the primary obstacles to ART distribution (Attaran 2004; Attaran and Gillespie-White 2001). Additionally, poor drug quality, inadequate public health infrastructure, understaffed clinics and hospitals, lack of political commitment, import tariffs on pharmaceuticals, and underfinancing of HIV treatment programs are cited as major factors obstructing the provision of ART.

While it is clear that these factors do impede access to antiretrovirals, patent law—because of its impact on drug prices—can't be left out of the equation in the creation of barriers to access to medicines. Current patent protection, by eliminating competition, generally leads to higher prices, which directly obstructs the promotion of global health equity (Dumoulin et al. 2003; Lucchini et al. 2003). Health activists point specifically to HIV treatment in this argument, charging that current intellectual property law and patent law allow pharmaceutical companies to monopolize the ART markets in developing nations (Rosenberg 2001; Stiglitz 2004; 't Hoen 2003). As a result, the cost of ARVs far exceeds personal and national budgets, and the development of more affordable generic alternatives is proscribed. The high cost of brand-name ART not only represents an insurmountable barrier to initiating treatment, but for those already on therapy, the unaffordable cost of medications may also hamper complete adherence and trigger drug resistance (Castro 2005).

As reflected in the circuitous history of efforts to bridge patent law and public health concerns, intellectual property obstacles—in addition to hurdles involving public health financing, medical and public health infrastructure, and drug quality—have encumbered efforts to scale up global ARV distribution. These obstacles represent a form of structural violence, which is the disadvantaging of certain populations through political, economic, and social structures that place individuals at a higher risk of encounter with disease and death (Farmer 2004). Understanding these barriers as structural violence is central to our conceptualization of commodity absence and the withholding of medicines from the poor. But this picture is far from complete. Unfortunately, but not surprisingly, the United States, backed by considerable pharmaceutical sector support, is now moving to strengthen IP law beyond the provisions of the TRIPS agreement.

U.S. Trade Policy and Access to Antiretrovirals

In January 2003, President George W. Bush announced his five-year plan that would allocate $15 billion to global programs aimed at HIV treatment and prevention (Office of the United States Global AIDS Coordinator 2004). Now referred to as the President's Emergency Plan for AIDS Relief (PEPFAR), this initiative endeavors, in 15 focus countries, to support treatment for two million people living with HIV/AIDS, to prevent seven million new infections, and to support care for ten million people infected and affected by HIV/AIDS by 2008. While PEPFAR has received many accolades for its progressive stance on promoting and funding global ART, the initiative has been sharply criticized for its exclusive, and therefore expensive, use of ART medications produced by major U.S. pharmaceutical companies and for its "go-it-alone" shunning of multilateral HIV treatment initiatives, such as the Global Fund to Fight AIDS, Tuberculosis and Malaria (United Nations Office for the Coordination of Humanitarian Affairs 2005). Despite these criticisms, after eight months of operation, PEPFAR reported rapid progress in achieving its aims—by March 2005, 155,000 people were receiving ART and 1.2 million women and infants had benefited from mother-to-child prevention measures (Office of the United States Global AIDS Coordinator 2005).

However, recent U.S. trade policy threatens to undermine these advancements in improving access to ARVs. After failing to convince other countries of embracing "free trade" at hemispheric and global levels, the United States has embarked on an aggressive campaign to liberalize trade through bilateral, regional, and multilateral trade agreements. These agreements have conditioned liberalized trade upon the expansion of intellectual property law for multinational pharmaceutical companies holding ARV patents, among other essential medicines. Specifically, these agreements extend the protection of patents beyond the 20-year period; freeze domestic, generic manufacturing of ARVs; protect the manufacturers' drug testing data for five years—known as data exclusivity—and limit options for compulsory licensing. Additional measures include a reduction in the number of inventions, such as "diagnostic, therapeutic, and surgical methods," that can be excluded from patent law, the allowance of known substances to be patented again for each new use, and provisions requiring national drug regulatory authorities to block registration of generic medications. Such broadened intellectual property rules beyond those negotiated in the WTO TRIPS agreement are now referred to as "TRIPS-plus" measures (Médecins Sans Frontières 2004).

TRIPS-plus measures are included in agreements recently signed and in others currently being negotiated. For example, in May 2004, the United States signed the Central American Free Trade Agreement (CAFTA) with Costa Rica, El Salvador, Guatemala, Honduras, and Nicaragua—the Dominican Republic was added in August 2004. CAFTA requires both data exclusivity for five years and patent extensions to offset delays in the granting of a patent (Office of the United States Trade Representative 2004:15–16 to 15–18). The United States and the Andean countries (Colombia, Ecuador, Peru, and potentially Bolivia) had discussed a similar agreement known as the U.S.-Andean Free Trade Agreement; however, the agreement, fell apart over issues related to intellectual property law. Following the collapse of the regional free trade agreement (FTA), the United States started to pursue bilateral FTAs with each Andean country. In December 2005, Peru broke with the caution exercised by the other Andean countries and signed an FTA with the United States that included strengthened patent law provisions, including five-year data exclusivity and permitted expansion of patent length beyond 20 years (Blustein 2005; Office of the United States Trade Representative 2005). Colombia followed suit in February 2006 and signed an FTA with the United States (Office of the United States Trade Representative 2006). The United States has signed similar trade agreements with Singapore, Chile, and Morocco, and is currently working on agreements with Panama and the Southern African Custom Union (Botswana, Lesotho, Namibia, South Africa, and Swaziland).

Concern exists among health activists, academics, developing country governments, and clinicians working in resource-poor settings that these agreements will greatly augment the power of research-based pharmaceutical companies in the markets of developing nations, thereby greatly compromising access to ARVs for the poor. The extension of patent law beyond the provisions delineated in the TRIPS agreement should warrant great unease. Trade agreements currently being negotiated may severely constrain generic production of drugs, when generics are the primary source of affordable medications in resource-poor settings. TRIPS-plus provisions continue a tradition of limiting access to ART for the poor by instituting measures that condone high drug prices.

In addition to the uneasiness expressed by activists, clinicians, and researchers, similar concerns have recently been voiced from within the U.S. government. On September 30, 2004, 12 Democrats of the U.S. House of Representatives submitted a letter to President Bush expressing opposition to the intellectual property provisions in CAFTA and the current "free" trade agreement negotiations with the Andean countries and Panama (Consumer Project on Technology 2004). Authors of the letter criticized the lack of specific language on the rights to compulsory licensing and parallel importation and the imposition of five-year blockades on drug testing data. They warned that these agreements could violate the TRIPS agreement and the Doha Declaration (Russell 2004).

Others have also waved warning flags. In June 2004, Catholic bishops from the United States and Latin America issued a joint statement in which they warned of the ill consequences of the intellectual property provisions in CAFTA (Bishops' Secretariat of Central America 2004). Former health ministers and academics from Ecuador recently sent an open letter to the president of Ecuador warning against agreeing to strengthened intellectual property rules with the United States (Consumer Project on Technology 2006). Most recently, the majority of current South American ministers of health drew up a pledge to resist TRIPS-plus measures in any trade deals (Khor 2006). Numerous organizations—such as the Consumer Project on Technology, Médecins Sans Frontières, Health Action International, Oxfam, Treatment Action Campaign, Act Up Paris, and the Health Gap Coalition—have carefully researched and documented current trade negotiations and the concerns associated with the provisions stipulated in trade agreements.

The poor and sick also have consistently raised voices of opposition to trade agreement negotiations in their respective countries. In mid-March 2006, Ecuadorian peasants erected roadblocks throughout the country in protest of U.S.-Ecuadorian free trade, thereby forcing the government to declare a state of emergency (Andrade 2005). When Guatemala's legislature passed measures to strengthen patent law in order to facilitate CAFTA's approval, Guatemalan HIV-positive patients protested that the measures would make the already arduous task of obtaining ARV medicines even harder (Daniel 2005). Whether or not to ratify CAFTA became the primary issue in Costa Rica's recent presidential elections between Otton Solís, an opponent of CAFTA, and Oscar Arias, an ardent CAFTA supporter (Dickerson and Iritani 2006). Whether through their votes or protests, the poor have raised consistent opposition to trade agreements that U.S. and foreign trade ministers and multinational corporations, in other words the elite, tout as "pro-poor."

Finally, TRIPS-plus measures may have deleterious consequences on PEPFAR, a program ostensibly predicated on a vision for improved global health. Professing a desire to ensure that the poor receive the best HIV treatment medications possible, PEPFAR utilizes a stringent system for determining which drugs could be used in the treatment program. Originally, only brand-name antiretrovirals were utilized in the start-up phases of PEPFAR. However, criticism about the exorbitant costs associated with brand-name drugs forced PEPFAR to consider using cheaper generic medications, thereby allowing for increased HIV treatment. Generic antiretrovirals—such as lamivudine, zidovudine, and nevirapine—produced by companies in South Africa and India, received FDA approval in 2005 with the hope that this would allow greater numbers of patients to be treated (Kaiser Daily HIV/AIDS Report 2005b; U.S. Food and Drug Administration 2005a, 2005b). Strengthened intellectual property provisions, such as TRIPS-plus measures, however, threaten to prevent future production of low-cost, generic antiretroviral alternatives for use in PEPFAR. The pursuit of TRIPS-plus measures stands counter to the lofty aims to address global health through initiatives such as PEPFAR.

Withholding Medicines from the Poor: A Reversible Tragedy

As evidenced by the millions who die each year of AIDS without access to ART, the absence of particular commodities can be deadly. Of course, to really gain a panoramic picture of the deadly scope of withholding medicines from the poor, a laundry list of treatable diseases must be added to AIDS, including malaria, tuberculosis, diarrhea, and pneumonia. Far too often, medications to treat these diseases are out of reach of the poor. Structural violence—inflicted upon the poor via structural adjustment policies, exorbitant military versus development spending, gender inequity, corruption among multinational corporations and governments worldwide, and unfair intellectual property law—deserves a large share of the blame for the tragedy of global health inequity. However, these human-made obstacles to delivering medicines to the poor can be reversed. Rigorous scientific and social research combined with well-informed advocacy offers a powerful tool to reverse the withholding of medicines from the poor.

In the case of intellectual property law, we pose four questions that deserve careful, cross-disciplinary attention if we are to work toward increased access to medicines. First, in what ways can patent regulation promote access to medicines for the poor? As medications generally serve to promote health and healing, a universal right agreed upon by most countries of the world, we ask if medicines can be regulated by intellectual property law in an ethical manner consistent with the promotion of social justice. Pharmaceutical product patents were long prohibited in many countries because health care was viewed as a public good, not a commodity. Today, pharmaceutical patents are viewed by many as a "right" rewarded to those who invest time and money into drug development. However, in an era where many drugs are actually developed through public tax funding (Angell 2004), it is unclear where recognition of the creation of an idea should actually start and stop. Further examination of the motives and ethics behind pharmaceutical patenting may allow for a recalibration of patent law in a manner that promotes medication access for all.

Second, does strengthened IP law make economic sense for low- and middle-income countries? Current attempts to standardize and strengthen IP law are done across disparate economic and social environments. Wealthy countries, such as the United States and those of the EU, have slowly strengthened patent law over centuries as their economies developed. Should a country like Guatemala suddenly be asked to fast-forward IP law while its economic development lags behind? What makes sense for the U.S. economy today may not make sense for Guatemala. We are told, most commonly by wealthy corporate owners or powerful trade ministers, that international trade agreements are in the interests of poor countries. Interestingly, it is often dispute over IP that persists until the end of international trade agreement negotiations and occasionally leads to a collapse of the talks, as happened in the U.S.-Andean negotiations. Most often, though, low-income countries are willing to give in to U.S.

demands for strengthened IP law in order to reap the other benefits of a trade agreement. In this light, it is clear that the separation of IP discussions from other aspects of trade agreements would allow for a more objective, fair playing field.

Third, where are the voices of the poor in this debate? And if we listen, what are they telling us? Trade agreement negotiations typically are the exclusive domain of wealthy, powerful government representatives from the United States and low-income countries. Rarely are the poor, who represent the majority of the population in low-income countries, ever invited into these discussions. The voices of the poor do surface occasionally in the form of media coverage of their protests against "free" trade agreements, as seen in Ecuador and Guatemala. Their message is clear: we desire health and economic prosperity and strengthened IP law will not help us achieve that. Despite these glimpses into their perspectives on trade agreements, their views are largely excluded from the purview of analysis. Expanded attention to the voices of the poor by policy makers, academics, pharmaceutical companies, and health activists would serve to promote the development of IP law in a manner that suits all.

Finally, what values drive the strengthening of IP law? And interestingly, does the concept of intellectual property in fact contradict the principles underlying "free" trade? Free trade is touted as the removal of restrictions on the movement of goods and services whereas current U.S. policy seeks to strengthen intellectual property law in ways that tighten regulations over pharmaceutical products. Under the surface, though, praise for free markets and the spread of bolstered intellectual property law do share a commonality—a disturbing valuation of profit. The perception that the bottom line and the interests of stockholders are paramount in the business world raises questions about the ethics of intellectual property "rights." In this debate, the right to health for the poor and property rights for the wealthy often appear opposed. Can these values be reoriented in a manner that promotes the right to health and economic opportunity for all? The values driving current changes in the global economic system must be explored with the UN Declaration of Human Rights, agreed upon by the majority of the world's nations, constantly in mind.

At a time when powerful countries use their financial leverage to negotiate trade agreements to expand their markets—dictating a new global economic order that has far-reaching public health implications—the promotion of global health rests upon a thorough consideration of these questions. Although poverty, public health infrastructure, lack of political commitment, and poor drug quality certainly contribute to inadequate HIV treatment and are issues with which to contend, international patent law becomes another structural factor with dire implications for ART in resource-poor settings. At a time when both massive expansion of ARV therapy and the restructuring of U.S. trade relations with many nations are occurring, the relationship between international patent law and its effect upon access to ARVs in the developing world needs urgent attention.

With both the intensification of trade negotiations and concern about the impact of trade liberalization on developing countries, it is vital to formulate alternative strategies that promise to mitigate the impact of strengthened intellectual property law upon poor patients. One such example is the Technological Network on HIV/AIDS, a consortium of seven countries, including Brazil, Cuba, China, Nigeria, Russia, Thailand, and Ukraine, that aim to achieve self-sufficiency in the research, development, production, and distribution of ARVs and other related medications (Morel et al. 2005). In addition, these countries aim to critically engage intellectual property law in order to ensure that patents do not prevent appropriate care of the sick. Brazil has led these efforts by repeatedly threatening to break patents in order to continue providing free ART for all HIV-positive Brazilians; such threats resulted in dramatic ART price reductions from brand-name pharmaceutical companies (British Broadcasting Corporation News 2001). Such courageous efforts must be publicly and financially supported.

Through interdisciplinary efforts, the strengthening of intellectual property law can be effectively challenged in the interests of promoting global health equity. Ultimately, increased research and advocacy must aim to effect concrete changes in the ways that intellectual property provisions are integrated into trade agreements. Such changes require that governments and pharmaceutical companies are held responsible for their self-proclaimed commitments to the common good. Numerous avenues exist for promoting these goals. The World Health Organization could serve as a participant in bilateral, regional, and multilateral trade negotiations to ensure that public health remains a priority. In addition, the WTO could create a Working Group on Health as has been suggested (Kimball 2006) whose recommendations would be based on WHO guidelines and recommendations. Low- and middle-income countries could simultaneously agree to restrict intellectual property law discussions to WTO forums, thereby preventing strong-arming of smaller governments in bilateral, regional, and multilateral trade negotiations. By supporting each other and working within the WTO, smaller countries will occupy a stronger negotiating position that will respect public health demands. Finally, partnerships such as the Global Alliance for TB Drug Development should be more actively supported to allow for the development of drugs that are free of patent restrictions and address the diseases of the poor.

This chapter stresses the importance of examining international patent law when considering global access to ARVs. During a time of rapid advancement in medical care and treatment, inequalities between the rich and the poor in accessing essential medicines are unacceptable. However, current bilateral, regional, and multilateral trade agreements threaten to construct additional obstacles in the provision of ARVs by strengthening patent law and thereby hindering the production of cheaper generic medications. Now more than ever, the potential for IP law to contribute to the withholding of medicines from the poor must be explored. In summarizing the hazards of pharmaceutical product patents over 100 years ago, Dr. Stewart noted: "Every substance used for the treatment of the sick should be left free from all control by secret processes and patents, so that they may be manufactured and dealt in at the least expense to the consumer, i.e., the sick; and be open to free investigation by all who desire knowledge concerning them" (Stewart 1897:816B). These words have not lost their salience in addressing the needs of the sick today. While various pharmaceutical products have proved to be killer commodities, the intentional control of pharmaceutical production and access, we argue, can be no less deadly. What both sides of this coin share is the valuing of profit over health, no doubt a lethal formula.

Acronyms

AIDS	acquired immunodeficiency syndrome
ART	antiretroviral therapy
CAFTA	Central American Free Trade Agreement

EU	European Union
FTA	Free Trade Agreement
HIV	human immunodeficiency virus
IP	intellectual property
MDR-TB	multidrug-resistant tuberculosis
MSF	Médecins Sans Frontières
NGOs	nongovernmental organizations
PEPFAR	President's Emergency Plan for AIDS Relief
PhRMA	Pharmaceutical Research and Manufacturers of America
TNCs	transnational corporations
TRIPS	trade-related aspects of intellectual property rights
UN	United Nations
U.S.	United States
WHO	World Health Organization
WIPO	World Intellectual Property Organization
WTO	World Trade Organization

References

Adelman, Ken
2005 Praise for Piracy? Washington Times, May 9.
AMFAR
2004 Expanded Availability of HIV/AIDS Drugs in Asia Creates Urgent Need for Trained Doctors. TREAT Asia special report. Electronic document, www.amfar.org/cgi-bin/iowa/asia/about/index.html?record=15, accessed November 21, 2005.
Andrade, Carlos
2005 Ecuador Calls Emergency to Quell Indian Protest. Washington Post, March 21.
Angell, Marcia
2004 The Truth about the Drug Companies. New York: Random House.
Attaran, Amir
2004 How Do Patents and Economic Policies Affect Access to Essential Medicines in Developing Countries? Health Affairs 23:155–166.
Attaran, Amir, and Lee Gillespie-White
2001 Do Patents for Antiretroviral Drugs Constrain Access to AIDS Treatment in Africa? Journal of the American Medical Association 286:1886–1892.

Bishops' Secretariat of Central America and the Chairmen of the Domestic and International Policy Committees of the United States Conference of Catholic Bishops
2004 Joint Statement Concerning the United States-Central American Free Trade Agreement (US-CAFTA). Electronic document, www.usccb.org, accessed January 15, 2004.

Blustein, Paul
2005 U.S., Peru Strike Free-Trade Agreement. Washington Post, December 5.

Boldrin, Michele, and David Levine
2005 Against Intellectual Monopoly. Electronic document, http://levine.sscnet.ucla.edu/general/intellectual/against.htm, accessed April 12, 2006.

British Broadcasting Corporation News
2001 Brazil to Break AIDS Patent. Electronic document, accessed June 19, 2006. http://news.bbc.co.uk/2/hi/business/1505163.stm.

Cage, Sam
2005 WTO OKs Measures to Improve Drug Access. Associated Press, December 6.

Castro, Arachu
2005 Adherence to Antiretroviral Therapy: Merging the Clinical and Social Course of AIDS. PLoS Medicine 2:1217–1221 (e1338).

Castro, Arachu, and Paul Farmer
2005 Understanding and Addressing AIDS-Related Stigma: From Anthropological Theory to Clinical Practice in Haiti. American Journal of Public Health 95(1):53–59.

Castro, Arachu, and Merrill Singer
2004 Unhealthy Health Policy. Walnut Creek, CA: AltaMira Press.

Chien, Colleen
2003 Cheap Drugs at What Price to Innovation: Does the Compulsory Licensing of Pharmaceuticals Hurt Innovation? Berkeley Technology Law Journal 18:1–57.

Consumer Project on Technology
2004 Letter from 12 Members of Congress to President Bush on Intellectual Property Provisions of CAFTA. Electronic document, www.cptech.org/ip/health/trade/cafta/congress09302004.html, accessed June 19, 2006.
2005 Recent Health-Related Compulsory Licenses and Disputes. Electronic document, www.cptech.org/ip/health/cl/recent-examples.html, accessed April 13, 2006.
2006 Open Letter to President of Ecuador Signed by Former Health Ministers, Academics, and NGO representatives. Electronic document,

www.cptech.org/ip/health/trade/andean/ecuadorletter03232006.html, accessed June 19, 2006.

Daniel, Frank
2005 Guatemalan HIV Patients Slam New Trade Rules. Electronic document, www.alertnet.org/thenews/newsdesk/N30211004.htm, accessed April 1, 2006.

Dickerson, Marla, and Evelyn Iritani
2006 Trade Accord with U.S. Splits Voters in Costa Rica. Los Angeles Times, February 7.

Dumoulin, Jérôme, Yves-Antoine Flori, Phillipe Vinard, and Thomas Borel
2003 World Market Strategies for Drugs to Fight AIDS. *In* Economics of AIDS and Access to HIV/AIDS Care in Developing Countries: Issues and Challenges. J. P. Moatti, B. Coriatt, and Y. Souteyrand, eds. Pp. 213–244. Paris: French Agency for AIDS Research.

Farmer, Paul
2003 Pathologies of Power: Health, Human Rights, and the New War on the Poor. Berkeley: University of California Press.
2004 On Suffering and Structural Violence: A View from Below. *In* Violence in War and Peace: An Anthology. Nancy Scheper-Hughes and Philippe Bourgois, eds. Pp. 281–289. Malden: Blackwell.

Farmer, Paul, Joia Mukherjee Léandre, Marie Claud, Patrice Nevil, Mary Smith-Fawzi, Serena Koenig, Arachu Castro, Mercedes Becerra, Jeffrey Sachs, Amir Attaran, and Jim Kim
2001 Community-Based Approaches to HIV Treatment in Resource-Poor Settings. Lancet 358(9279):404–409.

Hammer, Scott, Kathleen Squires, Michael Hughes, Janet Grimes, Lisa Demeter, Judith Currier, Joseph Eron, Judith Feinberg, Henry Balfour, Lawrence Deyton, Jeffrey Chodakewitz, and Margaret Fischl
1997 A Controlled Trial of Two Nucleoside Analogues Plus Indinavir in Persons with Human Immunodeficiency Virus Infection and CD4 Cell Counts of 200 per Cubic Millimeter or Less. New England Journal of Medicine 333(11):725–733.

Harries, A. D., D. S. Nyangulu, N. J. Hargreaves, O. Kaluwa, and F. M. Salaniponi
2001 Preventing Antiretroviral Anarchy in Sub-Saharan Africa. Lancet 358(9279):410–414.

Joint Action Committee against Amendment of the Indian Patents Act
2004 Declaration of the Joint Action Committee against Amendment of the Indian Patents Act. Electronic document, www.cptech.org/ip/health/c/india/ngodeclaration12292004.html, accessed April 14, 2005.

Kaiser Daily HIV/AIDS Report

2005a Brazil Requests Voluntary Licensing for AIDS Drugs to Treat More Patients, Reduce Costs of Importing Patented Drugs. Electronic document, www.kaisernetwork.org/daily_reports/rep_index.cfm?hint=1&DR_ID=28706, accessed November 21, 2005.

2005b Politics and Policy: FDA Approves Generic Antiretroviral Drug Combination, Allowing PEPFAR to Purchase Drugs for Use in Developing Countries. Electronic document, www.kaisernetwork.org/daily_reports/rep_index.cfm?DR_ID=27788, accessed March 23, 2006.

Khor, Martin

2005 Impasse on Talks on TRIPS and Health "Permanent Solution." Third World Network Service on Health Issues, no. 15. Geneva: Third World Network.

2006 South American Ministers Vow to Avoid TRIPS-Plus Measures. Third World Network Service on WTO and Trade Issues. Geneva: Third World Network.

Kim, Jim

2004 WHO Letter to India's Health Minister on Patent Legislation. Electronic document, www.cptech.org/ip/health/c/india/who12172004.html, accessed April 14, 2006.

Kimball, A. M.

2006 The Health of Nations: Happy Birthday WTO. Lancet 367:188–190.

Loff, Bebe

2002 No Agreement Reached in Talks on Access to Cheap Drugs. Lancet 360(9349):1951.

Lucchini, Stéphane, Boubou Cisse, Ségolène Duran, Marie de Cenival, Caroline Comiti, Marion Gaudry, and Jean-Paul Moatti

2003 Decrease in Prices of Antiretroviral Drugs for Developing Countries: From Political "Philanthropy" to Regulated Markets? *In* Economics of AIDS and Access to HIV/AIDS Care in Developing Countries: Issues and Challenges. Jean-Paul Moatti, B. Coriatt, and Y. Souteyrand, eds. Pp. 169–211. Paris: French Agency for AIDS Research.

May, Christopher, and Susan Sell

2006 Intellectual Property Rights: A Critical History. London: Lynne Rienner.

McNeil, Donald G.

2005 India Alters Law on Drug Patents. New York Times, March 24.

Médecins Sans Frontières

2004 Access to Medicines at Risk across the Globe: What to Watch Out for in the Free Trade Agreements with the United States. Electronic document, www.accessmed-msf.org/documents/ftabriefingenglish.pdf, accessed November 21, 2005.

2005a MSF to WTO: Re-think Access to Life-Saving Drugs Now. Electronic document, www.msf.org/msfinternational/invoke.cfm?objectid=224B1730-E018-0C72-091E8829E29F80E6&component=toolkit.article&method=full_html, accessed January 6, 2006.

2005b Sources of Affordable Generic Medicines Drying Up? India Should Ensure Global Access to Medicines When Amending Its Patent Law. New York: MSF.

Millen, Joyce, and Timothy Holtz

2000 Dying for Growth, Part I: Transnational Corporations and the Health of the Poor. *In* Dying for Growth: Global Inequality and the Health of the Poor. Jim Kim, Joyce Millen, Alec Irwin, and John Gershman, eds. Pp. 177–223. Monroe, ME: Common Courage Press.

Morel, Carlos, Tara Acharya, Denis Broun, Ajit Dangi, Christopher Elias, N. Ganguly, Charles Gardner, R. Gupta, Jane Haycock, Anthony Heher, Peter Hotez, Hannah Kettler, Gerald Keusch, Anatole Krattiger, Fernando Kreutz, Sanjaya Lall, Keun Lee, Richard Mahoney, Adolfo Martinez-Palomo, R. Mashelkar, Stephen Matlin, Mandi Mzimba, Joachim Oehler, Robert Ridley, Pramilla Senanayake, Peter Singer, and Mikyung Yun

2005 Health Innovation Networks to Help Developing Countries Address Neglected Diseases. Science 309:401–404.

Mukherjee, Joia, Michael Rich, Adrienne Socci, J. Keith Joseph, Felix Alcántara, Sonya Shin, Jennifer Furin, Mercedes Becerra, Donna Barry, Jim Kim, Jaime Bayona, Paul Farmer, Mary Smith Fawzi, and Kwonjune Seung

2004 Programmes and Principles in Treatment of Multidrug-Resistant Tuberculosis. Lancet 363(9407):474–481.

Müller, Olaf, Tumani Corrah, Elly Katabira, Frank Plummer, and David Mabey

1998 Antiretroviral Therapy in Sub-Saharan Africa. Lancet 351(9095):68.

New York Times

2005 India's Choice (editorial). New York Times, January 18.

Office of the United States Global AIDS Coordinator

2004 The President's Plan for AIDS Relief: U.S. Five-Year Global HIV/AIDS Strategy. Washington, DC: State Department.

2005 Engendering Bold Leadership. The President's Plan for Emergency AIDS Relief: First Annual Report to Congress. Washington, DC: State Department.

Office of the United States Trade Representative

2004 The Dominican Republic—Central America—United States Free Trade Agreement. Intellectual Property Rights. Electronic document, www.ustr.gov/assets/Trade_Agreements/Bilateral/CAFTA/CAFTA-DR_Final_Texts/asset_upload_file934_3935.pdf, accessed April 15, 2006.

2005 United States and Colombia Conclude Free Trade Agreement. Electronic document, www.ustr.gov/Document_Library/Press_Releases/2006/February/United_States_Colombia_Conclude_Free_Trade_Agreement.html, accessed April 1, 2006.

2006 US-Peru Free-Trade Agreement—Chapter 16, Intellectual Property Rights. Electronic document, www.ustr.gov/assets/Trade_Agreements/Bilateral/Peru_TPA/Final_Texts/asset_upload_file509_8706.pdf, accessed April 1, 2006.

Oliveira, Maria, Jorge Bermudez, Gabriela Chaves, and Germán Velásquez

2004 Has the Implementation of the TRIPS Agreement in Latin America and the Caribbean Produced Intellectual Property Legislation That Favours Public Health? Bulletin of the World Health Organization 82:815–821.

Pécoul, Bernard, Pierre Chirac, Patrice Trouiller, and Jacques Pinel

1999 Access to Essential Drugs in Developing Countries: A Lost Battle? Journal of the American Medical Association 281:361–367.

Pharmaceutical Research and Manufacturers of America

2005 PhRMA Welcomes TRIPS and Public Health Agreement. Electronic document, www.phrma.org/mediaroom/press/releases/06.12.2005.1335.cfmvia, accessed April 13, 2006.

Rosenberg, Tina

2001 Look at Brazil. New York Times, January 28.

Russell, Asia

2004 House Democrats Criticize Administration over IPR Provisions in FTAS. Electronic document, http://lists.essential.org/pipermail/ip-health/2004-October/007018.html,accessed April 15, 2006.

Severe, Patrice, Paul Leger, Charles Macarthur, Francine Noel, Gerry Bonhomme, Gyrlande Bois, Erik George, Stefan Kenel-Pierre, Peter Wright, Roy Gulick, Warren Johnson, Jean Pape, and Daniel Fitzgerald

2005 Antiretroviral Therapy in a Thousand Patients with AIDS in Haiti. New England Journal of Medicine 353(22):2325–2334.

Sterne, Jonathan, Miguel Hernán, Bruno Ledergerber, Kate Tilling, Rainer Weber, Pedram Sendi, Martin Rickenbach, James Robins, Matthias Egger, and the Swiss HIV Cohort Study

2005 Long-Term Effectiveness of Potent Antiretroviral Therapy in Preventing AIDS and Death: A Prospective Cohort Study. Lancet 366 (9483):378–384.

Stewart, F. E.
1897 Is It Ethical for Medical Men to Patent Medical Inventions? Journal of the American Medical Association 278(10):816B.
Stiglitz, Joseph
2004 New Trade Pacts Betray the Poorest Partners. New York Times, July 24.
't Hoen, Ellen
2003 TRIPS, Pharmaceutical Patents and Access to Essential Medicines: Seattle, Doha, and Beyond. *In* Economics of AIDS and Access to HIV/AIDS Care in Developing Countries: Issues and Challenges. J. P. Moatti, B. Coriatt, and Y. Souteyrand, eds. Pp. 39–67. Paris: French Agency for AIDS Research.
UNAIDS
2004 India, Epidemiological Fact Sheets on HIV and Sexually Transmitted Diseases—2004 Update. Geneva: UNAIDS.
2005 AIDS Epidemic Update December 2005. Geneva: UNAIDS.
United Nations Office for the Coordination of Humanitarian Affairs
2005 "Lazarus Drug": ARVs in the Treatment Era. Electronic document, www.irinnews.org/webspecials/ARV-era/48816.asp, accessed June 19, 2006.
U.S. Food and Drug Administration
2005a FDA Tentatively Approves First Generic Nevirapine under the President's Emergency Plan for AIDS Relief. Electronic document, www.fda.gov/bbs/topics/NEWS/2005/NEW01187.html, accessed March 23, 2006.
2005b HHS/FDA Tentatively Approves Another First-Time Generic AIDS Drug Associated with the President's Emergency Plan for AIDS Relief. Electronic document, www.fda.gov/bbs/topics/NEWS/2005/NEW01202.html, accessed March 23, 2006.
U.S. Patent and Trademark Office
2005 General Information Concerning Patents. Electronic document, www.uspto.gov/web/offices/pac/doc/general/#laws, accessed on April 12, 2006.
Weidle, Paul, Samuel Malamba, Raymond Mwebaze, Catherine Sozi, Gideon Rukondo, Robert Downing, Debra Hanson, Dorothy Ochola, Peter Mugyenyi, Jonathan Mermin, Badara Samb, and Eve Lackritz
2002 Assessment of a Pilot Antiretroviral Drug Therapy Programme in Uganda: Patients' Response, Survival, and Drug Resistance. Lancet 360(9326):34–40.
Weinberg, Stephanie
2006 US Congress letter to USTR on Guatemala & IP in CAFTA. Electronic document, http://lists.essential.org/pipermail/ip-health, accessed April 15, 2006.

Westerhaus, Michael, and Arachu Castro
2006 How Do Intellectual Property Law and International Trade Agreements Affect Access to Antiretroviral Therapy. PLoS Medicine 3(8):e332.
World Health Organization
2004 Antiretrovirals and Developing Countries: Report by the Secretariat. EB115/32. Geneva: World Health Organization.
2005a Coverage and Need for Antiretroviral Treatment—June 2005. Electronic document, www.who.int/hiv/facts/cov0605/en/index.html, accessed June 20, 2006.
2005b The WHO Model List of Essential Medicines: 14th Model List of Essential Medicines. Geneva: World Health Organization.
2006a Public Health, Innovation, and Intellectual Property Rights. Geneva: World Health Organization.
2006b Progress on Global Access to HIV Antiretroviral Therapy: A Report on "3 by 5" and Beyond. Geneva: World Health Organization.
World Intellectual Property Organization
1883 Paris Convention for the Protection of Industrial Property. Geneva.
2006 Contracting Parties of the Paris Convention. Electronic document, www.wipo.int/treaties/en/ShowResults.jsp?lang=en&treaty_id=2, accessed on April 10, 2006.
World Trade Organization
1994 Trade-Related Aspects of Intellectual Property Rights. Electronic document, www.wto.org/english/docs_e/legal_e/27-trips.pdf, accessed April 12, 2006.
2001 Declaration on the TRIPS Agreement and Public Health. Electronic document, www.wto.org/english/thewto_e/minist_e/min01_e/mindecl_trips_e.htm, accessed April 12, 2006.
2003a Implementation of Paragraph 6 of the Doha Declaration on the TRIPS Agreement and Public Health. Electronic document, www.wto.org/english/tratop_e/trips_e/implem_para6_e.htm, accessed April 13, 2006.
2003b The General Council Chairperson's Statement. Electronic document, www.wto.org/english/news_e/news03_e/trips_stat_28aug03_e.htm, accessed April 13, 2006.
2005 Members and Observers. Electronic document, www.wto.org/english/thewto_e/whatis_e/tif_e/org6_e.htm, accessed on April 11, 2006.

CONCLUSION

KILLER COMMODITIES AND SOCIETY

Fighting for Change

Hans Baer and Merrill Singer

Cumulatively, there can be no doubt that the killer commodity body count, in terms of actual deaths, but also all injuries and inflicted human suffering, is astronomical. Indeed, it is safe to say that killer commodities are a far greater threat to the lives and well-being of people in the United States and globally than has so far proved to be the case with terrorism, a menace that nonetheless attracts far greater government concern than the fight against harmful commercial products. Indeed, there appears to be a discernable pattern of inattention to killer commodities, with cases only attracting sustained and focused media consideration in extreme instances and rarely the notice of top government leaders without persistent reporting in the national media, and even then the attention of policy makers to dangerous products tends to be fleeting. There is something gravely wrong with this picture, a fundamental failure in what has come to be understood as a primary governmental responsibility: protecting the populace. The purpose of this book is to call attention to this fact; to show the broad range of deadly commodities on the market, in our communities and environments, in the cupboards of our homes, in the hands of our children, and in the cells of our bodies; to address the question of why our lives have come to be filled with and surrounded by perilous products; and to draw attention to popular efforts to turn the tide against the reigning culture of deregulation, corporate self-monitoring, and profits-above-people valuation driving the global killer commodity trend. While the array of killer commodities and their noxious impact is far greater than the specific topics and issues that could be covered by this book, the authors who contributed chapters have sought to illustrate some of the important sites on the global map of killer commodities. The picture collectively drawn by these accounts is chilling. It is intended, however, not to demoralize but to anger, not to frustrate but to build awareness of a clear and present danger. In short, it is intended as a call to arms and as fuel for social action.

Making the Connection between Killer Commodities and the Culture of Consumption

Global capitalism fosters a treadmill of commodity production and consumption primarily for the purpose of generating profits for the benefit of the few, and in the process, because they are rated of lesser importance to profit making, often sacrifices human safety, health, and even life. Consequently, a critical anthropology and broader social science of killer commodities must ultimately come to grips with the "culture of consumption" that is an integral component of global capitalism and the various processes of globalization, particularly in developed countries but also developing countries as well. As Slater (1997:121) aptly observes,

> culture as a whole has become consumer culture. All culture is now produced, exchanged and consumed in the form of commodities. . . . All consumption . . . has become compensatory, integrative and functional. It offers the illusions of freedom, choice and pleasure in exchange for the real loss of these qualities through alienated labor; or integrates people within the general system of exploitation by encouraging them to define their identities, desires and interests in terms of possessing commodities; and is functional in that consumer culture offers experiences ideally designed to reproduce workers in the form of alienated labour.

In order to survive, capitalism must generate an artificial need, namely the need to endlessly consume a diverse range of commodities, even potentially dangerous and lethal ones. Sinclair Lewis, a socialist novelist, satirized emergent consumerism in *Babbitt*, an early 20th-century novel in which he dramatically depicted a life of selling and consuming commodities as a one-way road to alienated mass conformity. As humanity enters the 21st century, we see not only the enormous expansion of consumerism in the developed world but also in developing countries, such as China and India—by far the two most populous countries in the world. While most of the commodities that the capitalist culture of consumption encourages people to purchase are not physically dangerous, as this volume emphasizes, some are quite deadly. More broadly, global capitalism and its associated ever-expanding cycle of production and consumption have fostered what Hofrichter (2000) terms "toxic culture," of which killer commodities are a part. According to Hofrichter (2000:1), "elements of toxic culture might include the unquestioned production of hazardous substances, tolerance for economic blight, dangerous technologies, substandard housing, chronic stress, and exploitative working conditions."

Global Trends in Killer Commodities

There is evidence that global capitalism manifests an ever-growing production of killer commodities. For example, despite rising gasoline or petrol prices around the globe, annual automobile production increased from 12.9 million vehicles in 1960 to 39.6 million vehicles in 2000 (Dicken 2003:358). The toxic exhaust produced by this ever-growing fleet is playing a significant role in triggering global warming. Ironically, another killer commodity that certain multinational corporations and states have begun to promote as a cure for global warming is the nuclear power plant. Like other commodities, the construction of these plants and the electricity they are intended to generate are of primary appeal to elements of the corporate sectors as another source of profits. As for the assertions that nuclear plants will help solve the problem of global warming, Green (n.d.:3) argues that

> claims that nuclear power is "greenhouse free" are incorrect as substantial greenhouse gas emissions are generated across the nuclear fuel cycle. Fossil-fuel generated electricity is more greenhouse intensive than nuclear power, but this comparative benefit will be eroded as higher-grade uranium ores are depleted. Most of the earth's uranium is found in very poor grade ores, and recovery of uranium from those ores is likely to be considerably more greenhouse intensive.

In her recent book, *Nuclear Power Is Not the Answer to Global Warming or Anything Else*, Helen Caldicott, a pediatrician, discusses not only the lethal dangers of nuclear power but also argues that it contributes to global warming and that there is not sufficient uranium in the world to sustain nuclear power over the long term. Like Green, she maintains (Caldicott 2006:xiii) that "nuclear power is not 'clean and green,' as the industry claims, because large amounts of traditional fossil fuels are required to mine and refine the uranium needed to run nuclear power reactors, to construct the massive concrete reactor buildings, and to transport and store the toxic radioactive waste created by the nuclear process." Furthermore, and of no small import in its own right, nuclear power plants produce plutonium which can be used to develop nuclear bombs, killer commodities of unparalleled lethality.

In addition to the massive dangers from the meltdown of a nuclear reactor, such as the ones that occurred at Three Mile Island and Chernobyl (Petryna 2003), nuclear power plants emit radiation which particularly impacts the health of workers in these facilities but also, vis-à-vis dissemination through air and water, the health of people residing in surrounding communities. Radiation also is released in the process of mining, milling, and enriching uranium to create nuclear energy (see Smith 2006). Last, but not least, the transportation and storage of nuclear wastes poses a massive health risk to humans and animals.

Yet another potential killer commodity of growing importance, at least in its discarded state, is the computer. Worn-out computer equipment, along with discarded cell phones, televisions, refrigerators, and other electronic devices, have become part and parcel of an entity referred to as *electronic waste* or *e-waste*. Computer equipment consists of more than 1,000 materials, many of which are highly toxic, including chlorinated and brominated substances, toxic gases, toxic metals, biologically active materials, acids, plastics, and plastic additives. Computer companies, such as Microsoft and Intel, continuously create new programs that require more speed, memory, and power, all of which have resulted in an industry characterized by fast-paced built-in obsolescence. While most defunct computers end up in storage, many find their way into landfills, incinerators, or on ships bound for developing countries, such as China, India, Pakistan, and various West African countries, where they will join the continually growing mound of hazardous waste on the planet. Simmons (2005:1) reports, for example:

> India's poor scrape a living by breaking down PCs and monitors. They boil, crush or burn parts in order to extract valuable materials like gold or platinum. But what they do not realize is that the toxic chemicals inside like cadmium and lead can pose serious health risks.

Toxic substances from e-waste eventually may leak into the air, water, and soil and contribute to lung complications and brain damage, signaling thereby the longevity of the threat inherent in killer commodities.

Why Don't Governments Protect Us Better?

An overview of the voluminous literature on the role of the state in advanced capitalist societies indicates that it facilitates the process of capital accumulation and legitimates this process in a variety of ways, including the creation of regulatory agencies ostensibly designed to protect the public but which, as seen in several chapters in this book, actually serve to distract and pacify its legitimate concerns (Freitag 1985). Despite the fact that regulatory agencies may conduct public hearings, these tend to be largely token gestures. According to Albert Szymanski (1978:205), a critical sociologist,

> although the regulatory commissions . . . are legally administrative agencies of the U.S. government, they function largely as parts of the industries they regulate. The private corporations dominate them by controlling appointments to the commissions and providing staff, through official advisory retiring commissioners and leading staff people.

There often exists a "revolving-door" syndrome in which there is an interchange of personnel between state regulatory agencies and the private enterprises that they purportedly regulate. Sociologist G. William Domhoff, for example, views regulatory agencies and rulings as part and parcel of what he terms the "special-interest process." He asserts (Domhoff 2006:173) that this "process is carried out by people with a wide range of experiences: former elected officials, experts who once served on congressional staffs or in regulatory agencies, employees of trade associations, corporate executives whose explicit function is government liaison, and an assortment of lawyers and public-relations specialists." For example, a U.S. General Accounting Office investigation revealed that about 10 percent of FDA senior staff "came directly from pharmaceutical firms, while about 10 percent of those who left the FDA immediately took up positions within the industry" (Abraham and Sheppard 1999:24).

Corporations routinely lobby, often successfully, for the insertion of special, self-serving loopholes in regulatory legislation. According to Domhoff (2006:175),

> when the Food and Drug Administration tried to regulate tobacco, Congress refused authorization in 2000 in deference to the tobacco industry. The FDA is now so lax with pharmaceutical companies that one-third of its scientific employees have less than full confidence that it tests new drugs adequately, and two-thirds expressed a lack of confidence in its market.

Although both the Republican and Democratic parties in the United States work within the parameters of a capitalist economy, the latter is somewhat more open to input from various social movements, such as labor, environmental, and consumer groups, all of which have lobbied for measures relating to occupational health, toxic wastes, and product safety. In some instances, regulatory agencies may be able to evade corporate influence to a limited degree, as happened when the FDA was able to impose some stringent regulations on the tobacco industry (Domhoff 2006). But this, of course, occurred in a climate in which the public credibility of the tobacco industry had been thoroughly damaged, as detailed in the introduction in this book.

Another problem with regulatory agencies is a duplication of effort, often resulting in varying and even conflicting guidelines. In terms of the asbestos regulation in the United States, for example, as discussed in the introduction, the Occupational Safety and Health Administration (OSHA) regulates workplace exposure to asbestos; the Mine Safety and Health Administration regulates the mining and milling of asbestos ore; the Food and Drug Administration oversees the use of asbestos in food, drugs, and cosmetics; and the Environmental Protection Agency, bearing the greatest responsibility, regulates the use of asbestos.

Ultimately, successful implementation of regulations requires imposition of enforcement strategies up to and including arresting, fining, and imprisoning violators. Further, the implementation of uniform national and international laws is needed to prevent industries from moving to regions or countries with limited regulation. As Turshen (1989:70) points out,

> the U.S. South owes its industrial growth to the relocation of factories before the passage of national legislation on clean air and water and occupational safety and health. Or, to take an international example, restrictions on the asbestos industry in the United States motivated its removal to Mexico, which an international convention banning asbestos production might have prevented. . . . Similarly, current concerns about the export of hazardous wastes by private firms located in industrial countries with strict laws to African nations with no protective legislation illustrate the role of international power relations in issues that affect national health and safety.

People's Struggles against Killer Commodities

Newspaper and magazine exposés of the meat industry and the publication of Upton Sinclair's *The Jungle*, which exposed unsanitary conditions in Chicago stockyards early in the 20th century, contributed to the development and passage of the Pure Food and Drugs Act of 1906 as well as the creation of the Food and Drug Administration, which was designed primarily to control the marketing of dubious and potentially dangerous foodstuffs. While the labor, environmental, ethnic rights, and women's movements have been involved in challenging the manufacture and marketing of killer commodities, historically, the foremost entity involved in this effort has been the consumer movement, a disparate collection of voluntary grassroots as well as professionalized advocacy groups. This movement has a long, if somewhat meandering, history. Florence Kelley spearheaded the creation of the National Consumers League in 1899 with the intention of abolishing sweatshops and improving manufacturing standards in the United States (Warne 1993). Beginning in the 1920s, figures such as sociologist Thorstein Veblen, Herbert Hoover (an engineer who went on to become U.S. president), Stuart Chase, and Frederick J. Schlink called for the standardized manufacturing procedures that would ensure that consumers were purchasing quality commodities (Warne 1993). Their efforts culminated with the establishment of Consumers Union of the United States in 1936. Consumers' International, formerly the International Organization of Consumers Unions, negotiated for UN ratification of the Code of Conduct for Transnational Corporations.

Consumer advocates have addressed a wide range of issues, including auto safety, food and drug safety, and the disclosure of product contents. For the most part, the consumer movement has had a liberal rather than radical agenda in that it seeks to function within existing institutions. It has attracted many professional people, including lawyers, scientists, and academics. Given that the consumer movement "consists of a loosely knit band of individuals, deriving its sustenance more from moral outrage and a desire for justice than from extensive financial resources," it has tended to eschew direct mass action (Mayer 1989:5).

The 1960s and the 1970s constituted the golden age of consumer advocacy in the United States. This era essentially came to a close with President Jimmy Carter's failure to persuade Congress to create the Agency for Consumer Advocacy and the subsequent election of Ronald Reagan to the presidency in 1980. Reagan's election, in effect, signaled the ascendancy of a probusiness anticonsumer initiative. President Gerald Ford vetoed the initial legislation designed to create the Agency for Consumer Advocacy, which had passed both houses of Congress in 1975, and a conservative coalition in the House managed to kill the bill in 1977 during the Carter years.

The Reagan administration had a significant adverse impact upon the proconsumer policies of the Consumer Product Safety Commission, the Federal Trade Commission, the National Highway Traffic Safety Administration, the Environmental Protection Agency, the Occupational Safety and Health Administration, the Legal Services Corporation, and the Freedom of Information Act. In this sense, the Reagan years constituted a corporate victory in the creation of a social and legal climate that was favorable to the expanded production, deregulation, and sale of killer commodities. The so-called Reagan revolution, in other words, from a class perspective, was revolution from above waged against those below.

The popular demand for commodity regulation and consumer safety, however, did not fade away. As Bykerk and Maney (1995:xi) point out,

> in this environment, consumer advocates and their allies resorted to traditional protest tactics like boycotts as a means to get the attention and cooperation of producers. Allies drawn from environmental, civil rights, women's and religious groups, and sympathetic media helped in boycotts of McDonald's, Nestle, 7-11 stores, and others. In comparison with the chilly reception from the White House, congressional committees continued to provide a forum for consumer grievances.

Organizations involved in consumer advocacy, of which there are many within the United States and worldwide, include Action on Smoking and Health, the Center for Auto Safety, the Consumer Federation of America, the Center for Science in the Public Interest, Partners in Health, the National Association of African Americans for Positive Imagery, the Marin Institute, Mothers Against Drunk Driving, the Center on Alcohol Marketing and Youth, Kids in Danger, WATCH, the National Coalition Against the Misuse of Pesticides, the National Toxics Campaign, and the Union of Concerned Scientists. As noted in the introduction, in 1971, consumer advocate Ralph Nader founded Public Citizen as a research, lobbying, and litigation organization which came to consist of five subsections, namely Buyers Up, Congress Watch, the Critical Mass Energy Project, the Health Research Group, and the Litigation Group (more recently, these have been reorganized to include Congress Watch, the Critical Mass Energy Program, the Health Research Group, the Auto Safety Group, Global Trade Watch, and the Litigation Group). The mission of Public Citizen is to advocate for openness and democratic accountability in government; for the right of consumers to seek redress in the courts; for clean, safe, and sustainable energy sources; for social and economic justice in trade policies; for strong health, safety, and environmental protections; and for safe, effective, and affordable prescription drugs and health care (Bykerk and Maney 1995; Public Citizen 2006).

One of the protest strategies that consumer groups have adopted, with mixed results, has been boycotts of products that they view as too expensive or unsafe. At an international level, the International Baby Action Network, for example, organized the famous Nestlé boycott, protesting the irresponsible marketing of baby formula in developing countries. In the case of the United States, efforts of the consumer movement have contributed to drug amendments to the Food, Drug, and Cosmetic Act of 1962, the Federal

Cigarette Labeling and Advertising Act of 1965, the Consumer Product Safety Act of 1972, the Infant Formula Act of 1984, and antismoking legislation in numerous communities around the country.

The consumer movement often overlaps with other social movements. An example of this overlap is seen in the work of environmental breast cancer activists who have expressed concern about various chemicals, particularly xenoestrogens that are present in plastics, pesticides, herbicides, cosmetics, dyes, and other synthetic products, which are believed to cause breast cancer by imitating natural estrogen (Ley 2006). An estimated one to two million Americans now purchase their medicines from Canadian drugstores over the Internet, despite the fact that Congress passed legislation prohibiting anyone other than manufacturers to import prescription drugs (Angell 2004). State governments have been exploring new ways to cut drug costs, including, in some instances, encouraging their populations to cross the border into Canada to purchase drugs (Angell 2004). Furthermore, Americans have been chartering buses destined for Canada and Mexico in order to purchase prescription drugs.

In large part, the consumer movement has become increasingly professionalized and institutionalized. Notes Mayer (1989:168),

> issues pertaining to workers' rights and environmental protection remain on the consumerist agenda, but clearly in a position of secondary importance. In terms of broader social goals, the movement tacitly supports the conventional objectives of economic growth and equality of opportunity, but not the more radical objective of income redistribution.

This assessment of the consumer movement continues to be accurate.

Nonetheless, grassroots consumer initiatives continue to emerge even in the most oppressed communities. In African American and Latino communities across the United States, struggles have developed against both the alcohol and tobacco industries in response to their continued and concerted efforts to market deadly products to ethnic minorities. With regard to the alcohol industry, a frequent target of community fight-back initiatives in both African American and Latino communities has been the marketing and aggressive promotion of malt liquor. Because of its high alcohol content (double that of regular beer and equivalent, in the common 40-ounce bottle, to five shots of whiskey), as well as its concentration of corn syrup and other sweeteners that are thought to accelerate intoxication, malt liquor has acquired the nickname "liquid crack." While advertisements for malt liquor never appear in suburban areas, they have been displayed in inner city communities across the country and in various media (TV, radio, magazines) with a high-minority audience, often involving the manipulation of ethnic cultural symbols for this purpose. An exemplary community fight-back against a malt liquor manufacturer targeting an ethnic minority population began in June 1991, when the G. Heileman Brewery announced the release of a new brand called PowerMaster in Chicago (Singer 2007). The community responded with sit-ins at the corporate office (which entailed travel to Wisconsin), community demonstrations, and a letter-writing campaign to the Bureau of Alcohol, Tobacco, Firearms and Explosives. Eventually, the latter responded revoking the product's license because its name violated the Federal Alcohol Administration Act of 1935, which banned the labeling or advertising of beer as being "strong, full strength, extra strength or high test," all words that could be construed as indicators of a product's alcohol potency. One of the key lessons learned by grassroots efforts to confront the legal drug industry (composed of Big Tobacco, Big Alcohol, and Big Pharma) is that winning individual battles does not mean that the war has been won. Corporate manufacturers continue to develop and introduce harmful products that are specially geared to oppressed populations.

A consumer movement also has emerged in developing countries, including groups that are specifically focused on the alcohol, tobacco, and pharmacy industries (e.g., Global Partnerships for Tobacco Control). In terms of killer commodities, the concerns of consumer organizations in developing countries "range from hazardous goods [e.g., asbestos] that are banned in industrialized nations, to products that are appropriate in the industrialized world but that pose immense risks for Third World populations [e.g., infant formula]" (Post 1986:167). Consumer groups in developing countries have monitored the practices and effects of multinational corporations and have lobbied their respective national governments for protection.

Overall, the consumer movement remains a somewhat amorphous array of often single issue–oriented groups that sometimes come together around common concerns. In order to become more effective, it may be necessary to form better linkages with other social movements, particularly the anticorporate globalization, labor, environmental, environmental justice, and indigenous rights movements. Indeed, the anti-SUV movement represents a convergence of the consumer advocacy and environmentalist movements. According to Vanderheiden (2006:24), "the anti-SUV movement crystallized as a grassroots revolt against an object of common disapprobation in which a wide variety of people invoke an equally wide variety of grievances against what is treated as either a cause or symbol of what is ailing society."

Readers may feel overwhelmed by the pervasiveness of "killer commodities" around the globe today, the power and size of the corporate manufacturers and promoters of these products, and the enormous hurdles faced by a disparate consumer movement and other small grassroots initiatives. The test facing consumer initiatives is how to collectively address these monumental challenges and participate in a large effort to create a just, environmentally sustainable, and healthy global community. The answers are not easy and require collaboration with many individuals and groups outside of the relatively small worlds of both medical anthropology and consumer advocacy. Critical anthropologists cannot create a world devoid of killer commodities, but we can point to the role of global capitalism in creating such products in its profit-making endeavors. We need to engage in "pragmatic solidarity" with a broad coalition of progressive people, ranging from health practitioners to academics in other disciplines (particularly sociology, political science, policy studies, and public health) and including the staffs of research institutes, government agencies, international health organizations, and nongovernmental organizations (NGOs), as well as people involved in peace, social justice, environmental issues, anticorporate globalization or global justice, health rights, women's rights, and other social and labor movements and progressive political parties around the world. Kenyon Stebbins, for example, is a critical anthropologist who embodies the notion of health praxis—the merger of theory and social action. He has conducted extensive research on smoking in Mexico and the impact of multinational tobacco corporations on the health of developing societies (Stebbins 1987). In addition, he was, prior to his retirement, an antiindustry activist in West Virginia while a faculty member at West Virginia University (Stebbins 1997).

The role of the scholar-activist is a double-edged sword. On the one hand, it may be exhilarating and offer a way to participate in making a difference in creating a healthier, safer, and more just world. On the other hand, social activism often is time-consuming, exhausting, and discouraging when the results of one's efforts are not apparent. Most social activism does not translate into large research grants and publications. Ultimately, social activism must be part and parcel of a critical anthropology that entails making research and analytic materials available to those people—namely the indigenous populations, peasants, proletariats, and ethnic minorities—who have been the traditional objects of our studies.

One possible starting point is to play a role in contributing to the array of information available to working-class people around the world, showing that the products, including the killer commodities, that they help to manufacture and consume serve as mechanisms for perpetuating their exploitation. The involvement of working-class people in the "pedagogy of the oppressed" as part of the larger struggle against killer commodities will require the unification of the labor movement with other progressive movements, including the consumer movement of which many working-class people are already a part.

Researching Killer Commodities in the Future: Pressing Questions for Praxis

In that capitalism ultimately views the production of commodities, regardless of their safety, as the bottom line in the generation of profits, in a sense it functions as a *global killing machine*. While this volume has not included any discussion of nuclear and conventional arms, they constitute the ultimate killer commodities in that, by design, their purpose is to inflict harm and death. Furthermore, there is more and more evidence that global warming is largely a by-product of the treadmill of production and consumption associated with capitalism as a global killing machine that not only impacts human beings but also animal and plant life. In their drive for profits, multinational corporations and state corporations in state capitalist societies such as China have created not only a global factory but also a new global ecosystem characterized by high levels of pollution, acid rain, toxic chemical and nuclear radioactive waste, desertification, defoliation, a buildup of greenhouse gases, and ozone depletion. Over the course of the 20th century, climate scientists estimate that the average global temperature rose about one degree Fahrenheit, or 1.8 degrees Centigrade. While this may not sound particularly serious, ongoing economic development coupled with the increasing demands of an ever-growing planet population—which, in part, is a response to the conditions of poverty that push people, particularly in developing countries, to have more children in order to have enough laborers to meet their subsistence needs—further aggravates the problem. The U.S. Environmental Protection Agency projects a rise in global temperature of between 1.6 and 6.3 degrees Fahrenheit by 2100, which, in turn, will result in a significant rise in the level of the seas and a devastating impact upon human populations living near coastlines and even further inland. The UN's Intergovernmental Panel on Climate Change (2007) projection of a rise of 1.8 to 6.4 degrees Centigrade by 2100 paints an even grimmer scenario for the planet and humanity. The World Health Organization estimates that the earth's continually warming climate already causes 150,000 deaths and five million illnesses each year, and this toll could double by the year 2020. According to Jonathan Patz of the Gaylord Nelson Institute for Environmental Studies at the University of Wisconsin in Madison, "those most vulnerable to climate change are not the ones responsible for causing it. . . . Our energy-consumptive lifestyles are having lethal impacts on other people around the globe, especially the poor" (Eilperin 2005:2).

As part of an effort to challenge the toxic culture associated with global capitalism, Steingraber (2000:32–33) proposes several guiding principles that could serve as a starting point for reversing the tide of killer commodity production and use. The first of these is the *precautionary principle* that stipulates that "*indication* of harm, rather the *proof* of harm, should be the trigger for action," as seen in the case of the production of dangerous and potentially lethal commodities. The second principle, the *principle of reverse onus*, requires that manufacturers must demonstrate why what they would like to produce and sell is unlikely to hurt anyone. Finally, the *principle of the least toxic alternative* "presumes that toxic substances will not be used as long as there is another way of accomplishing the task" (Steingraber 2000:33).

References

Abraham, John, and Julie Sheppard
1999 The Therapeutic Nightmare: The Battle over the World's Most Controversial Sleeping Pill. London: Earthscan Publications.

Angell, Marcia
2004 The Truth about the Drug Companies. New York: Random House.

Bykerk, Loree, and Ardith Maney
1995 U.S. Consumer Interest Groups: Institutional Profiles. Westport, CT: Greenwood Press.

Caldicott, Helen
2006 Nuclear Power Is Not the Answer to Global Warming or Anything Else. Carlton, Victoria: Melbourne University Press.

Dicken, Peter
2003 Global Shift: Reshaping the Global Economic Map, 4th ed. New York: Guilford Press.

Domhoff, G. William
2006 Who Rules America? Power, Politics, and Social Change. Boston: McGraw-Hill.

Eilperin, Juliet
2005 Scientists Link Global Warming, Disease. Hartford Courant, November 17: 2.

Freitag, P.
1985 Class Conflict and the Rise of Government Regulation. Insurgent Sociologist 12:65.

Green, Jim
N.d. Nuclear Power: No Solution to Climate Change. Paper prepared for Friends of the Earth (Australia), the Australian Conservation Foundation, Greenpeace Australia Pacific, the Medical Association for the Prevention of War, the Public Health Association of Australia, and Climate Action Network of Australia.

Hofrichter, Richard
2000 Introduction: Critical Perspectives on Human Health and the Environment. *In* Reclaiming the Environmental Debate: The Politics of Health in a Toxic Culture. Richard Hofrichter, ed. Pp. 1–15. Cambridge, MA: MIT Press.

Intergovernmental Panel on Climate Change
2007 Climate Change 2007: Synthesis Report. New York: United Nations.

Ley, Barbara L.
2006 Disease Categories and Disease Kinships: Classification Practices in the U.S. Environmental Breast Cancer Movement. Medical Anthropology 25:101–138.

Mayer, Robert N.
1989 The Consumer Movement: Guardians of the Marketplace. Boston: Twayne.

Petryna, Adriana
2003 Life Exposed: Biological Citizenship after Chernobyl. Princeton, NJ: Princeton University Press.

Post, James E.
1986 International Consumerism in the Aftermath of the Infant Formula Controversy. *In* The Future of Consumerism. Paul N. Bloom and Ruth Belk Smith, eds. Pp. 165–178. Lexington, MA: Lexington Books.

Public Citizen
2006 About Public Citizen. Electronic document, www.citizen.org/about.

Singer, Merrill
2007 Drugging the Poor: Legal and Illegal Drug Industries and the Structuring of Social Inequality. Long Grove, IL: Waveland Press.

Simmons, Dan
2005 India's Poor Tackle E-Waste. BBC News, October 14. Electronic document, http://news.bbc.co.uk.

Slater, Don
1997 Consumer Culture and Modernity. Cambridge, UK: Polity Press.

Smith, Bruce
2006 Insurmountable Risks: The Dangers of Using Nuclear Power to Combat Global Climate Change. Takoma Park, MD: Institute for Energy and Environmental Research Press.

Stebbins, Kenyon
1987 Tobacco or Health in the Third World? A Political-Economic Analysis with Special Reference to Mexico. International Journal of Health Services 17:523–538.
1997 Clearing the Air: Challenges to Introducing Smoking Restrictions in West Virginia. Social Science and Medicine 44:1395–1401.

Steingraber, Sandra
2000 Social Production of Cancer: A Walk Upstream. *In* Reclaiming the Environmental Debate: The Politics of Health in a Toxic Culture. Richard Hofrichter, ed. Pp. 19–38. Cambridge, MA: MIT Press.

Szymanski, Albert
1978 The Capitalist State and the Politics of Class. Cambridge, MA: Winthrop.

Turshen, Meredith
1989 The Politics of Public Health. New Brunswick, NJ: Rutgers University Press.

Vanderheiden, Steve
2006 Assessing the Case against the SUV. Environmental Politics 15(1):23–40.

Vincent, Eve
N.d. Yellowcake Country: Australia's Uranium Industry. Booklet. The Beyond Nuclear Energy Initiative, http://www.foe.org.au/resources/publications/anti-nuclear/Yellowcake.pdf.
Warne, Colston
1993 The Consumer Movement: Lectures by Colston E. Warne and edited by Richard L. D. Morse. Manhattan, KS: Family Economics Trust Press.

INDEX

ABOUT THE CONTRIBUTORS

Roberto Abadie, PhD, was born in Uruguay and received a BA in sociology from the Universidad de la Republica (UDELAR) in 1992 and an MA in anthropology from Université Laval (Canada) in 2000. Since 2000, he has resided in New York City, where he completed his doctoral studies in anthropology at the City University of New York (CUNY). Dr. Abadie is interested in the ethnographic study of clinical trials in America, focusing on the social construction of risks in biomedical research, ethics, and informed consent processes. Research leading to the chapter in this book was supported by grants from the Wenner-Gren Foundation for Anthropological Research and the Horowitz Foundation for Social Policy.

Hans Baer, PhD, is lecturer in the School of Philosophy, Anthropology, and Social Inquiry and the Centre for Health and Society at the University of Melbourne. He earned a PhD in anthropology at the University of Utah in 1976 and was a postdoctoral fellow in the Medical Anthropology Program at Michigan State University from 1979 to 1980. He held regular positions at Kearney State College, George Peabody College for Teachers, St. John's University, the University of Southern Mississippi, and the University of Arkansas at Little Rock. Dr. Baer has published 11 books, coedited several special journal issues, and published some 120 book chapters and journal articles. Some of his books include *The Black Spiritual Movement Recreating Utopia in the Desert*; *African American*

Religion (with Merrill Singer); *Encounters with Biomedicine: Critical Medical* (with Merrill Singer); *Medical Anthropology and the World System: A Critical Perspective* (with Merrill Singer and Ida Susser); *Crumbling Walls and Tarnished Ideals: An Ethnography of East Germany Before and After Unification*; *Biomedicine and Alternative Healing Systems in America: Issues of Class, Race, Ethnicity, and Gender*; and *Toward an Integrative Medicine.*

Arachu Castro, PhD, MPH, is assistant professor of social medicine in the Department of Social Medicine at Harvard Medical School, project manager for Mexico and Guatemala at Partners in Health, and medical anthropologist in the Division of Social Medicine and Health Inequalities in the Department of Medicine at Brigham and Women's Hospital in Boston, Massachusetts. Her major interests are how social inequalities are embodied as differential risk for pathologies common among the poor and how health policies may alter the course of epidemic disease and other pathologies afflicting populations living in poverty. Currently, she is involved in strategic research projects on AIDS in Latin America and the Caribbean. She is the recipient of the 2005 Rudolf Virchow Professional Award of the Critical Anthropology of Health Caucus of the Society for Medical Anthropology. She is a member of the steering committee on social, economic, and behavioral research at the UN Special Programme for Research and Training in Tropical Diseases (TDR), the World Health Organization (WHO)'s team on the development of appropriate research strategies for scale up of antiretroviral therapy in resource-constrained settings, TDR's scientific working group on tuberculosis, and the International Advisory Board of Public Health Watch (Open Society Institute). At the Society for Medical Anthropology, Dr. Castro was the secretary-treasurer (2003–2006) and chair of the Critical Anthropology of Health Caucus (1998–2002). She received her PhD in ethnology and social anthropology from the École des Hautes Études en Sciences Sociales in Paris, her PhD in sociology from the University of Barcelona, her master's in public health from the Harvard School of Public Health, and a professional degree in nutrition from the Polytechnic Institute of Barcelona. Dr. Castro published a book on social and nutritional anthropology (*Saber bien: Cultura y prácticas alimentarias en la Rioja*, Instituto de Estudios Riojanos 1998), an edited volume on medical anthropology (*Unhealthy Health Policy: A Critical Anthropological Examination*, Altamira Press 2004, with Merrill Singer), several articles in medical and social science journals, and is editor and coauthor of three international health policy documents on tuberculosis, AIDS, and access to health care in conjunction with WHO and the Pan-American Health Organization. She is currently writing a book titled *AIDS in the Pearls of the Antilles: The Social Structure of an Epidemic*, for the University of California Press.

Ann M. Cheney, MA, is a doctoral student in anthropology at the University of Connecticut (UCONN) with a concentration in medical anthropology and women's studies. Her research interests center on women's health, gender roles, gender identity, the theorization of the body, dietary habits, body image, and issues of control among young women and men. Her master's research investigated body image and weight control among university students, finding interesting parallels in male and female issues of body molding and control. Her doctoral research will look at culture change, transitional gender roles, and eating disorders among southern Italian women. She has done research on the dietary habits of student athletes as part of a larger research study funded by the National Collegiate Athletic Association to provide appropriate nutrition education for athletes. She has received Summer Research Funding from UCONN for preliminary dissertation research in southern Italy. She is the recipient of the State University of New York Chancellor's Award for Student Excellence, as well as an United States Achievement Academy All-American Scholar. She has a teaching assistantship as an instructor for Socio-Cultural Anthropology at UCONN as well as a graduate assistantship at the Undergraduate Writing Center.

Alexa S. Dietrich, MPH, is a PhD candidate in anthropology at Emory University, where, as a fellow with the Center for Health, Culture, and Society, she also received an MPH in epidemiology. Her interests draw from both grounded-theory and classical-theory approaches to community-based research in environmental and medical anthropology. She is particularly concerned with the role of so-called corporate citizens in their local worlds and their impact on both social and individual health and well-being. With training in both qualitative and quantitative methodologies, Dietrich is very interested in the means and methods through which grass-roots environmental movements in the Caribbean and the United

States assess risk and collect and deploy technical information about health and the environment. She is currently writing her dissertation based on the research project described in chapter 12. Funding for the project was provided by the National Science Foundation and the Wenner-Gren Foundation for Anthropological Research.

Pamela I. Erickson, DrPH, PhD, is a professor in the Department of Anthropology at the University of Connecticut. She is a medical anthropologist and teaches in both the Medical Anthropology Program and the School of Community Medicine. Her research interests include sexual and reproductive health and behavior; youth risk-taking behavior; maternal, adolescent, and child health; international health; health disparities; ethnomedicine; syndemics; and qualitative/quantitative research methods. She has done research and developed intervention and prevention programs in maternal and child health, adolescent sexual and reproductive behavior, and adolescent pregnancy and childbearing in the United States, Nepal, and the Philippines. She recently completed a collaborative study with EngenderHealth, a New York–based nongovernmental organization, aimed at increasing adolescent sexual and reproductive health knowledge, access to services, and male involvement in decision making in the Philippines. Her current research focuses on understanding sexual risk behaviors and the social and cultural context of sexual and romantic relationships among Puerto Rican and African American young adults in inner-city Hartford, an exploratory study of sex scholars (students who have sex for money for educational expenses) in the Philippines, and a collaborative study of fertility and warfare among the Waorani of Amazonian Ecuador. She has received research funding as principal investigator from the Centers for Disease Control and Prevention and the National Institute for Child Health and Development and as coinvestigator from the National Science Foundation, the Andrew W. Mellon Foundation, and the William and Flora Hewlett Foundation. She is a past editor of *Medical Anthropology Quarterly*.

Martine Hackett, PhD, received her PhD in sociology in 2007 from the Graduate Center of the City University of New York. She also holds a master's in public health from Hunter College. Her dissertation, which analyzed the Back to Sleep public health media campaign to reduce the risk of sudden infant death syndrome and its unintended consequences, reflects her research interest in health communication, racial disparities, and maternal and child health.

Jeff Howard, PhD, has been an assistant professor in the School of Urban and Public Affairs at the University of Texas at Arlington since 2004, when he earned a doctorate in science and technology studies at Rensselaer Polytechnic Institute. His research concerns environmental policy making, decision making, learning, planning, and sustainability theory. Grounded in "reconstructivist" scholarship on the political dimensions of science and technology, his work extends and applies theoretical writing on the democratic steering of technology. One cluster of his interests concerns the role of scientific and technical experts in environmental policy making and how this role can be made more compatible with "strong democratic" processes that involve the lay public in deliberation. A second cluster of interests concerns political processes of ecological/sustainable design, including programs to aggressively address global climate change, chemical pollution, and other pressing environmental threats. He has published articles in the *Journal of Industrial Ecology*, *Design Issues*, *Technology & Society*, and *Life Support: The Environment and Human Health* (MIT, 2002). Continuing a project he began in his dissertation, he is writing articles and a book on the need for the green-chemistry and the industrial-ecology movements to serve as vehicles for intelligent, democratic steering of industrial chemistry.

Martha Livingston, PhD, is associate professor of health and society at the State University of New York College at Old Westbury, where she teaches and researches U.S. health care, comparative health-care systems, international health, health policy, medical ethics, and women's health, and was the recipient of the 2003 SUNY Chancellor's Award for Excellence in Teaching. She is vice-chair of the board of directors of the New York metro chapter of Physicians for a National Health Program and a member of the editorial board of the *Journal of Public Health Policy*. She has spoken widely on the topic of health-care reform. Dr. Livingston lived and studied for several years in the province of Saskatchewan, Canada, and has conducted research and written on the Canadian health-care system. She was a recipient, in 1994, of the Canadian Embassy's Canadian Studies Research Grant.

Terence Love, PhD, is a research fellow at Curtin University of Technology, Western Australia. His research focus is on complex systems that involve social, ethical, environmental, and technical considerations. He is a fellow of the Design Research Society; a visiting fellow in the Institute of Entrepreneurship and Enterprise Development at Lancaster University, UK; and a visiting professor at UNIDCOM Institute of Design and Communication Research at IADE in Lisbon, Portugal.

Brian McKenna is a medical/environmental anthropologist and journalist with nearly two decades of experience as a public anthropologist. In the 1980s he worked in Philadelphia as a health-policy analyst for a number of nonprofits, including Temple University's Institute for Public Policy Studies and the United Way's Community Services Planning Council. Later he had a stint as developmental specialist for NPR's *Fresh Air*. He worked for six years (1992–1998) in medical education as an evaluator for the Kellogg Foundation to create community-oriented primary-care practitioners, the topic of his dissertation. He's written for more than a dozen journalistic outlets, including Lansing, Michigan's, *City Pulse*, where he wrote a weekly environmental health column. McKenna coordinated a study on Lansing's environmental health for the Ingham County Health Department between 1998 and 2001. He is currently writing a book titled *We All Live in Company Town USA*. McKenna teaches at the University of Michigan–Dearborn.

Michael Oldani, PhD, is an assistant professor of medical anthropology at the University of Wisconsin, Whitewater. He trained at Princeton University (PhD 2006) and the University of Wisconsin, Milwaukee (MS 1998). His overall project has been to follow prescriptions ("scripts") through their various life cycles in order to develop key ethnographic sites of inquiry. Initially, his ethnographic work described the impact of pharmaceutical sales practices (i.e., gift exchanges) on doctor prescribing habits at the site of the clinical encounter between reps and doctors. For part of this project, he drew upon his nine-year experience (1989–1998) within the pharmaceutical industry as a salesperson. His more recent work has followed scripts into the homes of families in order to ethnographically assess the impact of psychoactive medication on family life from a critical medical anthropological perspective. This work is divided into two overlapping research projects: the mainstream desire of using psychoactive medication to harmonize family relations and the continued use of psychoactive medication to control marginalized populations, namely Aboriginal children. He is currently working on a manuscript based on his dissertation, titled, *Filling Scripts: A Multisited Ethnography of Pharmaceutical Sales Practices, Psychiatric Prescribing, and Family Life in North America*, for submission to Cornell University Press.

Joan E. Paluzzi, PhD, is an assistant professor of medical anthropology at the University of North Carolina, Greensboro. From 2002 to 2005, while working at the nonprofit organization Partners in Health in Boston, she served as the administrative coordinator and a senior associate of the task force on HIV/AIDS, TB, malaria, and access to essential medicines within the United Nations Millennium Project. Her current research addresses issues of access to and quality of health services among Latino immigrants in North Carolina and the emergence of the promising health initiative, Barrio Adentro, in Venezuela.

Merrill Singer, PhD, is a senior researcher at the Center for Health, Intervention and Prevention (CHIP) and a professor in the Department of Anthropology, University of Connecticut, as well as a research affiliate of the Center for Interdisciplinary Research on AIDS (CIRA) at Yale University. Dr. Singer was director of research at the Hispanic Health Council from 1988 to 2007 and has been involved in community-based health research for over 25 years. He has conducted research on drinking, drug use, health disparities, reproductive health, and AIDS prevention in the United States, Brazil, China, Haiti, and the Virgin Islands, and has also done research in Israel. He is the author of over 190 articles and book chapters and author or editor of 16 books. Dr. Singer is the recipient of the 1991 Rudolf Virchow Professional Award of the Critical Anthropology of Health Caucus of the Society for Medical Anthropology, the AIDS and Anthropology Paper Prize, the George Foster Memorial Award for Practicing Anthropology from the Society for Medical Anthropology, and the Prize for Distinguished Achievement in the Critical Study of North America from the Society for the Anthropology of North America. He is on the board of directors of the Society for Applied Anthropology and a member of the Committee on Ethics of the American Anthropological Association.

Mike Westerhaus, MD, MA, is a 2006 graduate of Harvard Medical School and is currently doing an internal medicine residency at Brigham and Women's Hospital in Boston. During his medical studies, he obtained a master's in medical anthropology from the Department of Anthropology at Harvard University and worked in the Department of Social Medicine at Harvard Medical School on a project examining trade agreements, patent law, and access to antiretrovirals. He also spends considerable time working in northern Uganda on issues related to HIV transmission and health inequities in a war setting. Westerhaus is the recipient of the 2005 Rudolf Virchow Student Award of the Critical Anthropology of Health Caucus of the Society for Medical Anthropology.

Edward J. Woodhouse, PhD, is professor of political science in the Department of Science and Technology Studies at Rensselaer Polytechnic Institute. After earning a PhD from Yale and serving as associate director of the Institution for Policy Studies there, he spent a quarter-century studying how science and technology policy could become less unwise and less unfair. Woodhouse's current scholarship focuses on the runaway pace of technosocial change, misdirected and unfair scientific expertise, overconsumption by the world's affluent, democratizing nanotechnology, preparing for the age of androids, overcoming barriers to electric vehicles, environmentally conscious housing, and other socially beneficial innovations. Woodhouse's books include a classic policy text, *The Policy-Making Process* (with Charles Lindblom), and *The Demise of Nuclear Energy?: Lessons for Democratic Control of Technology* (with Joseph Morone). Forthcoming is *Detoxify the Planet: Why Environmentalists Must Demand Green Chemistry* (with Alastair Iles).